NEUROSCIENCE RESEARCH PROGRESS

STRIATUM

ANATOMY, FUNCTIONS AND ROLE IN DISEASE

NEUROSCIENCE RESEARCH PROGRESS

Additional books in this series can be found on Nova's website under the Series tab.

Additional E-books in this series can be found on Nova's website under the E-book tab.

CEREBROVASCULAR RESEARCH AND DISORDERS

Additional books in this series can be found on Nova's website under the Series tab.

Additional E-books in this series can be found on Nova's website under the E-book tab.

NEUROSCIENCE RESEARCH PROGRESS

STRIATUM

ANATOMY, FUNCTIONS AND ROLE IN DISEASE

HUGO T. MALDONADO
AND
IGNACIO M. ORTEGA
EDITORS

Nova Science Publishers, Inc.
New York

For permission to use material from this book please contact us:
Telephone 631-231-7269; Fax 631-231-8175
Web Site: http://www.novapublishers.com

Additional color graphics may be available in the e-book version of this book.

Library of Congress Cataloging-in-Publication Data

Striatum : anatomy, functions, and role in disease / [edited by] Hugo T. Maldonado and Ignacio M. Ortega.
p. cm.
Includes index.
ISBN 978-1-61942-384-8 (hardcover)
1. Neostriatum--Physiology. I. Maldonado, Hugo T. II. Ortega, Ignacio M.
QP383.9.S77 2011
612.825--dc23

2011046192

Published by Nova Science Publishers, Inc. † New York

Contents

Preface

In this book, the authors present current research in the study of the anatomy, functions and role in disease of the striatum. Topics discussed include the localization, processing and function of cholinesterases in striatum; impaired nigrostriatal dopaminergic neurotransmission in Huntington's disease; behavioral and neurochemical interrelations between the striatum and the cerebellum; striatal dysfunction and social cognition and the effects of experience on striatal morphology.

Chapter I - Acetylcholine is a key modulator of brain function and its action is well regulated, mainly through hydrolysis by acetylcholinesterase (AChE). The highest level of AChE in brain is localized in the striatum, and is expressed by cholinergic interneurons, somatostatinergic interneurons and by dopaminergic nigrostriatal neurons. AChE is localized at the membrane of the cholinergic cell body, axon and axonal varicosities. We have as well detected the enzyme throughout the entire secretory pathway in the cell body. AChE is present in brain predominantly as a tetrameric molecular form, associated to the outer neuronal membrane by the proline-rich membrane anchor (PRiMA). In this brief overview, the role of AChE in striatum is discussed based on the results obtained from three different mouse models in which AChE is absent in whole animal (AChE knockout; AChE -/-), AChE C-terminal is deleted and thus only soluble monomeric AChE is present (5+6 exon knockout; del AChE E5+6 -/-) or PRiMA is omitted (PRiMA knockout; PRiMA -/-). Lack of AChE tetramer increased acetylcholine levels in brain (in all studied AChE mutants), which was accompanied with intense changes of some cholinergic markers in the striatum. Deletion of the gene for AChE is not lethal, but the phenotype of AChE -/- mice is severely impaired. We showed that besides adaptation changes in the cholinergic system, the striatal dopaminergic system is as well clearly affected, which supports a hypothesis about the interconnectivity between these two neuronal systems in the striatum. Deletion of the gene encoding PRiMA and/or C-terminal of AChE removes 97-98% of AChE activity in brain. The residual activity is related to AChE that is retained in the endoplasmic reticulum in the case of PRiMA -/- striatum and endoplasmic reticulum and Golgi in del AChE E5+6 -/- striatum. This designates PRiMA to be essential for the AChE maturation and the assembly of PRiMA with AChE C-terminal for the targeting of AChE in the cholinergic neuron. Surprisingly, while the phenotype of del AChE E5+6 -/- mice is similar to AChE -/- phenotype, PRiMA -/- mice are indistinguishable from wild-type mice and detailed behavioral studies uncovered very slight differences between these two strains.

Chapter II - Parkinson's disease is the second most common neurodegenerative disorder following Alzheimer's disease, affecting approximately 1% of the population older than 50 years. Since the incidence of the disease increases with age (the most important risk factor), it is likely that the number of people suffering from Parkinson's disease will rise as improved health care lengthens the average life span. Classically, Parkinson's disease is considered to be a motor system disease and its diagnosis is based on the presence of a set of cardinal motor signs (e.g. rigidity, bradykinesia, rest tremor, and postural reflex disturbance). These symptoms of Parkinson's disease mainly result from the progressive degeneration of dopamine neurons of the *substantia nigra pars compacta* that project predominantly to the striatum. Today there is considerable evidence showing that deficits in olfactory and cognitive functions precede the classical motor symptoms seen in Parkinson's disease. The beneficial effects of the drugs currently available for the treatment of Parkinson's disease (such as levodopa) on improving the cognitive function affected in this disease is controversial. Thus, the management of non-motor symptoms of Parkinson's disease remains a challenge. Over the last decade, regular physical exercise has been implicated to an increased plasticity in the adult brain (such as increase in neurogenesis and cognitive processes and neurotrophic factors production). Research is now emerging on a possible influence of physical exercise in the neurodegenerative process associated to Parkinson's disease. The present chapter attempts to review results reported in different clinical studies and animal models to provide a comprehensive picture of the role of physical exercise in Parkinson's disease. Although many of the training programs investigated were accompanied by some degree of oxidative stress, which should be taken into account in physical training programs for this population, it is important to emphasize that this response did not promote any negative impact on the rehabilitation aspects of Parkinson's disease patients. Taken together, the current literature suggests that regular physical exercise can present beneficial effects in Parkinson's disease patients evaluated through different tests. It might also afford protection against dopaminergic neurons death and motor dysfunction elicited in experimental models. Finally, this chapter shows recent findings from our laboratory indicating that moderate physical exercise plays an important role into improvement cognitive deficits in an experimental model of Parkinson's disease, reinforcing the potential of physical exercise in the management of non-motor symptoms of Parkinson's disease.

Chapter III - *Background:* Huntington's disease (HD) is the most common polyglutamine neurodegenerative disorder. The mutation consists of an unstable expansion of CAG repeats within the coding region of the *HD* gene, which expresses the protein huntingtin. Although the abnormal protein is ubiquitously expressed throughout the organism, cell degeneration occurs mainly in the brain, particularly in the striatum. Motor disturbances, associated with the loss of voluntary movement coordination, are the classical symptoms of HD. Previous studies have shown that the nigrostriatal dopaminergic system is impaired in transgenic mouse models of HD. In this study, we have further characterized deficits in the regulation of the nigrostriatal dopaminergic pathway in R6/1 transgenic HD mice.

Results: We examined R6/1 mice at 18-19 weeks of age using *in vivo* microdialysis. Specifically, we analyzed the maximum capacity of the nigrostriatal neurons to release dopamine (DA) in the striatum following KCl-induced depolarization of the plasma membrane and after administration of amphetamine. We used high-performance liquid chromatography (HPLC) to measure the levels of DA and its metabolites 3,4-dihydroxy-phenylacetic acid (DOPAC) and homovanillic acid (HVA) in the dialysis perfusates.

Intrastriatal infusion of both KCl and amphetamine rapidly increased the extracellular levels of DA in the dialysates in both R6/1 and wild-type mice, but the increase was significantly greater in the wild-type animals. In addition, we assessed the total DA tissue levels in the striatum contralateral to the side where we had performed intracerebral dialysis. The striatal tissue levels of DA were significantly decreased in R6/1 mice as compared with their wild-type littermate controls. We also observed a significant and progressive reduction in the mRNA and protein levels of tyrosine hydroxylase (TH) in R6/1 mice compared to their wild-type littermates. This may be the underlying cause for the reduced levels of DA release and tissue content.

Conclusions: Our results support earlier observations indicating that the dopaminergic nigrostriatal pathway is severely affected in R6/1 transgenic HD mice. Based on the present study and previous literature that we review here, we suggest that a dysfunctional nigrostriatal dopaminergic pathway is likely to contribute to some of the symptoms associated with HD.

Chapter IV - Deep cerebellar nuclei project directly to the susbantia nigra pars compacta and ventral tegmental area, source of dopamine input to the striatum, nucleus accumbens, and prefrontal cortex. Behavioral tests sensitive to lesions of either region in mutant mice include limb-clasping, changes in motor activity, and deficits in motor coordination and spatial orientation. The ascending anatomical projections from the cerebellum to the striatum may explain some of the behavioral similarities, as well as disynaptic projections from the subthalamic nucleus to cerebellar cortex. This hypothesis is supported by findings of neurochemical changes in basal ganglia as a consequence of cerebellar atrophy and neurochemical changes in cerebellum of mice with basal ganglia lesions.

Chapter V - The last few decades of clinical research have revolutionised our view of the striatum, such that current understanding of the functions of this structure extend far beyond an exclusive influence on processes involved in motor control. By virtue of connections between the striatum and the prefrontal cortex, which form cortico-striato-thalamo-cortical circuits or frontostriatal pathways, changes in the functioning of the striatum can exert a critical influence on a range of aspects of human cognition. The study of cognitive functioning in patients with Movement Disorders has demonstrated how striatal dysfunction can impair memory, attention and executive functions. More recently, attention has turned towards the abilities of these patients to reason about aspects of social cognition. Research to date has revealed that individuals with disorders such as Parkinson's disease, Huntington's disease and Tourette syndrome can demonstrate difficulties in reasoning about human emotion and social interaction, including poor recognition of emotional facial expressions, misinterpretation of story character's intentions and difficulties in judging socially appropriate behaviours. These alterations in Theory of Mind implicate a role for the striatum in supporting cognitive processes which allow us to understand people's mental states, and emphasise the need to develop more precise and inclusive models of frontostriatal circuitry.

Chapter VI - The corpus striatum consists of the caudate nucleus, putamen and globus pallidus. the putamen and globus pallidus were once considered as an entity, termed the lentiform nucleus. However, it is now known that the caudate nucleus and the putamen both develop from the telencephalon, share a common chemocytoarchitecture connections, and sometimes are referred to as the neostriatum; while the globus pallidus develop from the diencephalon and is called as paleostriatum. However, the striatum can also be differentiated into dorsal and ventral striatum based on the limbic inputs and also on cyto- and chemoarchitectonic characteristics. The dorsal striatum forms a continuous and large mass including the caudate and the putamen; the ventral stritum contains the nucleus accumbens and the olfactory tubercle.

Neurons of striatum are mainly medium-sized multipolar cells, mixed with a smaller number of large multipolar cells, the dendrites of both medium and large cells may be either spiny or non-spiny. The most common neurons (usually 75% of the total) are medium-sized cells with spiny dendrites, containing γ-aminobutyric acid (GABA), enkephalin, or substance P/dynorphin as their transmitters. The remaining medium-sized striatal neurons are aspiny, these cells contain acetylcholinesterase (AChE), choline acetyltransferase (CAT), somatostatin and neuropeptide Y, and appear to synapse with striatal projection neurons. Large neurons with spiny dendrites contain AChE and CAT, and most of them are intrinsic neurons.

The major input and output pathways of the striatum have been well established. The most important afferent, in terms of quantities of axons, is the corticostriatal connections. Another well known afferent is the nigrostriatal connections. The striatum also receives afferents from the thalamus, subthalamic nucleus and the external globus pallidus. The output pathway is made up of the striato-pallidonigral bundle and this projection comprises successively the external and internal globus pallidus, the pars compacta of the substantia nigra, and the pars reticulate of substantia nigra. Among these targets upon, the external globus pallidus does not send axons outside the system, while the others send axons to the superior colliculus, passing through different parts of thalamus then, and reaching different parts of cortex finally.

Disorders of the striatum, such as Parkinson's disease and dyskinesias, are principally characterized by abnormalities of movement, muscle tone and posture. However, it is also thought that non motor functions (eg. learning, memory, drug addiction and Obsessive compulsive disorder and et al) are associated with the striatum.

Chapter VII - The neostriatum is considered a key-structure in the induction of goal-directed movements or in the suppression of movements. A complex neuronal network regulates these functions by involving different cell populations, such as spiny projection neurons and several types of aspiny interneurons. This chapter will focus on anatomical features of striatal cells and their circuitries to better understand how morphology sustains striatal activities.

Lifespan experience has been demonstrated to affect brain function inducing plastic remodelling of brain structure. Such a form of plasticity consists in cerebral adaptation to always changing information by means of generation of new synapses or reorganization of existing neuronal circuits in response to environmental experience. Moreover, brain plastic properties are heavily recruited to restore impaired abilities when damage occurs. This fundamental topic will be faced up in relation to experience-dependent morphological changes in striatal neurons, considering the involvement of the neostriatum in a number of motor-related diseases.

Chapter VIII - The striatum has been shown to play a critical role mediating cocaine addictive behavior. Functional and structural alterations in the striatum are a result of complex processes that are suggested to lead to drug craving and compulsive drug seeking in cocaine addicts. Single drug intake does not seem to produce stable structural or functional changes in the striatum, but the repetition of acute functional and behavioral drug-related effects produce later changes in brain structures linked to addiction until drug-taking transforms into a habit (Pierce and Vanderschuren 2010).

Three associated factors related to cocaine addiction are current topics of intense research interest: motivation, cognition and impulsivity. These three factors are functionally linked to the striatum, among other brain regions (Winstanley 2007). Within a neuropsychological perspective of cocaine addiction based on neuroimaging results, the functional and structural changes associated with cocaine addiction are reflected in addicts′ observable emotions, motivations, cognitions and their behavioral manifestations. Motivational changes in cocaine addiction directly involve or are mediated by the striatum (Childress et al., 1999; Garavan et al., 2000; Gu et al., 2010; Volkow et al., 2006; Wilcox et al. 2011). Although the research largely focused on understanding the reinforcing effects of cocaine, cognitive changes are also important to understand the generation and maintenance of addiction (Goldstein and Volkow 2002). Deficit in impulse control is a key feature of cocaine addiction and other psychiatric disorders (Baler and Volkow, 2006; Garavan et al., 2008). Likewise, individual differences in personality are suggested to modulate impulse control manifestation in cocaine addiction (Murray et al., 2003; Patkar et al., 2004; Winstanley, 2007). The review of neuroimaging literature regarding personality traits (Barrós-Loscertales et al., 2010; Hahn et al., 2009) and cocaine addiction (Barrós-Loscertales et al. 2011; Gu et al. 2010; Wilcox et al. 2011) suggests a common pattern of the striatum′s reduced structural volume and changing functionality underlying its cognitive manifestation.

In summary, the failure of control processes and the activation of implicit automatic ones by external and internal drug-related cues may be explained by the interaction between motivational and cognitive processes in cocaine addiction (Goldstein and Volkow 2002; Baler and Volkow 2006), taking into account modulating personality traits. For example, cocaine addicts under treatment may fail in their abstinence due to the lack of cognitive control over behavior, but this lack of control is probably caused by drug cues and the presence of the drug itself. Thus, given the reviewed literature, the striatum is suggested to be an important part of the neurobiological mechanism underlying the cognitive and motivational interactions in human cocaine addiction. The aim of this chapter is to review neuroimaging evidence regarding the human phenomenon of cocaine addiction within the striatum.

Chapter IX - The basal ganglia, generally accepted to be a motor control center, are not considered to be related to language function. However, recent detailed analyses of language in patients suffering from Parkinson's disease and Huntington's disease suggested that the basal ganglia circuitry might underlie the neural processing for language.

Recent human molecular genetic approaches have identified FOXP2, encoding a transcription factor, as a disease-causing gene for a rare inherited form of a speech and language disorder. More recently, mutations in FOXP1, another gene from the same subfamily, were found in individuals with autism spectrum disorders with speech and language deficits.

FOXP1 and FOXP2 are expressed in distinct but overlapping regions of the developing mouse, bird, non-human primate and human. Of importance, the expression of both genes is quite remarkable in the developing striatum, and to a lesser extent in the cerebral cortex. Thus, the spatio-temporal pattern of FOXP2 and FOXP1 expression suggests that the basic neural network underlying speech and language may include the cortico-striatal circuit. Moreover, morphometric and functional imaging studies in patients with FOXP2 mutations support this assumption. The fact that mice carrying mutations in Foxp2 show morphological and functional alterations in the striatum and a significant phenotypic change in ultrasonic vocalization also supports the importance of cortico-striatal circuits.

A better understanding of the role of the striatum in language may help the development of novel therapeutics for speech and language disturbances in various diseases.

Chapter X - Iron is essential for the normal central nervous system (CNS) growth and development. Now a lot of evidences point out that the iron levels in basal ganglia and substantia nigra are higher in PD brains than in normal brains. As a long term effect, iron chloride infusions into the rat SNc can decrease striatal dopamine (DA) levels. However, the striatal dopamine content after iron-dextran infusion into the rat SNc has not been completely elucidated. Thus, the aim of this work was to measure the striatal DA concentration after iron-dextran infusion into the SNc. 40 male Wistar rats that were used and divided into five groups to determine the striatal DA content. The groups consisted of control, saline infused at 7 and 30 days, and iron-dextran infused at 7 and 30 days. Motor performance was assessed in iron-dextran and saline infused groups at 30 days. The striatal DA levels were determined with HPLC. There was a significant ($P < 0.05$) decrease in DA concentrations in the striatum ipsilateral to the injury site. In contrast, there were no significant differences in DA concentration between the sham-operated and control groups. We also observed increased motor deficit in iron-dextran infused rats. In conclusion, the striatal DA reduction observed after iron-dextran infusion could be associated with oxidative injury in the SNc. On the other hand, the motor deficit could be a result of disturbances in striatal and cortical dopaminergic neuromodulation.

In: Striatum: Anatomy, Functions and Role in Disease
Editors: Hugo T. Maldonado and Ignacio M. Ortega
ISBN 978-1-61942-384-8

Chapter I

Localization, Processing and Function of Cholinesterases in Striatum

Anna Hrabovska
Department of Pharmacology and Toxicology, Faculty of Pharmacy,
Comenius University, Bratislava, Slovakia

Abstract

Acetylcholine is a key modulator of brain function and its action is well regulated, mainly through hydrolysis by acetylcholinesterase (AChE). The highest level of AChE in brain is localized in the striatum, and is expressed by cholinergic interneurons, somatostatinergic interneurons and by dopaminergic nigrostriatal neurons. AChE is localized at the membrane of the cholinergic cell body, axon and axonal varicosities. We have as well detected the enzyme throughout the entire secretory pathway in the cell body. AChE is present in brain predominantly as a tetrameric molecular form, associated to the outer neuronal membrane by the proline-rich membrane anchor (PRiMA). In this brief overview, the role of AChE in striatum is discussed based on the results obtained from three different mouse models in which AChE is absent in whole animal (AChE knockout; AChE -/-), AChE C-terminal is deleted and thus only soluble monomeric AChE is present (5+6 exon knockout; del AChE E5+6 -/-) or PRiMA is omitted (PRiMA knockout; PRiMA -/-). Lack of AChE tetramer increased acetylcholine levels in brain (in all studied AChE mutants), which was accompanied with intense changes of some cholinergic markers in the striatum. Deletion of the gene for AChE is not lethal, but the phenotype of AChE -/- mice is severely impaired. We showed that besides adaptation changes in the cholinergic system, the striatal dopaminergic system is as well clearly affected, which supports a hypothesis about the interconnectivity between these two neuronal systems in the striatum. Deletion of the gene encoding PRiMA and/or C-terminal of AChE removes 97-98% of AChE activity in brain. The residual activity is related to AChE that is retained in the endoplasmic reticulum in the case of PRiMA -/- striatum and endoplasmic reticulum and Golgi in del AChE E5+6 -/- striatum. This designates PRiMA to be essential for the AChE maturation and the assembly of PRiMA with AChE C-terminal for the targeting of AChE in the cholinergic neuron. Surprisingly, while the phenotype of del AChE E5+6 -/- mice is similar to AChE -/- phenotype,

PRiMA -/- mice are indistinguishable from wild-type mice and detailed behavioral studies uncovered very slight differences between these two strains.

Introduction

It is a widely accepted fact that the action of acetylcholinesterase is crucial for normal CNS function, while the highest acetylcholinesterase activity within the brain is in the striatum. The striatal cholinergic system was suggested to play an important role in cognition and learning, memory and movement. Impaired cholinergic mechanisms are linked to many diseases, e.g., Alzheimer's disease, Parkinson's disease, Huntington's disease and schizophrenia. However, current data obtained in this field and especially in regard to cholinesterases shed new light on the importance of this enzyme in CNS for physiological and pathological processes. Recently published results may, to some extent, change the current perspective of cholinesterases in CNS. Here I summarize the latest observations and conclusions about the cholinergic system in the striatum. All key players of cholinergic synapse are discussed, including the ones involved in the synthesis, storage, release and removal of acetylcholine. Special attention is paid to cholinesterases, distinctively in the striatum. For a better understanding of the discussed topics, cholinesterases are described thoroughly on the level of genetics, molecular and protein structure, kinetics and catalytic properties, processing and localization, their function in the body as well as the effect of the lack of cholinesterase activity either after inhibition or removal of the protein.

1. Why Striatum to Study the Cholinergic System?

The striatum is a convenient model to study the cholinergic system in brain due to several characteristics. It is a considerably well recognizable and easily dissectible structure. The striatum is the most extensive part of the basal ganglia (Brabec *et al.* 2003), i.e., the interconnective subcortical nuclei that are mostly involved in motoric and emotional regulatory functions (Bolam *et al.* 2000). The striatum is formed by clumps of gray matter, which determines its characteristic and easily identifiable appearance. In primates, white matter (or axonal fibers) projecting from the cortex - *capsula interna* divides the striatum into *nucleus caudatus* (consisting of head – *caput*, body – *corpus* and tail - *cauda*) and *putamen*. The striatum can be divided into two major anatomical parts – *matrix* and *striosomes* which have different histochemical and receptor makeup. The striatum contains an extremely high level of acetylcholine (ACh) and other cholinergic markers, e.g., cholinacetyltransferase, nicotinic and muscarinic cholinergic receptors (nAChR and mAChR). The highest level of acetylcholinesterase (AChE) was detected in the striatum (Dobbertin *et al.* 2009), while the majority of its activity was detected in *matrix*, which represents 85% of the whole striatum. The residual volume is formed by *striosomes*, which provide just trace AChE activity staining (Hrabovska *et al.* 2011). Both of these compartments are characterized by similar cytoarchitecture consisting of two major neuronal groups. Medium spiny sized neurons form the majority of the striatal mass and their main neurotransmitter is gamma-aminobutyric acid

(GABA). Striatal interneurons represent just 2-3% of striatal neurons. Besides three groups of GABA-ergic neurons (1. containing the calcium-binding protein parvalbumin; 2. containing the calcium-binding protein calretinine; and 3. containing somatostatin, neuropeptide Y, NADPH-diaphorase and nitric oxide (NO)-syntase) there are large cholinergic interneurons in the striatum that are rich in ACh synthesizing enzyme (cholinacetyltransferase). The size of the striatal cholinergic interneurons, the large volume of the cytoplasm and well developed intracellular organelles allow optimal conditions to study the cholinergic system at the subcellular level (Dobbertin *et al.* 2009). Finally, AChE gene is expressed by cholinergic interneurons, somatostatinergic interneurons and dopaminergic neurons of the substantia nigra (Bernard *et al.* 1995).

2. Cholinergic Synapse

Cholinergic transmission is essential for normal function of the autonomic nervous system and somatic neuromuscular junction. The cholinergic neurotransmitter ACh is the only low-molecular weight amine that is not an amino acid or its derivative. It is synthesized in the presynaptic neuron (or motor neuron). After release (for ACh synthesis, storage and release see section 3.), it activates presynaptic receptors or postsynaptic receptors on neurons, muscle or different effector organs.

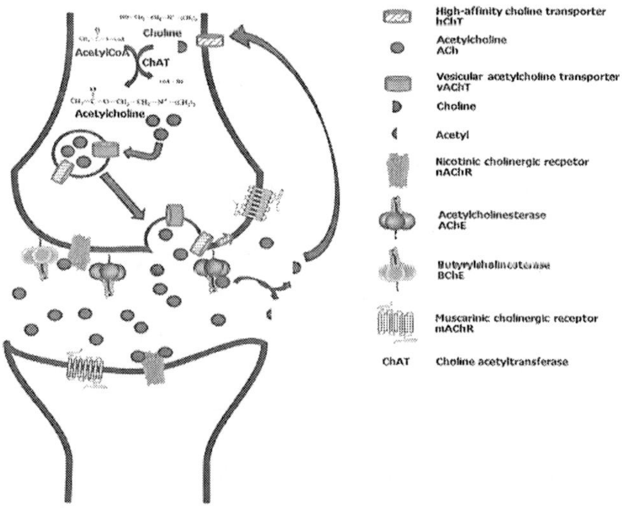

Figure 1. The schematic depicts the cholinergic synapse in brain. Acetylcholine is synthesized by choline acetyltransferase in the presynaptic neuron from choline and acetylCoA. The vesicular acetylcholine transporter facilitates uptake of acetylcholine into the vesicles, where it is stored until neuronal excitation. After exocytosis into the synaptic cleft, the released acetylcholine activates presynaptic and postsynaptic muscarinic and nicotinic acetylcholinergic receptors. Acetylcholine is hydrolyzed in the cholinergic synapse in brain by PRiMA-anchored cholinesterases into choline and acetate. The high affinity choline transporter mediates choline reuptake back into the presynaptic neuron. The level of the transporter on the cell membrane is regulated through synaptic trafficking.

Presynaptic receptors, also called autoreceptors, are located at the terminal from which neurotransmitter is released. Their activation usually modulates synaptic transmission, e.g., by regulating neurotransmitter release. Postsynaptic receptors are located at the membrane of the postsynaptic (receptive) cell. Neurotransmitter, through the activation of postsynaptic receptors, controls opening of the ion channels in the postsynaptic membrane, either directly or indirectly (Kandel E.R. *et al.* 2000). Receptors that gate ion channels directly are called ionotropic receptors (for more details about cholinergic ionotropic receptors see section 4.2.). Receptors that gate channels indirectly, through the intracellular metabolic reactions are called metabotropic receptors (for more details about cholinergic metabotropic receptors see section 4.1.) Cholinergic transmission is terminated by a decrease of the neurotransmitter in the synaptic cleft, by cholinesterases hydrolyzing ACh (ChE; for more information about ChE see section 5.). For a model architecture of the cholinergic synapse in brain, see Figure 1.

3. ACh Synthesis, Storage and Release

ACh is synthesized in a one-step reaction from choline and acetyl coenzyme A (AcetylCoA). The reaction is catalyzed by the enzyme choline acetyltransferase (ChAT). ChAT is the most common marker for identifying cholinergic neurons. Choline cannot be synthesized in neurons. It is obtained from diet and reuptaken from the synaptic cleft after enzymatic hydrolysis of ACh. Membranous phosphatidylcholine could possibly serve as a source of choline that could be released by phosphatase (Tucek 1985), but the contribution of these pathways to ACh synthesis has not been satisfactory documented. There are two choline transporters in neurons with different kinetic characteristics. Widely spread low-affinity transport (acting at high choline concentration) is believed to provide choline for a diversity of cellular needs, e.g., synthesis of phospohatidylcholine for membrane structure (Ferguson and Blakely 2004). High-affinity choline transport entails cotransport of sodium (Breer and Lueken 1983; Haga and Noda 1973; Simon and Kuhar 1976; Yamamura and Snyder 1972) and is devoted to ACh synthesis (Ferguson and Blakely 2004; Haga 1971). The transport is facilitated by high affinity choline transporter (hChT) that appears to be unique for cholinergic neurons (Breer 1983; Okuda *et al.* 2000). Transport of choline by hChT and its intracellular accumulation is believed to be a rate-limiting step for ACh synthesis (Jope and Jenden 1979; Kuhar and Murrin 1978; Tucek 1985). Neuronal stimulation potentiates high-affinity choline uptake (Murrin and Kuhar 1976; Simon and Kuhar 1975) that is provided by an increase in the number of hChT on the nerve terminal membrane (Murrin and Kuhar 1976; Newkirk *et al.* 1980; Roskoski, Jr. 1978). It was suggested that hChT traffics from plasma membrane through cytoplasmic compartments back to plasma membrane while some researchers claim that hChTacts as a transporter in synaptic vesicles (Ferguson*et al.* 2003; Ivy *et al.* 2010; Ribeiro *et al.* 2006; Ribeiro *et al.* 2003). Moreover it was suggested that hChT at steady-state is mainly localized intracellulary on presynaptic vesicles that store ACh and contain vAChT, synaptophysin, and Rab3A (Ferguson *et al.* 2011). This observation offered a regulatory function of vesicular exocytosis and thus ACh secretion in choline recycling and ACh synthesis.

The co-substrate for ACh synthesis, AcetylCoA that carries an acetyl group is, on the other hand, formed during different metabolic processes and is an abundant molecule in the majority of cells. Acetate might also be recycled at the cholinergic presynaptic terminal (Corthay *et al.* 1985).

ACh is synthesized in the cytoplasm. After uptake into synaptic vesicles it is stored until vesicular exocytosis, i.e., its release into the synaptic cleft. Vesicular uptake is facilitated through vesicular ACh transporter (vAChT), which is considered as a reliable marker for cholinergic neurons, fibers, and terminals (Gilmor *et al.* 1996). vAChT is believed to exchange ACh with intravesicular protons (Erickson *et al.* 1994), while the orientation of the ACh-binding site depends on the state of the vesicles. ACh-binding site in resting or energized vesicles is exposed but in the transporting vesicles it is oriented inside (Bravo *et al.* 2005; Nguyen *et al.* 1998).

4. Cholinergic Receptors

ACh can act as an agonist (i.e., has affinity and can generate a stimulus that leads to changes in cell) on cholinergic receptors. There are two major classes of cholinergic receptors which are named after their selective ligands, muscarinic receptors (mAChR; ligand muscarine) and nicotinic receptors (nAChR; ligand nicotine). All receptors are transmembrane proteins, however members in these two classes have different structure organization, mechanism of transduction and function.

4.1. Muscarinic Acetylcholine Receptors

Muscarinic receptors (mAChR) belong to the superfamily of G-protein coupled receptors. 5 receptor subtypes have been described so far, labeled M_1– M_5, which differ in their molecular structure, ligand specificity and signal transduction. mAChR can activate a wide range of second-messenger pathways while some of them are mediated by G-proteins and others are G-protein-independent. (Nathanson 2000; Tobin and Budd 2003; van Koppen and Kaiser 2003). The M_1, M_3 and M_5mAChR couple preferentially with the pertussis toxin-insensitive $G_{q/11}$and G_{13}G-proteinsubtypes that can activate phospholipase C (PLC) and phospholipase D (PLD). The M_2 and M_4mAChR are coupled to the pertussis-toxin sensitive G_i and G_0 G-protein coupled families, resulting in the inhibition of adenylyl cyclase (Caulfield 1993; Rumenapp *et al.* 2001). Coupling to alternative signaling pathways allows mAChR to control multiple distant effector cells. Indeed, mAChR are present throughout the whole body, in the CNS and peripheral organs, such as the heart, exocrine glands, and smooth muscle tissues (Caulfield 1993; Levey *et al.* 1991; Wess *et al.* 2007). Detailed study of the localization and physiology of mAChR is complicated due to the lack of mAChR subtype-selective ligands (agonist and antagonist), which is mostly due to a highly conserved amino-acid sequence at the ligand-binding site (i.e., orthosteric binding site) between the subtypes (Wess *et al.* 2007). However, mutant mouse strains deficient in each mAChR subtype (M_xR-/-) were generated, which helped to obtain much new information about mAChR subtypes. Some of the obtained results, however, could be disputable on the basis of possible adaptation mechanisms during early development.

All subtypes of mAChR are expressed throughout the brain, in neurons and glial cells (Wess *et al.* 2007). The striatum is equipped with all five mAChR, $M_1 – M_5$, with overlapping expression. (Bernard *et al.* 1992; Hersch *et al.* 1994; Levey *et al.* 1991; Weiner *et al.* 1990;

Yan *et al.* 2001; Yasuda *et al.* 1993). M_1mAChR are considered to be a key mAChR in brain. As it is significantly expressed in all major brain areas, it is believe to play an important role in many brain functions (Wess 2004). The main function of striatalM_1mAChR seems to be control of locomotor activity. Another function aligned to brain M_1mAChR is mediation of cognition-enhancing effects. However, only relatively mild and selective cognitive impairments were observed in M_1R -/- mice (Anagnostaras *et al.* 2003), part of which could possibly arise from the lack of the striatal M_1mAChR. Besides this receptor subtype, M_2mAChR and M_5mAChR were proposed to be involved in facilitation of cognitive functions (Wess *et al.* 2007). Striatal M_2mAChR were suggested to be responsible for some symptoms of Parkinson's disease, e.g., akinesia and whole-body tremor as these were not provoked after oxotremorine (a non-selective mAChR agonist) treatment in M_2R -/- mice (Gomeza *et al.* 1999a). Despite known expression of M_3mAChR in different brain regions (Wess 2004), only little is known about their CNS function. Recently, impairment of striatal M_3mAChR, together with M_1mAChR and α7 nicotinic receptors (nAChR) was reported in hypoglycemic and diabetic rats, which was concluded to be a predisposition to motor dysfunction (Sherin *et al.* 2011). Interestingly, at the periphery, ACh enhanced glucose-stimulated insulin secretion is mediated exclusively by the M_3mAChR in pancreatic β-cells (Wess *et al.* 2007). M_4mAChR were identified as the autoreceptors responsible for the inhibition of ACh release in the striatum (Bernard *et al.* 1999; Zhang *et al.* 2002). Additionally, as M_4mAChR are found at high concentrations in motor parts of the striatum, they were proposed for the treatment of Parkinson's disease and related movement disorders (Wess 2004). On the other hand, M_4mAChR were suggested to be responsible for the motor side effects of antipsychotics, and the alleviation of these side effects by anticholinergics (Fink-Jensen *et al.* 2011). The role of M_5mAChR in rewarding brain stimulation was documented by a lower response of M_5R -/- to morphine (Basile *et al.* 2002) and cocaine (Thomsen *et al.* 2005),morphine withdrawal symptoms were significantly attenuated (Basile *et al.* 2002).

4.2. Nicotinic Acetylcholine Receptors

Nicotinic receptors (nAChR) are distributed throughout the central nervous system (brain and spinal cord) and peripheral nervous system (in autonomic nervous system and at the neuromuscular junction). They have been studied extensively over past years and a lot of information is available that are summarized in many reviews, e.g., (Arias 1998; Changeux 2010; Corringer *et al.* 2000; Giniatullin *et al.* 2005; Lukas *et al.* 1999; Sine and Engel 2006; Taly *et al.* 2009; Unwin 2005; Yakel 2010) and many more. nAChR belong to the family of ligand-gated ion channels, with the channel being formed by five subunits around a central pore (Yakel 2010).nAChR are allosteric transmembrane proteins that are characterized by fast opening of the channel (microsecond to millisecond range) after stimulation by ACh or an exogenous agonist (such as nicotine). nAChR can be in three various states: the closed state (in the absence of ACh or agonist); the opened state (in the presence of ACh or agonist); and the desensitized state (ACh or high-affinity ligand is still bound but no conduction of the channel) (Arias 1998). The ACh binding sites are located at the extracellular interface between two subunits (Yakel 2010). Depending on the composition of the pentamer, two (in muscle nAChRs or brain α4β2 nAChRs) to five (in the α7 homopentamer) ACh binding sites are present in nAChR (Changeux 2010) (for subunit description and pentamer composition see further). The effect of ACh once bound to its binding site is the opening of a cationic channel that is permeable to Na^+, K^+ and in some cases Ca^{2+}. As mentioned above, at the molecular level, nAChR are formed by five subunits. The existence of a variety of different subunit variants gives rise to nAChR of different characteristics including pharmacological and kinetic properties and their cellular and subcellular localization (Changeux 2010; Gotti *et al.* 2009; Nashmi and Lester 2006). The nomenclature of nAChR is based on the subunit composition, stoichiometries if known (Taly *et al.* 2009). A total of 17 subunits of nAChR have been described so far: α1 –α10, β1 – β4, γ, δ, ε. The resulting nAChR can be either heteromeric (e.g., α4β2 and α1β1γδ) or homomeric (e.g., α7 and α8) pentamers. In contrast, skeletal muscle nAChR are made from α1, β1, γ, δ, ε subunits. nAChR of brain and spinal cord are made from α1 –α10 (in mammals, however, α8 subunit is not expressed) and β2 – β4, while predominant receptors α4β2 and α7 are being most abundant (Taly *et al.* 2009). The α4β2 hetero-oligomer shows high affinity and slow desensitization. The α7 homo-oligomer is characterized by a fast activation, a low affinity and a high Ca^{2+} permeability (Taly *et al.* 2009). In striatum, formation of α4β2; α4α5β2; α6β2β3 and α6α4β2β3 nAChR was reported so far (Changeux 2010). The nAChR in brain are believed to be involved in many behavioral processes, e.g., perception, cognition (learning and memory), attention, emotion, reduction in stress and anxiety, decreased appetite, relieved depression and succumbing to social pressures. They are responsible for nicotine addiction (especially α4β2) and moreover they seems to be linked to some other pathologies, like Alzheimer's disease, schizophrenia, depression, attention deficit hyperactivity disorder, epilepsy (Changeux 2010; Cordero-Erausquin *et al.* 2000; Lindstrom *et al.* 1996; Lukas *et al.* 1999; Picciotto *et al.* 1995; Picciotto 2003; Steinlein 2001; Taly *et al.* 2009).

5. Cholinesterases

An enzyme that hydrolyzes choline esters was discovered for the first time in 1917 in cat blood by Nobel Prize laureate Henry Hallet Dale. Sensitivity of the enzyme towards alkaloid serine (physostigmine), followed by a sustained ACh action was described in the 1920s. The laboratory of Stedman performed the first partial purification of the enzyme in 1932 and named it cholinesterase (ChE). The following years brought many important observations in the structure, mechanism of action, physical and chemical characteristics and localization of ChE.

5.1. Basic Characteristic of Cholinesterases

ChE belong to the small group of esterases (E.C. 3.1.1.). They are serine hydrolases which act preferentially on choline esters. Based on the affinity towards substrates and inhibitors, two enzymes can be recognized within ChE:

- acetylcholinesterase (AChE; E.C. 3.1.1.7), which favors hydrolysis of esters with short acyl moieties, e.g., ACh

- butyrylcholinesterase (BChE; E.C. 3.1.1.8), which prefers other types of esters, with longer aliphatic or aromatic acyl moieties, e.g., butyrylcholine and benzoylcholine.

AChE has high affinity toward ACh and its turnover with this substrate is extremely high. BChE is also able to hydrolyze ACh but less efficiently. On the other hand, BChE shows higher affinity towards butyrylcholine. In general one can say that BChE shows lower substrate specificity than AChE.

Beside hydrolytic activity, arylacylamidase activity (George and Balasubramanian 1980; George and Balasubramanian 1981) and weak proteolytic activity (Boopathy and Balasubramanian 1987; Chatonnet and Masson 1985; Chubb *et al.* 1980; Ismael *et al.* 1986; Lockridge 1982; Millar and Chubb 1984; Small *et al.*1987) were reported for ChE (Chatonnet and Lockridge 1989).

5.2. Catalytic Properties of Cholinesterases

Specificity and high turnover of ChE is partially determined by the architecture of the active site. The crystal structure revealed that the active site of ChE is localized within the core of the protein, protected from the surrounding environment. It is reachable through the long and narrow gorge that is lined by hydrophobic moieties (Sussman *et al.* 1991). At the bottom of the gorger, the catalytic triad (consisting of serine – histidine – glutamine) is present. Besides the catalytic triad, the oxyanion hole, choline binding site and acyl pocket are present in the active site. Differential BChE and AChE substrate selectivity was explained mostly by the different lining of the acyl pocket (Ordentlich *et al.* 1993; Radic *et al.* 1993; Vellom *et al.* 1993). The presence of smaller amino acid moieties in BChE allows penetration of bulkier substrates, e.g.,butyrylcholine or benzoylcholine into the active site (Cygler *et al.* 1993; Harel *et al.* 1992). There is a peripheral binding site on the surface of the protein at the entrance to the catalytic gorge which was suggested to be an initial substrate binding site (Mallender *et al.* 2000; Szegletes *et al.* 1999). A peripheral binding site exists in both ChE, however its precise location and response to ligand binding are different (Masson *et al.* 1997; Nachon *et al.* 1998). Different amino acid moiety composition participates in substrate specificity and sensitivity towards inhibitors (Harel *et al.* 1992; Kraut *et al.* 2000; Radic *et al.* 1993; Vellom *et al.* 1993). ChE do not follow the Michaelis-Menten kinetics with positively charged substrates. Excess of substrate at neutral pH and 25 °C inhibits AChE, while activates BChE (Masson *et al.* 2001). At low pH however, AChE is activated by excess of substrate (Masson *et al.* 2002). The peripheral binding site may play a role in substrate inhibition and substrate activation of ChE (Mallender *et al.* 2000; Szegletes *et al.* 1999). Binding of a second molecule of substrate to this site can induce conformational changes that would alternate the kinetic characteristics.

Besides pH-dependent substrate inhibition/activation (Johnson *et al.* 2003; Masson *et al.* 2002; Masson *et al.* 2003), other complexities in the approach to steady-state were observed for certain substrates. Pre-steady-state induction phase detected for AChE (Sadar and Laidler 1975) and BChE (Masson *et al.* 2002) with neutral substrate N-methylindoxyl acetate was explained by a slow transition from form E to form E' and enzyme-substrate complexes ES to E'S, while only E'S forms the product (Masson *et al.* 2005). More complex hysteresis was observed for BChE with benzoylcholine as a substrate when damped oscillations superimposed on the hysteretic lag (Hrabovska *et al.* 2006; Masson *et al.* 2005). This was explained by the presence of two forms of enzyme in equilibrium, and multiple conformational substrate clusters. For exemplary recordings capturing hysteretic behavior of BChE and its schematic explanation, see Figure 2.

These observations are in concert with the protein dynamic theory, which states that proteins exist in equilibrium between pre-existing, functional and nonfunctional forms, while the equilibrium is shifted towards the functional form once a ligand binds (James and Tawfik 2003). There is no evidence of hysteretic behavior of ChE *in vivo*; however it was suggested that slow equilibria between enzyme forms may be responsible for hysteresis in response to carbamates and may play a role in damping out cholinergic response to a rapid change in inhibitory concentration (Hrabovska *et al.* 2006).

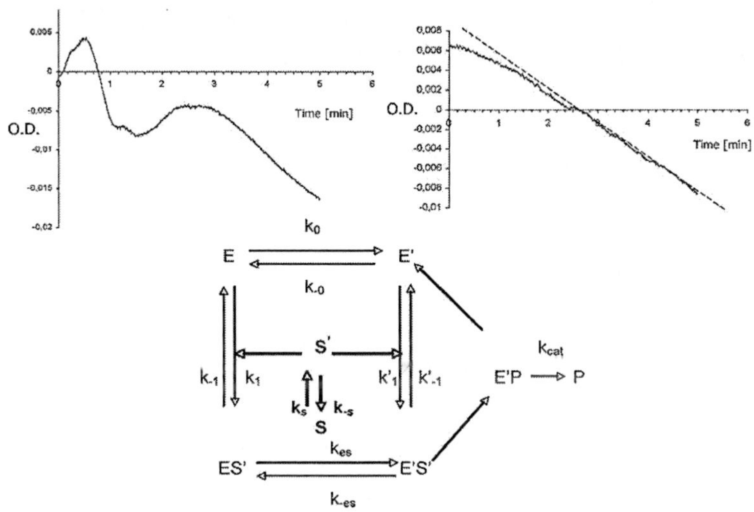

Figure 2. Hysteretic behavior of butyrylcholinesterase in the hydrolysis of N-alkyl derivatives of benzoylcholine. Pictures above show an exemplary recording of the substrate decrease in the incubation mixture during the enzyme hydrolysis. Hysteretic behaviour was detected in the approach to steady-state and hysteresis consisted of a long lag phase (above, left) and damped oscillations (above, right). The pre-steady-state induction phase can be explained (bottom) by slow transition from a form E to a form E' and enzyme–substrate complexes ES to E'S, while only E'S leads to product (P) formation. Damped oscillations were explained by the time-dependent change in substrate concentration caused by the presence of multiple substrate forms (aggregates and conformers; S) in slow equilibrium, and only one of these forms interacts with enzyme (S'). k_0 and k_{-0}, k_{es} and k_{-es}, k_s and k_{-s} k_1 and k'_1, are the first-order rate constants for the reversible transition between E and E', ES'and E'S', S and S'', S binding to E and E' rexpectivelly. k_{cat} is the turnover number, O.D. stands for optical density.

5.3. Genetic and Molecular Aspects of Cholinesterases

Cholinergic components are present in plantae, fungi, bacteria and animal kingdoms. The ubiquitousness of ChEs suggests descent from an ancestral ChE, possibly concurring with the beginning of life (Karczmar 2010). Extensive duplications brought on multiple ChE genes, e.g., two AChE genes are possessed by hexapods (Bourguet *et al.* 1996; Li and Han 2002; Malcolm *et al.* 1998); four AChE genes were described in nematodes (Combes *et al.* 2000). Duplication in the lineage prominent to vertebrates gave rise to two sister enzymes – AChE and BChE (Massoulie *et al.* 2008; Sutherland *et al.* 1997), however phylogenic origin of this duplication is still unknown (Pezzementi and Chatonnet 2010). Until today, a single gene was described for AChE and a single gene for BChE in vertebrates, which seem to carry several transcriptional start sites (Massoulie *et al.* 2008). Besides exons 2-4 that encode the catalytic domain, there are alternative exons 5 and 6 in the AChE gene. The BChE gene contains 4 exons while exon 2 encodes 83% of the coding sequence for the mature protein, including the N-terminal and the active-site serine (Arpagaus *et al.* 1990). AChE exists in multiple molecular forms in the body due to an alternative splicing on the C-terminal and its association with structural proteins (Massoulie 2002). The mature protein therefore always carries an identical catalytic domain while the C-terminal can be distinct for different molecular forms. The ratio of different molecular forms is organ specific. If no exons are spliced, readthrough or R-transcript is formed. The resulting catalytic subunit is soluble and monomeric. Interestingly, the sequence shows high interspecies variability and is not well preserved in mammalians, where it varies noticeably in composition and length (Massoulie *et al.* 2008). The R-transcript was detected so far in *Torpedo* (marine electric ray), in mouse erythrocytes (not human) and mouse brain (Massoulie 2002). It was hypothesized to be present in other species e.g., rat, bovine, cat, dog and primates (Massoulie *et al.* 2008). Moreover, this transcript was suggested to be inducible by stress (Massoulie 2002). Hydrophobic or H-transcript produce $AChE_H$ in which C-terminal peptide holds a GPI-addition signal (Massoulie *et al.* 2008). The resulting protein forms GPI-anchored AChE dimers (Massoulie 2002). H-transcript was described throughout the animal kingdom but its absence was reported for some classes e.g., amphibians, reptiles, birds. In mammals, $AChE_H$ is predominantly expressed in hematopoietic cells. The h-peptide is relatively divergent and it may show some variations even between closely related species (e.g., in rodents) (Massoulie *et al.* 2008). $AChE_T$ ("T" stands for tailed, describing the ability to assemble with anchoring proteins) is present in all vertebrates while it is the only variant expressed in brain and muscle of the healthy adult mammals (Legay *et al.* 1995). Based on recent data, BChE is represented uniquely by this variant. It forms monomers, dimers, tetramers and anchored heterooligomers, while the latter are the functional form in the cholinergic synapse of the vertebrate (Bon *et al.* 1997). The t-peptides of AChE and BChE are strongly conserved within the species, carrying seven aromatic residues. Soluble or secreted S-variant was detected in venom glands of the snake family *Elapidea*, where it is produced and secreted. Presence of AChE does not seem to participate in toxicity of the venom (Massoulie 2002).

5.4. Anchoring Proteins of Cholinesterases and Their Assembly

In addition to alternative splicing at the C-terminus (see section 5.3.), association with structural proteins determines the existence of multiple molecular forms of AChE in the body. The $AChE_T$ subunit forms mostly intracellular amphiphilic monomers (G_1^a) and dimers (G_2^a) that probably serve as precursors of functional forms, secreted non-amphiphilic tetramers (G_4^{na}) and amphiphilic tetramers (G_4^a) that are attached to the cell surface (amphiphilic and non-amphiphilic forms can be distinguished in sucrose gradients containing either 1% Triton X-100 or 1% Brij 96, while amphiphilic forms sediment slower in Brij96 and non-amphiphilic forms have the same sedimentation coefficient in the two conditions) (Bon *et al.* 1990). The last mentioned ones are the functional forms of ChE at the vertebrate cholinergic synapses. Their formation in AChE is dependent on the presence of the t-peptide, i.e., 40 amino acid residues in AChE and 41 residues in BChE (Blong *et al.* 1997; Cousin *et al.* 1996; Cousin *et al.* 1998), also called Tryptophan (***W***) **A**mphiphilic **T**etramerisation (WAT) domain based on the participating four C-terminal tryptophan moieties. It is encoded by alternatively spliced exon 6 of the AChE gene. WAT domain functions as an autonomous interaction domain. Cysteine residues that are present in this domain form di-sulfide bonds between catalytic subunits or between catalytic subunits and anchoring proteins that stabilize the complexes. But these bonds are not essential for the complex assembly (Arpagaus *et al.* 1994; Blong *et al.* 1997). Two proteins anchoring ChE have been identified so far, a specific collagen (ColQ) (Krejci *et al.* 1991b; Krejci *et al.* 1991a; Krejci *et al.* 1997) and a **P**roline-**R**ich **M**embrane **A**nchor (PRiMA) (Perrier *et al.* 2002). Assembly of ChE_T with an anchor is achieved by an interaction of WAT domain with a **P**roline-**R**ich **A**ttachment **D**omain (PRAD) of the anchoring proteins (Bon *et al.* 1997; Simon *et al.* 1998). In both anchoring proteins, PRAD organizes $AChE_T$ subunits into tetramers ($(WAT)_4$PRAD). ColQ is a triple helical collagen tail that attaches one to three tetramers on the basal lamina forming asymmetric forms (A4, A8, A12) (Massoulie and Bon 1982). It is a predominant molecular form in the neuromuscular junction (Feng *et al.* 1999). PRiMA is a transmembrane anchor that attaches one tetramer to the plasma membrane and forms a principal ChE molecular form in CNS (Dobbertin *et al.* 2009; Fernandez *et al.* 1996; Perrier *et al.* 2002).

The crystallization of the WAT/PRAD complex uncovered the supercoil structure with four parallel WAT chains in a left-handed superhelix surrounding an antiparallel left-handed PRAD helix. Mutation in PRAD of ColQ that disrupts crucial WAT-WAT and WAT-PRAD interactions leads to the congenital endplate AChE deficiency (Dvir *et al.* 2004).

5.5. Localization and Targeting of Acetylcholinesterase in Striatum

AChE is organized as a PRiMA-linked amphiphilic tetramer in striatum. AChE activity is localized in neurons, located on the membrane of the cholinergic cell body, axon and axonal varicosities (Dobbertin *et al.* 2009). Production of an active striatal AChE is dependent on the WAT-PRAD interaction, as described in section 5.4. This assembly is essential for processing through the secretory pathway, AChE targeting and stabilization in the axon.

If any of the interacting domains is missing (WAT and/or PRAD), amphiphilic (anchored) tetramer is not produced. Indeed, this molecular form is missing in the striatum of genetically modified mice with deleted PRiMA gene (PRiMA -/-; for more detailed description see section 5.8.). However, very low AChE activity (2-3% of wild-type value) is still detectable in striatal homogenates (accompanied by normal mRNA level), linked to the cell bodies of scattered interneurons (neurons that produce AChE in healthy striatum). This low activity arises from the nonamphiphilic tetramer, amphiphilic monomer and amphiphilic dimer (Dobbertin *et al.* 2009).A similar observation was made in transfected cell lines: while cotransfection of $AChE_T$ with PRiMA leads to production of membrane-anchored AChE, expression of $AChE_T$ alone gives rise to mature monomers, dimers and tetramers. These are however efficiently secreted (Massoulie 2002) which is not the case of striatal neurons of PRiMA -/- mouse in which AChE protein is restricted to the cytoplasm of cell bodies and no AChE is present extracellularly (Dobbertin *et al.* 2009). In correlation with the absence of

PRiMA-anchored molecular form, AChE is not detectable in axonal varicosities. In healthy striatum, AChE is detected throughout the whole secretory pathway of the cell body (outer nuclear membrane, endoplasmic reticulum, Golgi apparatus and plasma membrane). In PRiMA -/- striatum, the enzyme is captured in endoplasmic reticulum and is prevented from proceeding to the Golgi apparatus (Dobbertin *et al.* 2009).

Lack of WAT domain of $AChE_T$ prevents tetramerization thus cells transfected with this mutant DNA produce only monomers. Interestingly, secretion of AChE is increased. In agreement with this observation, in the striatum of mutant mouse in which exons encoding the C-terminal domain are deleted (del AChE E5+6 -/-;(Camp *et al.* 2008); for more detailed description see section 5.8.) only non-amphiphilic, soluble monomers are produced (Dobbertin *et al.* 2009).Contrary to transfected cells, AChE in del AChE E5+6 -/- striatum is not secreted but retained in the cell bodies. Striatum lacking WAT domain of AChE shares some similarities with an absence of PRiMA (that is described above) however, AChE processing in striatum of these two cases is clearly not same. Even if AChE activity in both genotypes is comparably low (2-3% of wild-type value) and linked strictly to the cell bodies of scattered interneurons, the mRNA level in del AChE E5+6 -/- striatum is reduced by 35% whereas mRNA levels are normal in PRiMA -/-(Dobbertin *et al.* 2009). The most important observation, however, is that in the absence of WAT domain AChE is not retained in endoplasmic reticulum but protein is detected at physiological level in Golgi apparatus. If both peptides (WAT and PRiMA) are missing (double knock-outs), AChE is still completely absent in axonal varicosities but detectable in endoplasmic reticulum and Golgi apparatus at the levels comparable to wild-type mice. It is clear then that the assembly between PRAD of PRiMA and WAT of AChE is accomplished in endoplasmic reticulum and that presence of an unassembled WAT domain restrains AChE protein in this organelle. Moreover, PRiMA is essential for stabilization of AChE and targeting of AChE to the membrane of axonal varicosities (Dobbertin *et al.* 2009).

5.6. Function of Cholinesterases

Based on substrate specificity, high ACh turnover and on the high concentration of AChE in the cholinergic synapse, AChE is considered to be the key enzyme of ACh hydrolysis. It is believed that the main physiological function of AChE is to protect cholinergic receptors in cholinergic synapses from overstimulation by ACh and thus it contributes to the proper physiology of both the central and peripheral nervous systems. The physiological function of the sister enzyme, BChE, is so far unknown. Its ability to hydrolyze ACh suggests a possible role in substitution of AChE cholinergic action, albeit its lower turnover in comparison to AChE. On the other hand, higher affinity towards esters with longer aliphatic (e.g., butyrylcholine) or aromatic (e.g., benzoylcholine) acyl moieties and wider substrate specificity together with its presence in tissues of the first contact (skin, blood, lung) suggest a protective and detoxification function of BChE.

Non-cholinergic function of ChE was as well suggested. This includes the catalytic hydrolysis of ACh outside the synapse, e.g., cell associated and soluble ChE in blood circulation. In CNS, ACh can act as a neuromodulator rather than a common neurotransmitter (Descarries 1998). It was suggested that both ChE have a significant role in neuronal proliferation and differentiation based on structural interaction (Bigbee *et al.* 1999; Brimijoin and Koenigsberger 1999). Brimijoin (Brimijoin 2005) compiled existing evidence that could suggest or even support involvement of ChE in neuronal development: 1. homology of AChE with chosen molecules involved in neuronal development; 2. correspondence of developmental switch from BChE to AChE with neuronal differentiation in mammals and birds; 3. interference of suppression of BChE expression with developmental processes in organotypic retinal cultures; 4. correspondence of transient AChE expression in many neural pathways to the period of axonal outgrowth; 5. inhibition potential of anticholinesterases to neurite outgrowth; 6. enhanced differentiation in neuronal cells overexpressing AChE and depressed neurite outgrowth in cells underexpressing AChE; 7. interference of specific anti-AChE antibodies with extension of neural processes and 8.promotion of axonal elongation by AChE constructs with no enzyme activity. On the other hand Brimijoin correctly underscores that no structural or neurochemical abnormalities are observed in the brain of genetically modified mice totally deficient in AChE (AChE -/-; for closer characteristic of the mutant see section 5.8.). Moreover, no anatomical changes were seen in brain of mutant mice in which ChE transmembrane anchor PRiMA is missing (for closer characteristic of the PRiMA -/- mouse see section 5.8.) (Dobbertin *et al.* 2009; Farar *et al.* 2011). One can conclude than that lack of AChE or AChE and BChE in brain during the embryonic period does not have an influence on neural outgrowth, neuronal proliferation and differentiation. However, one cannot omit possible adaptation changes that could develop during pre-natal or early post-natal development that could facilitate normal neuronal development. Indeed many adaptation changes were described in the striatum of AChE -/- and PRiMA -/- mice that were used to explain the survival and phenotype of these mutants (Dobbertin *et al.* 2009; Hrabovska *et al.* 2010; Volpicelli-Daley *et al.* 2003b). The impact of exposure to ChE inhibitors (blocking its activity and/or protein interaction) on normal neuronal development cannot therefore be ruled out. However, based on the recent results from Lockridge's research group, the action of anticholinesterase cannot be assigned exclusively to ChE as these agents interact with a variety of molecules in brain (Grigoryan *et al.* 2008). AChE -/- mice, despite the lack of AChE, are hypersensitive towards organophosphates (Xie *et al.* 2000) and thus it was suggested that organophosphates act through non-AChE mechanisms (Duysen *et al.* 2001).

Recently AChE and BChE in relation to Alzheimer's disease receives a lot of attention. Four medications are currently approved by the U.S. Food and Drug Administration and the European Medicines Agency in the therapy of the cognitive alteration, three of which are AChE and/or BChE inhibitors. Unfortunately, the mechanisms by which these drugs improve the clinical profile of patients are unknown. However, there are at least two rationales: 1.a reduction in ACh level is compensated by inhibition of AChE (Geula and Mesulam 1995) and/or 2. blockade of the AChE peripheral anionic site inhibits formation of amyloid plaques (Alvarez *et al.* 1997; Reyes *et al.* 1997). AChE facilitates aggregation of ß-amyloid peptides, probably through the interaction with the peripheral anionic site (Alvarez *et al.* 1997; Inestrosa *et al.* 2000) and thus increases toxicity of this protein towards nervous cell cultures (Alvarez *et al.* 1998; Calderon *et al.* 1998). AChE and BChE are associated with amyloid plaques and neurofibrillary tangles in Alzheimer's disease (Carson *et al.* 1991; Wright *et al.* 1993) and can participate in the development of this disease. Indeed, double transgenic mouse overexpressing both human amyloid precursor protein and human $AChE_T$, formed amyloid plaques earlier and in a larger amount and size than mouse overexpressing human amyloid precursor protein alone (Inestrosa *et al.* 2008). In contrast to $AChE_T$, overexpression of $AChE_R$, a stress variant, did not contribute to amyloid plaque formation and even reduced toxicity of the complex, possibly due to different C-terminals. Interestingly, human BChE and its C-terminus prevent formation of toxic amyloid fibril *in vitro*. This was explained by an inverse association of peptide with soluble amyloid-beta conformers (Diamant *et al.* 2006) that is toxic with AChE but not with BChE.

5.7. Inhibition of Cholinesterases

Inhibition of ChE is important from two aspects – pharmacological and toxicological. Pharmacologically, inhibition of ChE is used in therapy, e.g., in case of insufficient cholinergic stimulation in the neuromuscular junction or the lack of ACh neurotransmitter in the synaptic junction (Alzheimer's disease). Toxicologically, inhibition of ChE is the reason for the toxicity of pesticides (paraoxon, parathion and chlorpyrifos) and nerve paralytic agents (sarin, soman, tabun and VX).

ChE inhibitors can be divided into two classes: 1. short-term acting inhibitors, implying carbamate compounds e.g., physostigmine and neostigmine and 2. long-term inhibitors involving organophosphates e.g., paraoxon and parathion. ChE inhibitors from both classes act as false substrates, whereas carbamates acylate and organophosphates phosphylate catalytic serine (Radic *et al.* 2010). While deacetylation of the AChE active site after ACh hydrolysis occurs within a few milliseconds, decarbaminoylation takes hours to days and spontaneous dephosphorylation is impossible. Phosphylated ChEs can be reactivated by oximes, e.g., 2-PAM, HI-6, TMB-4, MMB-4 and obidoxime (Worek *et al.* 2004). However phosphylated ChE undergoes "aging", a side reaction that progressively decreases their reactivatability. Some chemical compounds (atropine, fasciculine, tacrine, decamethonium and huperizine) can act through the non-acylating mechanism. They are directed to a site distant to the active site and prevent ACh hydrolysis through an allosteric mechanism (Greenblatt *et al.* 2003; Radic *et al.* 1995; Weiner *et al.* 2009).

Inhibitors of ChE are pharmacologically classified as indirect parasympathomimetics (Lullmann H. *et al.* 2000). This arises from the prolonged stimulation of cholinergic receptors by ACh that accumulates in cholinergic synapse as a consequence of its decreased breakdown. The quaternary carbamates (contain quaternary ammonium groups in the chemical structure, hence carry a positive charge) in contrast to tertiary carbamates (contain tertiary ammonium groups, hence not charged) cannot cross the blood-brain barrier and thus they act only at the periphery. The quaternary carbamate neostigmine is thus used in postoperative atonia of the bowel or bladder. The tertiary carbamate physostigmine, based on its ability to enter the brain can be used as an antidote in poisoning with parasympatholytic drugs and tricyclic antidepressants (Crome 1986). Paradoxically, pyridostigmine can protect against the toxicity of other ChE inhibitors and it has been used by the US military to protect against potential exposures to organophosphorus nerve agents (Gunderson *et al.* 1992; Lee 1997). Neostigmine and pyridostigmine have been used in pharmacology of Myasthenia gravis, a neuromuscular disease of autoimmune origin (Pope *et al.* 2005), or to reverse the neuromuscular blockade by nondepolarizing muscle relaxants. Carbamates (e.g., neostigmine, pyridostigmine and physostigmine) and organophosphates (e.g., paraoxon and ecothiopate) have a local effect on the eye in the treatment of glaucoma (long-term use is however not recommended due to possible cataract formation). Tacrine, donepezil, galantamine and rivastigmine have been approved for treatment of some subtypes of Alzheimer's disease, to improve the cognitive functions in dementia (Homma *et al.* 2008; Rogers *et al.* 1998). However, based on some clinical studies there is skepticism about the beneficial effect of these drugs on symptoms and retardation of disease progress (Allain *et al.* 2007). Controversy and uncertainty about the clinical benefit of ChE inhibitors for patients with Alzheimer's disease seem to contribute to their lower prescription over the past few years (Franchi *et al.* 2011).

Besides pharmacological importance, carbamates (e.g., aldicarb, carbaryl, propoxur, oxamyl and terbucarb) and organophospates (e.g., malathion, dibrom, chlorpyrifos, temephos, diazinon and terbufos) can be used as pesticides. The compounds at the dose used in farming are highly toxic towards target organisms but less toxic to humans. However, toxicity is possible from exposure during handling of the pesticide (inhalation or ingestion) or due to suicidal attempt. Intoxication by pesticides is followed by one or more cholinergic toxicity symptoms. These are even more profound in case of exposure to more potent organophospates (sarin, soman, tabun and VX) that can be misused as nerve paralytic agents (e.g., terrorist attack using sarin on the Tokyo subway in 1995; (Satoh and Hosokawa 2000)). Miosis (resulting from ciliary muscle contraction) is one of the most sensitive indicators of aerosol exposures to the most potent organophosphates, e.g., soman (Benschop *et al.* 1998; Pope *et al.* 2005; Soli *et al.* 1980). Stimulation of exocrine glands and contraction of smooth musculature develops symptoms that can be abbreviated as SLUD (salivation, lacrimation, urination and defecation) (Pope *et al.* 2005). Muscle twitching as a sign of muscle fibrillations and fasciculations can result in complete muscle paralysis. Other signs of short-term exposure to ChE inhibitors are headache, nausea, dizziness, loss of memory, bradycardia (slowed heartbeat), seizures and convulsions and hypothermia. Respiratory failure is considered to be the primary cause of death after exposure to a lethal dose (Pope *et al.* 2005). Long-term exposure can produce delayed neurotoxicity which may result in paralysis; damage to the liver, kidney, immune system and bone marrow. Some carbamates and organophosphates are suspected carcinogens.

Organophosphates are of importance in laboratory use as well. They are the most commonly used tool to quantify active AChE. The AChE active sites are titrated by determination of residual activity after chlorpyrifos oxon (DFP) inhibition (Amitai *et al.* 1998). As DFP irreversibly phosphorylates serine of the catalytic triad in the AChE active site, it binds to AChE subunits in equimolar ratio. In spite of successful applications of this method in studies of isolated and purified enzyme (Hrabovska *et al.* 2006), it has serious limitations for examination of AChE in biological systems, e.g., unspecific binding towards any serine hydrolase and low sensitivity restraining detection of low density AChE.

5.8. Adaptation Changes in Striatum to the Lack of Cholinesterases

Many mouse models that lack ChE or their particular molecular forms are available nowadays. Preparation of these animals established the model of acute or chronic organophosphate intoxication and started the opportunity to search for effective ways of protection and therapy against chemical warfare and pesticides of this type. Moreover, genetic approaches enable detailed study of the distinct localization of ChE molecular forms within the body, their localization at the subcellular level, their role in physiology and pathology, as well as ChE processing and targeting within the cell. Genetically modified mice brought important information about striatal cholinergic functions and organization of the striatal cholinergic system.

The first work describing a knocked out AChE gene allele in mouse was published in 1999 (Xie *et al.* 1999). One year later, surprisingly it was described that the animals with no AChE activity survived for up to three weeks after birth (Xie *et al.* 2000). Special care (e.g., replacing pellets with nutritionally balanced liquid food, temperature regulation, cage bedding) led to an increase in the time of survival of these mice to more than one year (Duysen *et al.* 2002; Sun *et al.* 2007).

Generation of a genetically modified, AChE -/-, mouse, in which the AChE gene is knocked out and thus no AChE protein is synthesized ruled out the dogma about the essential role of AChE for survival. Mice can survive until adulthood, yet they show a severely changed phenotype. Compared to the wild-type siblings, nullizygous animals show muscle weakness, tremor, late development and inability to reproduce. Mutants develop tonic-clonic seizures, which are a usual cause of death, with a mortality peak around postnatal day 30 (Hrabovska *et al.* 2005). Probably the main question regarding AChE -/- mice was about adaptation mechanisms allowing survival of these animals. One of the first hypotheses was a substitution role of BChE. Indeed, it was confirmed that BChE plays an important role in the biodegradation of ACh, in both wild-type and AChE-/- animals (Li *et al.* 2000) however, expected overexpression or changed activity was not confirmed. As a consequence, a 60-fold increase in ACh level was determined by *in vivo* microdialysis in the hippocampus accompanied by changes in the level of cholinergic receptors. Most recent results obtained in AChE -/- mice showed significantly changed responses to drugs targeting mAChR, e.g., hypersensitivity to scopolamine and atropine (Volpicelli-Daley *et al.* 2003b); downregulation of these receptors in the brain (Li *et al.* 2003), specifically in *nucleus basalis, magnocellularis*, frontal cortex (Bernard *et al.* 2003; Decossas *et al.* 2003), *hippocampus* (Volpicelli-Daley *et al.* 2003a), striatum (Volpicelli-Daley *et al.* 2003b) and even at the periphery, e.g., in the lungs (Myslivecek *et al.* 2007).

Many features of the impaired phenotype of AChE -/- mouse, e.g., body tremor, cocaine and scopolamine induced hyperlocomotion, impaired movement coordination could be assigned to the disrupted cholinergic system or cholinergic/dopaminergic imbalance in the striatum. Special attention was therefore paid to further study of this brain compartment. Three key proteins of ACh synthesis and release were examined. Choline acetyltransferase activity and vesicular ACh transporter levels (for healthy striatum description, see section 2. and Figure 1) were the same for AChE -/- and wild-type mice. The level of high-affinity choline transporter (which facilitates presynaptic reuptake of choline after ACh hydrolysis) was significantly elevated in the striatum of AChE -/-mice (Volpicelli-Daley *et al.* 2003b). Moreover, changes in the cholinergic system due to the lack of AChE reflected in adaptation changes of linked receptor systems. Dramatic changes in the level of dopaminergic receptors (DR) in the striatum of AChE -/- mouse (28-fold decrease of D_1-like and more than 37-fold decrease of D_2-like DR) were described (for more details on the link between cholinergic and dopaminergic receptor systems in striatum see section 6.1.) (Hrabovska *et al.* 2010).

Recently, PRiMA -/- mouse in which the PRiMA gene is knocked-out was generated. Deletion of the PRiMA gene prevents maturation of AChE and BChE in brain. Histochemical analysis of PRiMA -/- striatum showed that the AChE level was severely decreased and protein was localized strictly in the cell body. Despite a normal level of mRNA in the striatum, only 2-3% of the AChE activity can be detected and is localized in the endoplasmic reticulum; thus, no active form of AChE and/or BChE is present in the striatum. One could therefore expect a phenotype similar to AChE -/- mouse, especially regarding features that were assigned to the lack of AChE in the striatum. PRiMA mutant mice, however, are undistinguishable from their wild-type littermates (Dobbertin *et al.* 2009). Behavioral studies revealed no differences in spatial learning ability (tested in Morris water maze), locomotor activity (open field) and gait (analyzed with Catwalk system) between PRiMA -/- and wild-type siblings (Farar *et al.* 2011). No changes in choline acetyltransferase, vesicular ACh transporter or high-affinity choline transporter were detected. The level of ACh in the striatum of PRiMA -/- mice is still more than 50 times that of wild-type mice. In accordance, the total number of muscarinic receptors is decreased throughout the whole brain, while the highest decrease within the studied brain compartments was observed in the striatum (a 58% reduction). Results obtained from binding studies were confirmed by a pharmacological approach where PRiMA -/- mice responded differently to cholinergic receptor agonists and antagonists (Farar *et al.* 2011). These surprising results suggest that: 1. the role of AChE in CNS is not of such an importance as it has once been believed; 2. the decreased number of mAChRs is sufficient to cope with the high level of ACh in brain; 3. the cholinergic changes solitarily in the striatum (as in the whole brain), without contribution from the periphery, are not sufficient to affect movement coordination, cause body tremor and pharmacologically induced hyperlocomotion. Indeed, two other mutant mice with deficits of ChE at the periphery confirm the last hypothesis. The del AChE E5+6 -/- mouse, in which exons encoding the C-terminal domain are deleted and thus only the soluble ChE form exists (Camp *et al.* 2008), closely resembles the AChE -/- phenotype. In this mutant mouse, both amphiphilic tetramers (G_4^a), anchored by PRiMA and ColQ are absent. That means that no active AChE (or BChE) is present in brain (Dobbertin *et al.* 2009), and based on recent data about ChE at the neuromuscular junction (Bernard *et al.* 2011), no active ChE is present at the neuromuscular junction either. Based on this model, one could assume that presence of ChE at both CNS and periphery is essential for a “healthy” phenotype. However, another mutant mouse in which the gene for ColQ anchor was deleted (ColQ -/-) and thus has no ColQ-anchored ChEs at the neuromuscular junction (Bernard *et al.* 2011) argue against this hypothesis. Surprisingly, this mutant has, despite undetectable changes in ChE activity in brain, a phenotype that is very similar, yet not the same, to the AChE -/- mouse. Homozygous ColQ -/-mice exhibit tremor when moving, grow at a slower rate than wild-type siblings (Feng *et al.* 1999) and they benefit from special liquid food. Based on the aforementioned, one can conclude that the phenotype of AChE -/- is mostly due to the lack of AChE activity at the periphery and not in CNS.

6. Role of Striatal Cholinergic System

The fact that the striatum is a brain region that is the richest in AChE (see section 1.) suggests that the regulation of the level of ACh or the non-hydrolytic action of AChE in the striatum is of very high importance. But this has not been sufficiently explained so far.

Participation in many important regulatory mechanisms was assigned to the striatal cholinergic system based on results from physiological recordings, selective lesioning of cholinergic neurons and pharmacological *in vivo* studies. Many of these actions, however, seem to result from the orchestra of interacting neurotransmitter and neuromodulator systems, especially dopaminergic systems. A number of diseases, e.g., Parkinson's disease, Alzheimer's disease, and Huntington's chorea, may result from imbalances in the main neurotransmitters of the forebrain, particularly dopamine and ACh.

6.1. Cooperation of Cholinergic and Dopaminergic Systems

The dopaminergic and cholinergic systems show a tight connection in the striatum and they seem to control the activity of each other. Complex modulation of the cholinergic *tonus* (activation or inhibition) is achieved by D_1-like and D_2-like DR that are expressed on the cholinergic interneurons (Pisani *et al.* 2000). On the other hand, dopamine release is controlled through the cholinergic receptors that are expressed on striatal dopaminergic terminals (Zhou *et al.* 2001). A balance between these two neurotransmitter systems is involved mostly in many physiological functions. Challenging one system can reflect in a reaction arising from the other system. For example, cholinergic receptors stimulated by nicotine cause dopamine-mediated addiction to this agonist (Basile *et al.* 2002; Exley and Cragg 2008; Thomsen *et al.* 2005; Zhou *et al.* 2001). On the other hand, activation of D_2 DR causes inhibition of N-type Ca^{2+} channel opening and the Ca^{2+}-dependent release of ACh (Bertorelli *et al.* 1992; DeBoer *et al.* 1993; Di *et al.* 1994; Lehmann and Langer 1983; Maurice *et al.* 2004; Stoof *et al.* 1992; Yan *et al.* 1997). For many years, it has been believed that the character of the striatal balance between cholinergic and dopaminergic interaction is purely antagonistic (Bon *et al.* 1990; Calabresi *et al.* 1998; Calabresi *et al.* 2000; Centonze *et al.* 2003; Kerr and Wickens 2001; Reynolds *et al.* 2001; Zhou *et al.* 2002; Zhou *et al.* 2003); however, recent studies uncover higher complexity of this interaction (Maurice *et al.* 2004; Rice and Cragg 2004; Salminen *et al.* 2004; Zhang and Sulzer 2004), e.g., activating/inhibiting action of ACh on dopamine release through the nAChR located on presynaptic dopaminergic terminals (Cragg 2006; Salminen *et al.* 2004; Zoli *et al.* 2002).

Expression of all mAChR subtypes (for more information on mAChR subtypes see section 4.1.) in the striatum suggests that dopamine release in the striatum may be controlled by multiple members of the mAChR family. Indeed, mutant M_1R -/- mice show double the concentration of extracellular dopamine in the striatum that is probably due to increased dopamine release (Gerber *et al.* 2001). However, dopamine release studies (in the absence and presence of a non-selective mAChR agonist, oxotremorine) in superfused striatal slices from M_1R -/- mouse ruled out the participation of striatal M_1mAChR on this action (Zhang *et al.* 2002). This suggests that M_1mAChR control of dopamine release in the striatum originates extrastriataly. On the other hand, participation of striatal M_3, M_4 and M_5mAChRs in regulation of striatal dopamine release was confirmed while the effect of striatal M_2mAChR activation on dopamine release in striatum was disproved. It is believed that the control of striatal dopamine release by M_4mAChR is accomplished by a "subpopulation" of M_4mAChR expressed on GABAergic neurons. Activation of these receptors inhibits GABA release and thus consequently decreases the activation of $GABA_A$ receptors located on dopaminergic neurons, which leads to reduced inhibition of dopamine release, resulting in increased extracellular dopamine levels (Wess *et al.* 2007). M_5mAChR are colocalized with DR and it is the only mAChR subtype mRNA of which was detectable in the dopaminergic cells of substantia nigra pars compacta and ventral tegmental area. Oxotremorine reduces dopamine release from the striatal slices of M_5R -/- mice (Zhang *et al.* 2002). Controversially, oxotremorine has an opposite effect on the striatal slices of M_3R -/- mice.

A variety of nAChR is suggested to control striatal dopamine transmission based on the existence of different subunits on the striatal dopaminergic neurons (Threlfell and Cragg 2011). The α4, α5, α6, β2 and β3 nAChR subunits are expressed in the striatum, while α7 and β4 subunits are not, despite their abundance in other brain regions. The α3 exists in the primate striatum, but not in the rodent striatum. Based on a study with α-Conotoxin MII, it was concluded that the striatal nAChR population consists of α6-containing nAChR (comprising α6α4β2β3 and α6β2) and non-α6-containing nAChRs (comprising α4β2 and α4α5β2). The β2 subunit is believed to be present in every nAChR on striatal dopaminergic terminals (Threlfell and Cragg 2011). Striatal cholinergic interneurons, with their regular tonic firing, could control dopamine release in the striatum by activating (excitatory) nAChRs on the dopaminergic terminals. Prolonged nicotine exposure (a nAChR agonist) leads to nAChR desensitization, which enhances striatal dopamine release from bursts (phasic firing).

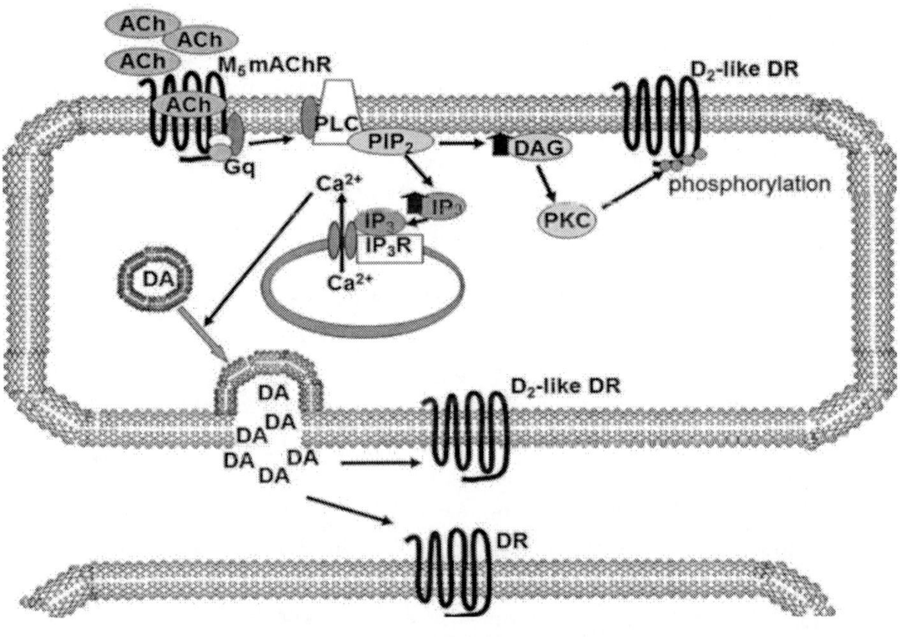

Figure 3. Diagram proposing the mechanism of dopaminergic receptor downregulation in striatal dopaminergic neuron of mutant mouse with deleted gene for acetylcholinesterase. 1. In homologous regulation, overstimulation of muscarinic receptors (mAChR; M_5 subtype has been detected on striatal dopaminergic neurons so far) on the cell body of the dopaminergic neuron leads to increased release of dopamine (DA). Consequently, overstimulation of (pre- and post-synaptic) dopamine receptors (DR) leads to their desensitization or down-regulation. 2. In heterologous regulation, overstimulation of mAChR activates protein kinase C (PKC) through a secondary intracellular pathway and PKC phosphorylates pre-synaptic DR. Such a modification in the receptor structure can lead to changes in its binding characteristic or in receptor number. PLC is phospholipase C, PIP_2 is phosphatidylinositol 4,5-bisphosphate, DAG is diacylglycerol, IP_3 is inositol 1,4,5- trisphosphate, IP_3R is IP_3 receptor, CA^{2+} is intracellular calcium.

The increased level of physiological ACh at the cholinergic synapse leads to a dramatic decrease in the number of cholinergic receptors as observed in brain of mouse with knocked out AChE and thus no AChE present in the body (AChE -/- mouse); and in brain of mouse with deleted PRiMA and thus no AChE and BChE in brain (PRiMA -/- mouse; for more information on AChE -/- mouse and PRiMA -/- mouse and the adaptation changes that occur in them in order to cope with the lack of ChE in brain see section 5.8.) (Hartmann *et al.* 2007; Hrabovska *et al.* 2010; Li *et al.* 2003; Volpicelli-Daley *et al.* 2003b).The reduction of cholinergic receptors in the striatum of AChE -/- mouse is accompanied by an intense decrease in the number of D_1-like and D_2-like DR (Hrabovska *et al.* 2010). It is, however, unclear whether these changes happen due to the increased release of dopamine in this hypercholinergic state (homologous regulation) and/or whether the number of DR on the cell surface is controlled through the intracellular secondary pathways that are shared by mAChR and DR (heterologous regulation) (Hrabovska *et al.* 2010). A schematic explanation of homologous and heterologous regulation of DR by mAChRis shown in Figure 3.

Moreover, it is uncertain whether changes in dopaminergic receptor systems arise from the impaired cholinergic functions in CNS and/or from the periphery as no changes in DR numbers were observed in the striatum of PRiMA -/- mouse, despite more than 50-fold higher ACh levels compared to wild-type littermates (Farar *et al.* 2011).

6.2. Role of Striatal Cholinergic System in Control of Motor Functions, Cognitive Functions and Reward Functions

A balance between cholinergic and dopaminergic neurotransmitter systems in the striatum is believed to be involved mostly in motor functions, cognitive functions and reward (linked to addiction). Challenging the striatal cholinergic system was reported to disturb control of attention through sensory systems (Shapovalova 1999), sensory integration and movement coordination (Aliane *et al.* 2011; Bonsi *et al.* 2011; Dubrovskaya and Zhuravin 1998). The *nucleus accumbens* is believed to be involved in control of locomotor activity (Delfs *et al.* 1990; Plaznik *et al.* 1989), while the *caudate putamen* in stereotyped behaviors (Bordi *et al.* 1989; Carr and White 1984; Kelley *et al.* 1988) in rats. In accordance, the M_4R -/- mice show an increase in basal locomotor activity and are more sensitive to the stimulatory locomotor effects of D_1 DR activation (Gomeza *et al.* 1999b). AChE -/- mice showed a trend of decreased locomotion (Volpicelli-Daley *et al.* 2003b) in comparison to wild-type littermates, which may arise from the generalized muscle weakness (Duysen *et al.* 2001) in AChE -/- mice. Nevertheless, mutant mice showed enhanced sensitivity to the effect of mAChR antagonist on locomotor activity, which was concluded based on significantly increased locomotion after the low dose that did not cause any effect in wild-type littermates (Volpicelli-Daley *et al.* 2003b). No difference in locomotion, exploration and anxiety parameters tested in the open-field were observed in heterozygous AChE knockout mice, despite significant decreased AChE activity throughout the brain (as measured in the hippocampus and cortex) (Espallergues *et al.* 2010).

The striatal cholinergic system is believed to be crucial for the proper functioning of memory and learning processes. Inhibition of ChE is a main pharmacological intervention for dementia, e.g., in Alzheimer's disease patients. ChE inhibitors have been proposed as additional treatment to antipsychotic medication in patients with cognitive deficits (Risch *et al.* 2007), e.g., schizophrenia, major depression, bipolar disorder and to cognitive impairment due to other brain injuries, like alcohol abuse and hypoxia. The beneficial effect of these drugs has been questioned lately (Allain *et al.* 2007). Our recent data does not show any behavioral changes in the memory and learning of mutant PRiMA -/- mice in which no functional ChE is present in brain (Farar *et al.* 2011). On the other hand, we cannot omit the adaptation changes that occur during pre-natal or early post-natal age of PRiMA -/- mouse, which help to cope with elevated ACh in the striatum and may save the memory and learning functions. Contradicting to the usage of ChE inhibitors in order to ameliorate cognitive functions, are the observations from multiple labs that prolonged exposure to ChE inhibitors at the level that does not cause any cholinergic symptoms leads to cognitive impairments (Grigoryan *et al.* 2008; Mearns *et al.* 1994; Roldan-Tapia *et al.* 2005).

The striatal cholinergic system is considered to play a critical role in natural reward-related behaviors and responses to drugs (Ferguson *et al.* 2011; Witten *et al.* 2010). For example, cholinergic receptors stimulated by nicotine cause dopamine-mediated addiction to this agonist (Exley and Cragg 2008; Zhou *et al.* 2001). It was shown that nicotine application intravenously at doses known to maintain self-administration (Chen *et al.* 2010) as well as local administration (Quarta *et al.* 2007) increases the level of extracellular dopamine in the striatum (*nucleus accumbens)*, measured by brain microdialysis. Two possible mechanisms were proposed: 1. a direct stimulation of dopamine release through the activation of nAChR not containing α7 subunits; 2. an indirect stimulation of dopamine release by activation of α7-containing receptors that are localized on glutamatergic terminals and consequent stimulation of glutamate receptors on the dopaminergic terminals (Quarta *et al.* 2007). Based on results from self-administration of nicotine in nAChR subunits knock-outs, it was concluded that nAChR containing α4ß2 subunits and α6ß2 subunits, but not α7 containing nAChR, are crucial in the rewarding effects of nicotine in drug-naïve mice. On the other hand, deletion of α5 subunit or overexpression of ß4 subunits enhanced nicotine self-administration (Changeux 2010). The effect of chronic nicotine exposure on the brain reward system is unique and does not show the same characteristics as in the case of other drugs of abuse. Chronically, self-administered nicotine causes increased sensitivity to nicotine in dopamine rewards circuits. This process, also called sensitization, seems to be crucial for development of nicotine addiction (Changeux 2010). Changeux has proposed three hypotheses to explain the nicotine-caused change in sensitivity of dopaminergic reward circuits: 1. upregulation of high-affinity nAChR, mostly α4β2-containing, in the ventral tegmental area or on midbrain dopaminergic and GABA-ergic neurons; 2. changes in cholinergic transmission in brain circuits at the presynaptic level, possibly downregulation of β2-containing nAChRs, followed by an enhanced α7-containing nAChR-mediated cholinergic transmission; 3. potentiation of activity in anterior regions of the brain (infralimbic cortex and bed nucleus of the *stria terminalis*) that would increase the bursting activity of dopaminergic neurons by enhancing glutamatergic input to the ventral tegmental area (Changeux 2010).

The role of cholinergic interneurons in reward-related responses to drugs such as cocaine is even nowadays full of contradicting observations. Some authors claim cholinergic transmission in the *nucleus accumbens* to be required for reward learning while others report enhanced reward learning after distortion of cholinergic interneurons in this striatal structure (Witten *et al.* 2010).

The rewarding effect of cocaine is based on enhanced dopamine action by inhibition of its reuptake by the dopamine transporter. It was however suggested that reward-predictive conditioned stimuli, which elevate extracellular dopamine levels are responsible for the ultrafast rewarding action of cocaine. Input from these stimuli reaches the dopaminergic system partially through excitatory glutamatergic and cholinergic afferents. A similar fast acting rewarding mechanism was proposed for other addictive drugs, e.g. nicotine, heroin, opiates and amphetamines (Wise and Kiyatkin 2011).

Conclusion

ChE in brain have for a long time been believed to be essential for life. However, our discoveries over past decade revealed that the brain has regulatory mechanisms that enable coping with the lack of ChE functions and adjustment to the excess of ACh in the cholinergic synapse. Moreover, we uncovered that the local absence of ChE in brain does not necessary reflect in the dramatic changes of the phenotype. This could either confirm a strong adaptation capability of the nervous system in the regulation of body functions or suggest little importance of the striatal cholinergic system (and central cholinergic system) in the physiological functions than we have so far believed. On the other hand, lack of ChE activity at the periphery is linked to severely changed phenotype and requires special handling, which could mean that the regulatory mechanisms to the absence of ChE activity at the periphery are less sufficient or that the importance of ChE at the periphery is of higher importance than we have so far believed.

Existence of diverse molecular forms of ChE in the body has not been satisfactory explained so far. As localization of different ChE molecular forms within the body is strict, they may serve some important role in specific cholinergic and non-cholinergic functions or hypothetically this diversity may be a tool for selective control of ChE activity. Adaptation mechanisms in the striatum as well as the existence of a variety of specifically localized ChE molecular forms in the striatum may serve as future pharmacological intervention for selected striatum related pathologies. Moreover, striatal cholinergic receptors may be pharmacological targeted based on the specific localization and fine physiological role of different receptor subtypes. However, while the role of different mAChR subtypes in striatal function has been pretty well described, the role of striatal nAChR subtypes in brain functions is still full of question marks.

Acknowledgments

The author thanks Dr. Lotte de Groote and Dr. Zsolt Csaba for their comments and suggestions on this manuscript; and grant agencies AFM, ANR Neuroscience and APVV (SK-FR-0031-09 a SK-CZ-0028-09) for financial support.

References

Aliane V., Perez S., Bohren Y., Deniau J. M. and Kemel M. L. (2011) Key role of striatal cholinergic interneurons in processes leading to arrest of motor stereotypies. *Brain 134*, 110-118.

Allain H., Akwa Y., Lacomblez L., Lieury A. and tue-Ferrer D. (2007) Impaired cognition and attention in adults: pharmacological management strategies. *Neuropsychiatr. Dis. Treat.3*, 103-116.

Alvarez A., Alarcon R., Opazo C., Campos E. O., Munoz F. J., Calderon F. H., Dajas F., Gentry M. K., Doctor B. P., De Mello F. G. and Inestrosa N. C. (1998) Stable complexes involving acetylcholinesterase and amyloid-beta peptide change the biochemical properties of the enzyme and increase the neurotoxicity of Alzheimer's fibrils. *J. Neurosci. 18*, 3213-3223.

Alvarez A., Opazo C., Alarcon R., Garrido J. and Inestrosa N. C. (1997) Acetylcholinesterase promotes the aggregation of amyloid-beta-peptide fragments by forming a complex with the growing fibrils. *J.. Mol. Biol. 272*, 348-361.

Amitai G., Moorad D., Adani R. and Doctor B. P. (1998) Inhibition of acetylcholinesterase and butyrylcholinesterase by chlorpyrifos-oxon. *Biochem. Pharmacol. 56*, 293-299.

Anagnostaras S. G., Murphy G. G., Hamilton S. E., Mitchell S. L., Rahnama N. P., Nathanson N. M. and Silva A. J. (2003) Selective cognitive dysfunction in acetylcholine M1 muscarinic receptor mutant mice. *Nat. Neurosci. 6*, 51-58.

Arias H. R. (1998) Binding sites for exogenous and endogenous non-competitive inhibitors of the nicotinic acetylcholine receptor. *Biochim. Biophys. Acta 1376*, 173-220.

Arpagaus M., Fedon Y., Cousin X., Chatonnet A., Berge J. B., Fournier D. and Toutant J. P. (1994) cDNA sequence, gene structure, and in vitro expression of ace-1, the gene encoding acetylcholinesterase of class A in the nematode Caenorhabditis elegans. *J. Biol. Chem. 269*, 9957-9965.

Arpagaus M., Kott M., Vatsis K. P., Bartels C. F., La Du B. N. and Lockridge O. (1990) Structure of the gene for human butyrylcholinesterase. Evidence for a single copy. *Biochemistry 29*, 124-131.

Basile A. S., Fedorova I., Zapata A., Liu X., Shippenberg T., Duttaroy A., Yamada M. and Wess J. (2002) Deletion of the M5 muscarinic acetylcholine receptor attenuates morphine reinforcement and withdrawal but not morphine analgesia. *Proc. Natl. Acad. Sci. U S A 99*, 11452-11457.

Benschop H. P., Trap H. C., Spruit H. E., van der Wiel H. J., Langenberg J. P. and de Jong L. P. (1998) Low level nose-only exposure to the nerve agent soman: toxicokinetics of soman stereoisomers and cholinesterase inhibition in atropinized guinea pigs. *Toxicol. Appl. Pharmacol. 153*, 179-185.

Bernard V., Brana C., Liste I., Lockridge O. and Bloch B. (2003) Dramatic depletion of cell surface m2 muscarinic receptor due to limited delivery from intracytoplasmic stores in neurons of acetylcholinesterase-deficient mice. *Mol. Cell Neurosci. 23*, 121-133.

Bernard V., Girard E., Hrabovska A., Camp S., Taylor P., Plaud B. and Krejci E. (2011) Distinct localization of collagen Q and PRiMA forms of acetylcholinesterase at the neuromuscular junction. *Mol. Cell Neurosci. 46*, 272-281.

Bernard V., Legay C., Massoulie J. and Bloch B. (1995) Anatomical analysis of the neurons expressing the acetylcholinesterase gene in the rat brain, with special reference to the striatum. *Neuroscience 64*, 995-1005.

Bernard V., Levey A. I. and Bloch B. (1999) Regulation of the subcellular distribution of m4 muscarinic acetylcholine receptors in striatal neurons in vivo by the cholinergic environment: evidence for regulation of cell surface receptors by endogenous and exogenous stimulation. *J. Neurosci. 19*, 10237-10249.

Bernard V., Normand E. and Bloch B. (1992) Phenotypical characterization of the rat striatal neurons expressing muscarinic receptor genes. *J. Neurosci. 12*, 3591-3600.

Bertorelli R., Zambelli M., Di C. G. and Consolo S. (1992) Dopamine depletion preferentially impairs D1- over D2-receptor regulation of striatal in vivo acetylcholine release. *J. Neurochem. 59*, 353-357.

Bigbee J. W., Sharma K. V., Gupta J. J. and Dupree J. L. (1999) Morphogenic role for acetylcholinesterase in axonal outgrowth during neural development. *Environ. Health Perspect. 107 Suppl 1*, 81-87.

Blong R. M., Bedows E. and Lockridge O. (1997) Tetramerization domain of human butyrylcholinesterase is at the C-terminus. *Biochem. J327 (Pt 3)*, 747-757.

Bolam J. P., Hanley J. J., Booth P. A. and Bevan M. D. (2000) Synaptic organisation of the basal ganglia. *J. Anat. 196 (Pt 4)*, 527-542.

Bon S., Bader M. F., Aunis D., Massoulie J. and Henry J. P. (1990) Subcellular distribution of acetylcholinesterase forms in chromaffin cells. Do chromaffin granules contain a specific secretory acetylcholinesterase? *Eur. J. Biochem. 190*, 221-232.

Bon S., Coussen F. and Massoulie J. (1997) Quaternary associations of acetylcholinesterase. II. The polyproline attachment domain of the collagen tail. *J. Biol. Chem. 272*, 3016-3021.

Bonsi P., Cuomo D., Martella G., Madeo G., Schirinzi T., Puglisi F., Ponterio G. and Pisani A. (2011) Centrality of striatal cholinergic transmission in Basal Ganglia function. *Front Neuroanat.5*, 6.

Boopathy R. and Balasubramanian A. S. (1987) A peptidase activity exhibited by human serum pseudocholinesterase. *Eur. J. Biochem. 162*, 191-197.

Bordi F., Carr K. D. and Meller E. (1989) Stereotypies elicited by injection of N-propylnorapomorphine into striatal subregions and nucleus accumbens. *Brain Res. 489*, 205-215.

Bourguet D., Raymond M., Fournier D., Malcolm C. A., Toutant J. P. and Arpagaus M. (1996) Existence of two acetylcholinesterases in the mosquito Culex pipiens (Diptera:Culicidae). *J. Neurochem. 67*, 2115-2123.

Brabec J., Kraseny J. and Petrovicky P. (2003) Volumetry of striatum and pallidum in man--anatomy, cytoarchitecture, connections, MRI and aging. *Sb. Lek.104*, 13-65.

Bravo D. T., Kolmakova N. G. and Parsons S. M. (2005) New transport assay demonstrates vesicular acetylcholine transporter has many alternative substrates. *Neurochem. Int. 47*, 243-247.

Breer H. (1983) Choline transport by synaptosomal membrane vesicles isolated from insect nervous tissue. *FEBS Lett. 153*, 345-348.

Breer H. and Lueken W. (1983) Transport of choline by membrane vesicles prepared from synaptosomes of insect nervous tissue. *Neurochem. Int. 5*, 713-720.

Brimijoin S. (2005) Can cholinesterase inhibitors affect neural development? *Environ. Toxicol. Pharmacol. 19*, 429-432.

Brimijoin S. and Koenigsberger C. (1999) Cholinesterases in neural development: new findings and toxicologic implications. *Environ. Health Perspect. 107 Suppl 1*, 59-64.

Calabresi P., Centonze D., Gubellini P., Pisani A. and Bernardi G. (1998) Blockade of M2-like muscarinic receptors enhances long-term potentiation at corticostriatal synapses. *Eur. J. Neurosci. 10*, 3020-3023.

Calabresi P., Centonze D., Gubellini P., Pisani A. and Bernardi G. (2000) Acetylcholine-mediated modulation of striatal function. *Trends Neurosci. 23*, 120-126.

Calderon F. H., von B. R., De F. G., Luza S., Aldunate R. and Inestrosa N. C. (1998) Toxic effects of acetylcholinesterase on neuronal and glial-like cells in vitro. *Mol. Psychiatry 3*, 247-255.

Camp S., De J. A., Zhang L., Marquez M., De la T. B. and Taylor P. (2008) Acetylcholinesterase expression in muscle is specifically controlled by a promoter-selective enhancesome in the first intron. *J. Neurosci. 28*, 2459-2470.

Carr G. D. and White N. M. (1984) The relationship between stereotypy and memory improvement produced by amphetamine. *Psychopharmacology (Berl)82*, 203-209.

Carson K. A., Geula C. and Mesulam M. M. (1991) Electron microscopic localization of cholinesterase activity in Alzheimer brain tissue. *Brain Res. 540*, 204-208.

Caulfield M. P. (1993) Muscarinic receptors--characterization, coupling and function. *Pharmacol. Ther. 58*, 319-379.

Centonze D., Gubellini P., Pisani A., Bernardi G. and Calabresi P. (2003) Dopamine, acetylcholine and nitric oxide systems interact to induce corticostriatal synaptic plasticity. *Rev. Neurosci. 14*, 207-216.

Changeux J. P. (2010) Nicotine addiction and nicotinic receptors: lessons from genetically modified mice. *Nat. Rev. Neurosci. 11*, 389-401.

Chatonnet A. and Lockridge O. (1989) Comparison of butyrylcholinesterase and acetylcholinesterase. *Biochem. J. 260*, 625-634.

Chatonnet A. and Masson P. (1985) Study of the peptidasic site of cholinesterase: preliminary results. *FEBS Lett. 182*, 493-498.

Chen B. T., Hopf F. W. and Bonci A. (2010) Synaptic plasticity in the mesolimbic system: therapeutic implications for substance abuse. *Ann. N Y Acad. Sci. 1187*, 129-139.

Chubb I. W., Hodgson A. J. and White G. H. (1980) Acetylcholinesterase hydrolyzes substance P. *Neuroscience 5*, 2065-2072.

Combes D., Fedon Y., Grauso M., Toutant J. P. and Arpagaus M. (2000) Four genes encode acetylcholinesterases in the nematodes Caenorhabditis elegans and Caenorhabditis briggsae. cDNA sequences, genomic structures, mutations and in vivo expression. *J. Mol. Biol. 300*, 727-742.

Cordero-Erausquin M., Marubio L. M., Klink R. and Changeux J. P. (2000) Nicotinic receptor function: new perspectives from knockout mice. *Trends Pharmacol. Sci. 21*, 211-217.

Corringer P. J., Le N. N. and Changeux J. P. (2000) Nicotinic receptors at the amino acid level. *Annu. Rev. Pharmacol. Toxicol. 40*, 431-458.

Corthay J., Dunant Y., Eder L. and Loctin F. (1985) Incorporation of acetate into acetylcholine, acetylcarnitine, and amino acids in the Torpedo electric organ. *J. Neurochem. 45*, 1809-1819.

Cousin X., Hotelier T., Giles K., Toutant J. P. and Chatonnet A. (1998) aCHEdb: the database system for ESTHER, the alpha/beta fold family of proteins and the Cholinesterase gene server. *Nucleic Acids Res. 26*, 226-228.

Cousin X., Hotelier T., Lievin P., Toutant J. P. and Chatonnet A. (1996) A cholinesterase genes server (ESTHER): a database of cholinesterase-related sequences for multiple alignments, phylogenetic relationships, mutations and structural data retrieval. *Nucleic Acids Res. 24*, 132-136.

Cragg S. J. (2006) Meaningful silences: how dopamine listens to the ACh pause. *Trends Neurosci. 29*, 125-131.

Crome P. (1986) Poisoning due to tricyclic antidepressant overdosage. Clinical presentation and treatment. *Med. Toxicol. 1*, 261-285.

Cygler M., Schrag J. D., Sussman J. L., Harel M., Silman I., Gentry M. K. and Doctor B. P. (1993) Relationship between sequence conservation and three-dimensional structure in a large family of esterases, lipases, and related proteins. *Protein Sci. 2*, 366-382.

DeBoer P., Abercrombie E. D., Heeringa M. and Westerink B. H. (1993) Differential effect of systemic administration of bromocriptine and L-dopa on the release of acetylcholine from striatum of intact and 6-OHDA-treated rats. *Brain Res. 608*, 198-203.

Decossas M., Bloch B. and Bernard V. (2003) Trafficking of the muscarinic m2 autoreceptor in cholinergic basalocortical neurons in vivo: differential regulation of plasma membrane receptor availability and intraneuronal localization in acetylcholinesterase-deficient and -inhibited mice. *J. Comp. Neurol. 462*, 302-314.

Delfs J. M., Schreiber L. and Kelley A. E. (1990) Microinjection of cocaine into the nucleus accumbens elicits locomotor activation in the rat. *J. Neurosci. 10*, 303-310.

Descarries L. (1998) The hypothesis of an ambient level of acetylcholine in the central nervous system. *J. Physiol. Paris 92*, 215-220.

Di C. G., Morelli M. and Consolo S. (1994) Modulatory functions of neurotransmitters in the striatum: ACh/dopamine/NMDA interactions. *Trends Neurosci. 17*, 228-233.

Diamant S., Podoly E., Friedler A., Ligumsky H., Livnah O. and Soreq H. (2006) Butyrylcholinesterase attenuates amyloid fibril formation in vitro. *Proc. Natl. Acad. Sci. U S A 103*, 8628-8633.

Dobbertin A., Hrabovska A., Dembele K., Camp S., Taylor P., Krejci E. and Bernard V. (2009) Targeting of acetylcholinesterase in neurons in vivo: a dual processing function for the proline-rich membrane anchor subunit and the attachment domain on the catalytic subunit. *J. Neurosci. 29*, 4519-4530.

Dubrovskaya N. M. and Zhuravin I. A. (1998) Role of the cholinergic systems of the dorsal and ventral striatum of the rat brain in controlling learned movements. *Neurosci. Behav. Physiol. 28*, 386-391.

Duysen E. G., Li B., Xie W., Schopfer L. M., Anderson R. S., Broomfield C. A. and Lockridge O. (2001) Evidence for nonacetylcholinesterase targets of organophosphorus nerve agent: supersensitivity of acetylcholinesterase knockout mouse to VX lethality. *J. Pharmacol. Exp. Ther. 299*, 528-535.

Duysen E. G., Stribley J. A., Fry D. L., Hinrichs S. H. and Lockridge O. (2002) Rescue of the acetylcholinesterase knockout mouse by feeding a liquid diet; phenotype of the adult acetylcholinesterase deficient mouse. *Brain Res. Dev. Brain Res. 137*, 43-54.

Dvir H., Harel M., Bon S., Liu W. Q., Vidal M., Garbay C., Sussman J. L., Massoulie J. and Silman I. (2004) The synaptic acetylcholinesterase tetramer assembles around a polyproline II helix. *EMBO J. 23*, 4394-4405.

Erickson J. D., Varoqui H., Schafer M. K., Modi W., Diebler M. F., Weihe E., Rand J., Eiden L. E., Bonner T. I. and Usdin T. B. (1994) Functional identification of a vesicular acetylcholine transporter and its expression from a "cholinergic" gene locus. *J. Biol. Chem. 269*, 21929-21932.

Espallergues J., Galvan L., Sabatier F., Rana-Poussine V., Maurice T. and Chatonnet A. (2010) Behavioral phenotyping of heterozygous acetylcholinesterase knockout (AChE+/-

) mice showed no memory enhancement but hyposensitivity to amnesic drugs. *Behav. Brain Res. 206*, 263-273.

Exley R. and Cragg S. J. (2008) Presynaptic nicotinic receptors: a dynamic and diverse cholinergic filter of striatal dopamine neurotransmission. *Br. J. Pharmacol. 153 Suppl 1*, S283-S297.

Farar V., Mohr F., LegrandM., Bernard V., Martre M.P., Baud, Klein J, Houze, Hrabovska A., Myslivecek J. and Krejci E. (2011) *Absence of impairment of respiratory and body temperature control despite the absence of any cholinesterase in the Central Nervous System.*

Feng G., Krejci E., Molgo J., Cunningham J. M., Massoulie J. and Sanes J. R. (1999) Genetic analysis of collagen Q: roles in acetylcholinesterase and butyrylcholinesterase assembly and in synaptic structure and function. *J. Cell Biol. 144*, 1349-1360.

Ferguson S. M. and Blakely R. D. (2004) The choline transporter resurfaces: new roles for synaptic vesicles? *Mol. Interv. 4*, 22-37.

Ferguson S. M., Eskenazi D., Ishikawa M., Wanat M. J., Phillips P. E., Dong Y., Roth B. L. and Neumaier J. F. (2011) Transient neuronal inhibition reveals opposing roles of indirect and direct pathways in sensitization. *Nat. Neurosci. 14*, 22-24.

Ferguson S. M., Savchenko V., Apparsundaram S., Zwick M., Wright J., Heilman C. J., Yi H., Levey A. I. and Blakely R. D. (2003) Vesicular localization and activity-dependent trafficking of presynaptic choline transporters. *J Neurosci23*, 9697-9709.

Fernandez H. L., Moreno R. D. and Inestrosa N. C. (1996) Tetrameric (G4) acetylcholinesterase: structure, localization, and physiological regulation. *J. Neurochem. 66*, 1335-1346.

Fink-Jensen A., Schmidt L. S., Dencker D., Schulein C., Wess J., Wortwein G. and Woldbye D. P. (2011) Antipsychotic-induced catalepsy is attenuated in mice lacking the M4 muscarinic acetylcholine receptor. *Eur. J. Pharmacol. 656*, 39-44.

Franchi C., Lucca U., Tettamanti M., Riva E., Fortino I., Bortolotti A., Merlino L., Pasina L. and Nobili A. (2011) Cholinesterase inhibitor use in Alzheimer's disease: the EPIFARM-Elderly Project. *Pharmacoepidemiol. Drug Saf. 20*, 497-505.

George S. T. and Balasubramanian A. S. (1980) The identity of the serotonin-sensitive aryl acylamidase with acetylcholinesterase from human erythrocytes, sheep basal ganglia and electric eel. *Eur. J. Biochem. 111*, 511-524.

George S. T. and Balasubramanian A. S. (1981) The aryl acylamidases and their relationship to cholinesterases in human serum, erythrocyte and liver. *Eur. J. Biochem. 121*, 177-186.

Gerber D. J., Sotnikova T. D., Gainetdinov R. R., Huang S. Y., Caron M. G. and Tonegawa S. (2001) Hyperactivity, elevated dopaminergic transmission, and response to amphetamine in M1 muscarinic acetylcholine receptor-deficient mice. *Proc. Natl. Acad. Sci. U S A98*, 15312-15317.

Geula C. and Mesulam M. M. (1995) Cholinesterases and the pathology of Alzheimer disease. *Alzheimer Dis. Assoc. Disord. 9 Suppl 2*, 23-28.

Gilmor M. L., Nash N. R., Roghani A., Edwards R. H., Yi H., Hersch S. M. and Levey A. I. (1996) Expression of the putative vesicular acetylcholine transporter in rat brain and localization in cholinergic synaptic vesicles. *J. Neurosci. 16*, 2179-2190.

Giniatullin R., Nistri A. and Yakel J. L. (2005) Desensitization of nicotinic ACh receptors: shaping cholinergic signaling. *Trends Neurosci. 28*, 371-378.

Gomeza J., Shannon H., Kostenis E., Felder C., Zhang L., Brodkin J., Grinberg A., Sheng H. and Wess J. (1999a) Pronounced pharmacologic deficits in M2 muscarinic acetylcholine receptor knockout mice. *Proc. Natl. Acad. Sci. U S A 96*, 1692-1697.

Gomeza J., Zhang L., Kostenis E., Felder C., Bymaster F., Brodkin J., Shannon H., Xia B., Deng C. and Wess J. (1999b) Enhancement of D1 dopamine receptor-mediated locomotor stimulation in M(4) muscarinic acetylcholine receptor knockout mice. *Proc. Natl. Acad. Sci. U S A 96*, 10483-10488.

Gotti C., Clementi F., Fornari A., Gaimarri A., Guiducci S., Manfredi I., Moretti M., Pedrazzi P., Pucci L. and Zoli M. (2009) Structural and functional diversity of native brain neuronal nicotinic receptors. *Biochem. Pharmacol. 78*, 703-711.

Greenblatt H. M., Dvir H., Silman I. and Sussman J. L. (2003) Acetylcholinesterase: a multifaceted target for structure-based drug design of anticholinesterase agents for the treatment of Alzheimer's disease. *J. Mol. Neurosci. 20*, 369-383.

Grigoryan H., Schopfer L. M., Thompson C. M., Terry A. V., Masson P. and Lockridge O. (2008) Mass spectrometry identifies covalent binding of soman, sarin, chlorpyrifos oxon, diisopropyl fluorophosphate, and FP-biotin to tyrosines on tubulin: a potential mechanism of long term toxicity by organophosphorus agents. *Chem. Biol. Interact. 175*, 180-186.

Gunderson C. H., Lehmann C. R., Sidell F. R. and Jabbari B. (1992) Nerve agents: a review. *Neurology 42*, 946-950.

Haga T. (1971) Synthesis and release of (14 C)acetylcholine in synaptosomes. *J. Neurochem. 18*, 781-798.

Haga T. and Noda H. (1973) Choline uptake systems of rat brain synaptosomes. *Biochim. Biophys. Acta 291*, 564-575.

Harel M., Sussman J. L., Krejci E., Bon S., Chanal P., Massoulie J. and Silman I. (1992) Conversion of acetylcholinesterase to butyrylcholinesterase: modeling and mutagenesis. *Proc. Natl. Acad. Sci. U S A 89*, 10827-10831.

Hartmann J., Kiewert C., Duysen E. G., Lockridge O., Greig N. H. and Klein J. (2007) Excessive hippocampal acetylcholine levels in acetylcholinesterase-deficient mice are moderated by butyrylcholinesterase activity. *J. Neurochem. 100*, 1421-1429.

Hersch S. M., Gutekunst C. A., Rees H. D., Heilman C. J. and Levey A. I. (1994) Distribution of m1-m4 muscarinic receptor proteins in the rat striatum: light and electron microscopic immunocytochemistry using subtype-specific antibodies. *J. Neurosci. 14*, 3351-3363.

Homma A., Imai Y., Tago H., Asada T., Shigeta M., Iwamoto T., Takita M., Arimoto I., Koma H. and Ohbayashi T. (2008) Donepezil treatment of patients with severe Alzheimer's disease in a Japanese population: results from a 24-week, double-blind, placebo-controlled, randomized trial. *Dement. Geriatr. Cogn. Disord. 25*, 399-407.

Hrabovska A., Debouzy J. C., Froment M. T., Devinsky F., Paulikova I. and Masson P. (2006) Rat butyrylcholinesterase-catalysed hydrolysis of N-alkyl homologues of benzoylcholine. *FEBS J. 273*, 1185-1197.

Hrabovska A., Duysen E. G., Sanders J. D., Murrin L. C. and Lockridge O. (2005) Delivery of human acetylcholinesterase by adeno-associated virus to the acetylcholinesterase knockout mouse. *Chem. Biol. Interact. 157-158*, 71-78.

Hrabovska A., Farar V., Bernard V., Duysen E. G., Brabec J., Lockridge O. and Myslivecek J. (2010) Drastic decrease in dopamine receptor levels in the striatum of acetylcholinesterase knock-out mouse. *Chem. Biol. Interact. 183*, 194-201.

Hrabovska A., Krejci E. and Bernard V. (2011) Subcellular addressing of Acetylcholinesterase in cholinergic and non cholinergic neurons with a special reference to the striatum.

Inestrosa N. C., Alvarez A., Godoy J., Reyes A. and De Ferrari G. V. (2000) Acetylcholinesterase-amyloid-beta-peptide interaction and Wnt signaling involvement in Abeta neurotoxicity. *Acta Neurol. Scand. Suppl. 176*, 53-59.

Inestrosa N. C., Dinamarca M. C. and Alvarez A. (2008) Amyloid-cholinesterase interactions. Implications for Alzheimer's disease. *FEBS J275*, 625-632.

Ismael Z., Millar T. J., Small D. H. and Chubb I. W. (1986) Acetylcholinesterase generates enkephalin-like immunoreactivity when it degrades the soluble proteins (chromogranins) from adrenal chromaffin granules. *Brain Res. 376*, 230-238.

Ivy M. T., Newkirk R. F., Wang Y. and Townsel J. G. (2010) A novel choline cotransporter sequestration compartment in cholinergic neurons revealed by selective endosomal ablation. *J. Neurochem. 112*, 1295-1304.

James L. C. and Tawfik D. S. (2003) Conformational diversity and protein evolution--a 60-year-old hypothesis revisited. *Trends Biochem. Sci. 28*, 361-368.

Johnson J. L., Cusack B., Davies M. P., Fauq A. and Rosenberry T. L. (2003) Unmasking tandem site interaction in human acetylcholinesterase. Substrate activation with a cationic acetanilide substrate. *Biochemistry 42*, 5438-5452.

Jope R. S. and Jenden D. J. (1979) Dimethylaminoethanol (deanol) metabolism in rat brain and its effect on acetylcholine synthesis. *J. Pharmacol. Exp. Ther. 211*, 472-479.

Kandel E.R., Schwartz J.H. and Jessell T.M. (2000) *Principles of Neural Science*. McGraw-Hill, New York.

Karczmar A. G. (2010) Cholinesterases (ChEs) and the cholinergic system in ontogenesis and phylogenesis, and non-classical roles of cholinesterases - a review. *Chem. Biol. Interact. 187*, 34-43.

Kelley A. E., Lang C. G. and Gauthier A. M. (1988) Induction of oral stereotypy following amphetamine microinjection into a discrete subregion of the striatum. *Psychopharmacology (Berl)95*, 556-559.

Kerr J. N. and Wickens J. R. (2001) Dopamine D-1/D-5 receptor activation is required for long-term potentiation in the rat neostriatum in vitro. *J. Neurophysiol. 85*, 117-124.

Kraut D., Goff H., Pai R. K., Hosea N. A., Silman I., Sussman J. L., Taylor P. and Voet J. G. (2000) Inactivation studies of acetylcholinesterase with phenylmethylsulfonyl fluoride. *Mol. Pharmacol. 57*, 1243-1248.

Krejci E., Coussen F., Duval N., Chatel J. M., Legay C., Puype M., Vandekerckhove J., Cartaud J., Bon S. and Massoulie J. (1991a) Primary structure of a collagenic tail peptide of Torpedo acetylcholinesterase: co-expression with catalytic subunit induces the production of collagen-tailed forms in transfected cells. *EMBO J. 10*, 1285-1293.

Krejci E., Duval N., Chatonnet A., Vincens P. and Massoulie J. (1991b) Cholinesterase-like domains in enzymes and structural proteins: functional and evolutionary relationships and identification of a catalytically essential aspartic acid. *Proc. Natl. Acad. Sci. U S A 88*, 6647-6651.

Krejci E., Thomine S., Boschetti N., Legay C., Sketelj J. and Massoulie J. (1997) The mammalian gene of acetylcholinesterase-associated collagen. *J. Biol. Chem. 272*, 22840-22847.

Kuhar M. J. and Murrin L. C. (1978) Sodium-dependent, high affinity choline uptake. *J. Neurochem. 30*, 15-21.

Lee E. J. (1997) Pharmacology and toxicology of chemical warfare agents. *Ann. Acad. Med. Singapore 26*, 104-107.

Legay C., Huchet M., Massoulie J. and Changeux J. P. (1995) Developmental regulation of acetylcholinesterase transcripts in the mouse diaphragm: alternative splicing and focalization. *Eur. J. Neurosci. 7*, 1803-1809.

Lehmann J. and Langer S. Z. (1983) The striatal cholinergic interneuron: synaptic target of dopaminergic terminals? *Neuroscience 10*, 1105-1120.

Levey A. I., Kitt C. A., Simonds W. F., Price D. L. and Brann M. R. (1991) Identification and localization of muscarinic acetylcholine receptor proteins in brain with subtype-specific antibodies. *J. Neurosci. 11*, 3218-3226.

Li B., Duysen E. G., Volpicelli-Daley L. A., Levey A. I. and Lockridge O. (2003) Regulation of muscarinic acetylcholine receptor function in acetylcholinesterase knockout mice. *Pharmacol. Biochem. Behav. 74*, 977-986.

Li B., Stribley J. A., Ticu A., Xie W., Schopfer L. M., Hammond P., Brimijoin S., Hinrichs S. H. and Lockridge O. (2000) Abundant tissue butyrylcholinesterase and its possible function in the acetylcholinesterase knockout mouse. *J. Neurochem. 75*, 1320-1331.

Li F. and Han Z. J. (2002) Two different genes encoding acetylcholinesterase existing in cotton aphid (Aphis gossypii). *Genome 45*, 1134-1141.

Lindstrom J., Anand R., Gerzanich V., Peng X., Wang F. and Wells G. (1996) Structure and function of neuronal nicotinic acetylcholine receptors. *Prog. Brain Res. 109*, 125-137.

Lockridge O. (1982) Substance P hydrolysis by human serum cholinesterase. *J. Neurochem. 39*, 106-110.

Lukas R. J., Changeux J. P., Le N. N., Albuquerque E. X., Balfour D. J., Berg D. K., Bertrand D., Chiappinelli V. A., Clarke P. B., Collins A. C., Dani J. A., Grady S. R., Kellar K. J., Lindstrom J. M., Marks M. J., Quik M., Taylor P. W. and Wonnacott S. (1999) International Union of Pharmacology. XX. Current status of the nomenclature for nicotinic acetylcholine receptors and their subunits. *Pharmacol. Rev. 51*, 397-401.

Lullmann H., Mohr K., Ziegler A. and Bieger D. (2000) *Color Atlas of Pharmacology*. Thieme, New York.

Malcolm C. A., Bourguet D., Ascolillo A., Rooker S. J., Garvey C. F., Hall L. M., Pasteur N. and Raymond M. (1998) A sex-linked Ace gene, not linked to insensitive acetylcholinesterase-mediated insecticide resistance in Culex pipiens. *Insect. Mol. Biol. 7*, 107-120.

Mallender W. D., Szegletes T. and Rosenberry T. L. (2000) Acetylthiocholine binds to asp74 at the peripheral site of human acetylcholinesterase as the first step in the catalytic pathway. *Biochemistry 39*, 7753-7763.

Masson P., Froment M. T., Bartels C. F. and Lockridge O. (1997) Importance of aspartate-70 in organophosphate inhibition, oxime re-activation and aging of human butyrylcholinesterase. *Biochem. J. 325 (Pt 1)*, 53-61.

Masson P., Nachon F., Bartels C. F., Froment M. T., Ribes F., Matthews C. and Lockridge O. (2003) High activity of human butyrylcholinesterase at low pH in the presence of excess butyrylthiocholine. *Eur. J. Biochem. 270*, 315-324.

Masson P., Schopfer L. M., Bartels C. F., Froment M. T., Ribes F., Nachon F. and Lockridge O. (2002) Substrate activation in acetylcholinesterase induced by low pH or mutation in the pi-cation subsite. *Biochim. Biophys. Acta 1594*, 313-324.

Masson P., Schopfer L. M., Froment M. T., Debouzy J. C., Nachon F., Gillon E., Lockridge O., Hrabovska A. and Goldstein B. N. (2005) Hysteresis of butyrylcholinesterase in the approach to steady-state kinetics. *Chem. Biol. Interact. 157-158*, 143-152.

Masson P., Xie W., Froment M. T. and Lockridge O. (2001) Effects of mutations of active site residues and amino acids interacting with the Omega loop on substrate activation of butyrylcholinesterase. *Biochim. Biophys. Acta 1544*, 166-176.

Massoulie J. (2002) The origin of the molecular diversity and functional anchoring of cholinesterases. *Neurosignals 11*, 130-143.

Massoulie J. and Bon S. (1982) The molecular forms of cholinesterase and acetylcholinesterase in vertebrates. *Annu. Rev. Neurosci. 5*, 57-106.

Massoulie J., Perrier N., Noureddine H., Liang D. and Bon S. (2008) Old and new questions about cholinesterases. *Chem. Biol. Interact. 175*, 30-44.

Maurice N., Mercer J., Chan C. S., Hernandez-Lopez S., Held J., Tkatch T. and Surmeier D. J. (2004) D2 dopamine receptor-mediated modulation of voltage-dependent Na+ channels reduces autonomous activity in striatal cholinergic interneurons. *J. Neurosci. 24*, 10289-10301.

Mearns J., Dunn J. and Lees-Haley P. R. (1994) Psychological effects of organophosphate pesticides: a review and call for research by psychologists. *J. Clin. Psychol. 50*, 286-294.

Millar T. J. and Chubb I. W. (1984) Treatment of sections of chick retina with acetylcholinesterase increases the enkephalin and substance P immunoreactivity. *Neuroscience 12*, 441-451.

Murrin L. C. and Kuhar M. J. (1976) Activation of high-affinity choline uptake in vitro by depolarizing agents. *Mol. Pharmacol. 12*, 1082-1090.

Myslivecek J., Duysen E. G. and Lockridge O. (2007) Adaptation to excess acetylcholine by downregulation of adrenoceptors and muscarinic receptors in lungs of acetylcholinesterase knockout mice. *Naunyn. Schmiedebergs Arch. Pharmacol. 376*, 83-92.

Nachon F., Ehret-Sabatier L., Loew D., Colas C., van D. A. and Goeldner M. (1998) Trp82 and Tyr332 are involved in two quaternary ammonium binding domains of human butyrylcholinesterase as revealed by photoaffinity labeling with (3H)DDF. *Biochemistry 37*, 10507-10513.

Nashmi R. and Lester H. A. (2006) CNS localization of neuronal nicotinic receptors. *J. Mol. Neurosci. 30*, 181-184.

Nathanson N. M. (2000) A multiplicity of muscarinic mechanisms: enough signaling pathways to take your breath away. *Proc. Natl. Acad. Sci. U S A97*, 6245-6247.

Newkirk R. F., Maleque M. A. and Townsel J. G. (1980) Choline uptake, acetylcholine synthesis and release by Limulus abdominal ganglia. *Neuroscience 5*, 303-311.

Nguyen M. L., Cox G. D. and Parsons S. M. (1998) Kinetic parameters for the vesicular acetylcholine transporter: two protons are exchanged for one acetylcholine. *Biochemistry 37*, 13400-13410.

Okuda T., Haga T., Kanai Y., Endou H., Ishihara T. and Katsura I. (2000) Identification and characterization of the high-affinity choline transporter. *Nat. Neurosci. 3*, 120-125.

Ordentlich A., Barak D., Kronman C., Flashner Y., Leitner M., Segall Y., Ariel N., Cohen S., Velan B. and Shafferman A. (1993) Dissection of the human acetylcholinesterase active center determinants of substrate specificity. Identification of residues constituting the anionic site, the hydrophobic site, and the acyl pocket. *J. Biol. Chem. 268*, 17083-17095.

Perrier A. L., Massoulie J. and Krejci E. (2002) PRiMA: the membrane anchor of acetylcholinesterase in the brain. *Neuron 33*, 275-285.

Pezzementi L. and Chatonnet A. (2010) Evolution of cholinesterases in the animal kingdom. *Chem. Biol. Interact. 187*, 27-33.

Picciotto M. R. (2003) Nicotine as a modulator of behavior: beyond the inverted U. *Trends Pharmacol. Sci. 24*, 493-499.

Picciotto M. R., Zoli M., Lena C., Bessis A., Lallemand Y., Le N. N., Vincent P., Pich E. M., Brulet P. and Changeux J. P. (1995) Abnormal avoidance learning in mice lacking functional high-affinity nicotine receptor in the brain. *Nature 374*, 65-67.

Pisani A., Bonsi P., Centonze D., Calabresi P. and Bernardi G. (2000) Activation of D2-like dopamine receptors reduces synaptic inputs to striatal cholinergic interneurons. *J. Neurosci. 20*, RC69.

Plaznik A., Stefanski R. and Kostowski W. (1989) Interaction between accumbens D1 and D2 receptors regulating rat locomotor activity. *Psychopharmacology (Berl) 99*, 558-562.

Pope C., Karanth S. and Liu J. (2005) Pharmacology and toxicology of cholinesterase inhibitors: uses and misuses of a common mechanism of action. *Environ. Toxicol. Pharmacol. 19*, 433-446.

Quarta D., Ciruela F., Patkar K., Borycz J., Solinas M., Lluis C., Franco R., Wise R. A., Goldberg S. R., Hope B. T., Woods A. S. and Ferre S. (2007) Heteromeric nicotinic acetylcholine-dopamine autoreceptor complexes modulate striatal dopamine release. *Neuropsychopharmacology 32*, 35-42.

Radic Z., Kalisiak J., Fokin V. V., Sharpless K. B. and Taylor P. (2010) Interaction kinetics of oximes with native, phosphylated and aged human acetylcholinesterase. *Chem. Biol. Interact. 187*, 163-166.

Radic Z., Pickering N. A., Vellom D. C., Camp S. and Taylor P. (1993) Three distinct domains in the cholinesterase molecule confer selectivity for acetyl- and butyrylcholinesterase inhibitors. *Biochemistry 32*, 12074-12084.

Radic Z., Quinn D. M., Vellom D. C., Camp S. and Taylor P. (1995) Allosteric control of acetylcholinesterase catalysis by fasciculin. *J. Biol. Chem. 270*, 20391-20399.

Reyes A. E., Perez D. R., Alvarez A., Garrido J., Gentry M. K., Doctor B. P. and Inestrosa N. C. (1997) A monoclonal antibody against acetylcholinesterase inhibits the formation of amyloid fibrils induced by the enzyme. *Biochem. Biophys. Res. Commun. 232*, 652-655.

Reynolds J. N., Hyland B. I. and Wickens J. R. (2001) A cellular mechanism of reward-related learning. *Nature 413*, 67-70.

Ribeiro F. M., Black S. A., Prado V. F., Rylett R. J., Ferguson S. S. and Prado M. A. (2006) The "ins" and "outs" of the high-affinity choline transporter CHT1. *J. Neurochem. 97*, 1-12.

Ribeiro F. M., ves-Silva J., Volknandt W., Martins-Silva C., Mahmud H., Wilhelm A., Gomez M. V., Rylett R. J., Ferguson S. S., Prado V. F. and Prado M. A. (2003) The hemicholinium-3 sensitive high affinity choline transporter is internalized by clathrin-mediated endocytosis and is present in endosomes and synaptic vesicles. *J. Neurochem. 87*, 136-146.

Rice M. E. and Cragg S. J. (2004) Nicotine amplifies reward-related dopamine signals in striatum. *Nat. Neurosci. 7*, 583-584.

Risch S. C., Horner M. D., McGurk S. R., Palecko S., Markowitz J. S., Nahas Z. and DeVane C. L. (2007) Double-blind donepezil-placebo crossover augmentation study of atypical antipsychotics in chronic, stable schizophrenia: a pilot study. *Schizophr. Res. 93*, 131-135.

Rogers S. L., Doody R. S., Mohs R. C. and Friedhoff L. T. (1998) Donepezil improves cognition and global function in Alzheimer disease: a 15-week, double-blind, placebo-controlled study. Donepezil Study Group. *Arch. Intern. Med. 158*, 1021-1031.

Roldan-Tapia L., Parron T. and Sanchez-Santed F. (2005) Neuropsychological effects of long-term exposure to organophosphate pesticides. *Neurotoxicol. Teratol. 27*, 259-266.

Roskoski R., Jr. (1978) Acceleration of choline uptake after depolarization-induced acetylcholine release in rat cortical synaptosomes. *J. Neurochem. 30*, 1357-1361.

Rumenapp U., Asmus M., Schablowski H., Woznicki M., Han L., Jakobs K. H., Fahimi-Vahid M., Michalek C., Wieland T. and Schmidt M. (2001) The M3 muscarinic acetylcholine receptor expressed in HEK-293 cells signals to phospholipase D via G12 but not Gq-type G proteins: regulators of G proteins as tools to dissect pertussis toxin-resistant G proteins in receptor-effector coupling. *J. Biol. Chem. 276*, 2474-2479.

Sadar M. H. and Laidler K. J. (1975) Transient kinetics of the acetylcholinesterase catalyzed hydrolysis of N-methylindoxyl acetate. *Can. J. Biochem. 53*, 380-387.

Salminen O., Murphy K. L., McIntosh J. M., Drago J., Marks M. J., Collins A. C. and Grady S. R. (2004) Subunit composition and pharmacology of two classes of striatal presynaptic nicotinic acetylcholine receptors mediating dopamine release in mice. *Mol. Pharmacol. 65*, 1526-1535.

Satoh T. and Hosokawa M. (2000) Organophosphates and their impact on the global environment. *Neurotoxicology 21*, 223-227.

Shapovalova K. B. (1999) Activation of the cholinergic system of the striatum improves attention to conditioned reflex stimuli. *Neurosci. Behav. Physiol. 29*, 493-503.

Sherin A., Peeyush K. T., Jayanarayanan S., Amee K. K. and Paulose C. S. (2011) Decreased Cholinergic Receptor Expression in the Striatum: Motor Function Deficit in Hypoglycemic and Diabetic Rats. *Cell Mol. Neurobiol.*

Simon J. R. and Kuhar M. G. (1975) Impulse-flow regulation of high affinity choline uptake in brain cholinergic nerve terminals. *Nature 255*, 162-163.

Simon J. R. and Kuhar M. J. (1976) High affinity choline uptake: ionic and energy requirements. *J. Neurochem. 27*, 93-99.

Simon S., Krejci E. and Massoulie J. (1998) A four-to-one association between peptide motifs: four C-terminal domains from cholinesterase assemble with one proline-rich attachment domain (PRAD) in the secretory pathway. *EMBO J. 17*, 6178-6187.

Sine S. M. and Engel A. G. (2006) Recent advances in Cys-loop receptor structure and function. *Nature 440*, 448-455.

Small D. H., Ismael Z. and Chubb I. W. (1987) Acetylcholinesterase exhibits trypsin-like and metalloexopeptidase-like activity in cleaving a model peptide. *Neuroscience 21*, 991-995.

Soli N. E., Karlsen R. L., Opsahl M. and Fonnum F. (1980) Correlations between acetylcholinesterase activity in guinea-pig iris and pupillary function: a biochemical and pupillographic study. *J. Neurochem. 35*, 723-728.

Steinlein O. K. (2001) Genes and mutations in idiopathic epilepsy. *Am. J. Med. Genet. 106*, 139-145.

Stoof J. C., Drukarch B., de B. P. and Westerink B. H. (1992) In vitro and in vivo acetylcholine release from rat striatum as a functional paradigm of signal transduction via a D-2 dopamine receptor. *Neurochem. Int. 20 Suppl*, 201S-205S.

Sun M., Lee C. J. and Shin H. S. (2007) Reduced nicotinic receptor function in sympathetic ganglia is responsible for the hypothermia in the acetylcholinesterase knockout mouse. *J. Physiol. 578*, 751-764.

Sussman J. L., Harel M., Frolow F., Oefner C., Goldman A., Toker L. and Silman I. (1991) Atomic structure of acetylcholinesterase from Torpedo californica: a prototypic acetylcholine-binding protein. *Science 253*, 872-879.

Sutherland D., McClellan J. S., Milner D., Soong W., Axon N., Sanders M., Hester A., Kao Y. H., Poczatek T., Routt S. and Pezzementi L. (1997) Two cholinesterase activities and genes are present in amphioxus. *J. Exp. Zool. 277*, 213-229.

Szegletes T., Mallender W. D., Thomas P. J. and Rosenberry T. L. (1999) Substrate binding to the peripheral site of acetylcholinesterase initiates enzymatic catalysis. Substrate inhibition arises as a secondary effect. *Biochemistry 38*, 122-133.

Taly A., Corringer P. J., Guedin D., Lestage P. and Changeux J. P. (2009) Nicotinic receptors: allosteric transitions and therapeutic targets in the nervous system. *Nat. Rev. Drug Discov. 8*, 733-750.

Thomsen M., Woldbye D. P., Wortwein G., Fink-Jensen A., Wess J. and Caine S. B. (2005) Reduced cocaine self-administration in muscarinic M5 acetylcholine receptor-deficient mice. *J. Neurosci. 25*, 8141-8149.

Threlfell S. and Cragg S. J. (2011) Dopamine signaling in dorsal versus ventral striatum: the dynamic role of cholinergic interneurons. *Front. Syst. Neurosci. 5*, 11.

Tobin A. B. and Budd D. C. (2003) The anti-apoptotic response of the Gq/11-coupled muscarinic receptor family. *Biochem. Soc. Trans. 31*, 1182-1185.

Tucek S. (1985) Regulation of acetylcholine synthesis in the brain. *J. Neurochem. 44*, 11-24.

Unwin N. (2005) Refined structure of the nicotinic acetylcholine receptor at 4A resolution. *J. Mol. Biol. 346*, 967-989.

van Koppen C. J. and Kaiser B. (2003) Regulation of muscarinic acetylcholine receptor signaling. *Pharmacol. Ther. 98*, 197-220.

Vellom D. C., Radic Z., Li Y., Pickering N. A., Camp S. and Taylor P. (1993) Amino acid residues controlling acetylcholinesterase and butyrylcholinesterase specificity. *Biochemistry 32*, 12-17.

Volpicelli-Daley L. A., Duysen E. G., Lockridge O. and Levey A. I. (2003a) Altered hippocampal muscarinic receptors in acetylcholinesterase-deficient mice. *Ann. Neurol. 53*, 788-796.

Volpicelli-Daley L. A., Hrabovska A., Duysen E. G., Ferguson S. M., Blakely R. D., Lockridge O. and Levey A. I. (2003b) Altered striatal function and muscarinic cholinergic receptors in acetylcholinesterase knockout mice. *Mol. Pharmacol. 64*, 1309-1316.

Weiner D. M., Levey A. I. and Brann M. R. (1990) Expression of muscarinic acetylcholine and dopamine receptor mRNAs in rat basal ganglia. *Proc. Natl. Acad. Sci. U S A 87*, 7050-7054.

Weiner L., Shnyrov V. L., Konstantinovskii L., Roth E., Ashani Y. and Silman I. (2009) Stabilization of Torpedo californica acetylcholinesterase by reversible inhibitors. *Biochemistry 48*, 563-574.

Wess J. (2004) Muscarinic acetylcholine receptor knockout mice: novel phenotypes and clinical implications. *Annu. Rev. Pharmacol. Toxicol. 44*, 423-450.

Wess J., Eglen R. M. and Gautam D. (2007) Muscarinic acetylcholine receptors: mutant mice provide new insights for drug development. *Nat. Rev. Drug Discov. 6*, 721-733.

Wise R. A. and Kiyatkin E. A. (2011) Differentiating the rapid actions of cocaine. *Nat. Rev. Neurosci. 12*, 479-484.

Witten I. B., Lin S. C., Brodsky M., Prakash R., Diester I., Anikeeva P., Gradinaru V., Ramakrishnan C. and Deisseroth K. (2010) Cholinergic interneurons control local circuit activity and cocaine conditioning. *Science 330*, 1677-1681.

Worek F., Thiermann H., Szinicz L. and Eyer P. (2004) Kinetic analysis of interactions between human acetylcholinesterase, structurally different organophosphorus compounds and oximes. *Biochem. Pharmacol. 68*, 2237-2248.

Wright C. I., Geula C. and Mesulam M. M. (1993) Protease inhibitors and indolamines selectively inhibit cholinesterases in the histopathologic structures of Alzheimer's disease. *Ann. N Y Acad. Sci. 695*, 65-68.

Xie W., Stribley J. A., Chatonnet A., Wilder P. J., Rizzino A., McComb R. D., Taylor P., Hinrichs S. H. and Lockridge O. (2000) Postnatal developmental delay and supersensitivity to organophosphate in gene-targeted mice lacking acetylcholinesterase. *J. Pharmacol. Exp. Ther. 293*, 896-902.

Xie W., Wilder P. J., Stribley J., Chatonnet A., Rizzino A., Taylor P., Hinrichs S. H. and Lockridge O. (1999) Knockout of one acetylcholinesterase allele in the mouse. *Chem. Biol. Interact. 119-120*, 289-299.

Yakel J. L. (2010) Gating of nicotinic ACh receptors: latest insights into ligand binding and function. *J. Physiol. 588*, 597-602.

Yamamura H. I. and Snyder S. H. (1972) Choline: high-affinity uptake by rat brain synaptosomes. *Science 178*, 626-628.

Yan Z., Flores-Hernandez J. and Surmeier D. J. (2001) Coordinated expression of muscarinic receptor messenger RNAs in striatal medium spiny neurons. *Neuroscience103*, 1017-1024.

Yan Z., Song W. J. and Surmeier J. (1997) D2 dopamine receptors reduce N-type Ca2+ currents in rat neostriatal cholinergic interneurons through a membrane-delimited, protein-kinase-C-insensitive pathway. *J. Neurophysiol. 77*, 1003-1015.

Yasuda R. P., Ciesla W., Flores L. R., Wall S. J., Li M., Satkus S. A., Weisstein J. S., Spagnola B. V. and Wolfe B. B. (1993) Development of antisera selective for m4 and m5 muscarinic cholinergic receptors: distribution of m4 and m5 receptors in rat brain. *Mol. Pharmacol. 43*, 149-157.

Zhang H. and Sulzer D. (2004) Frequency-dependent modulation of dopamine release by nicotine. *Nat. Neurosci. 7*, 581-582.

Zhang W., Yamada M., Gomeza J., Basile A. S. and Wess J. (2002) Multiple muscarinic acetylcholine receptor subtypes modulate striatal dopamine release, as studied with M1-M5 muscarinic receptor knock-out mice. *J. Neurosci. 22*, 6347-6352.

Zhou F. M., Liang Y. and Dani J. A. (2001) Endogenous nicotinic cholinergic activity regulates dopamine release in the striatum. *Nat. Neurosci. 4*, 1224-1229.

Zhou F. M., Wilson C. and Dani J. A. (2003) Muscarinic and nicotinic cholinergic mechanisms in the mesostriatal dopamine systems. *Neuroscientist. 9*, 23-36.

Zhou F. M., Wilson C. J. and Dani J. A. (2002) Cholinergic interneuron characteristics and nicotinic properties in the striatum. *J. Neurobiol. 53*, 590-605.

Zoli M., Moretti M., Zanardi A., McIntosh J. M., Clementi F. and Gotti C. (2002) Identification of the nicotinic receptor subtypes expressed on dopaminergic terminals in the rat striatum. *J. Neurosci. 22*, 8785-8789.

In: Striatum: Anatomy, Functions and Role in Disease
Editors: Hugo T. Maldonado and Ignacio M. Ortega
ISBN 978-1-61942-384-8

Chapter II

Physical Therapy, Exercise and Parkinson's Disease

Aderbal S. Aguiar Jr.* and Rui Daniel S. Prediger
Laboratório Experimental de Doenças Neurodegenerativas, Departamento de Farmacologia, Universidade Federal de Santa Catarina (UFSC), Florianópolis-SC, Brazil

Abstract

Parkinson's disease is the second most common neurodegenerative disorder following Alzheimer's disease, affecting approximately 1% of the population older than 50 years. Since the incidence of the disease increases with age (the most important risk factor), it is likely that the number of people suffering from Parkinson's disease will rise as improved health care lengthens the average life span. Classically, Parkinson's disease is considered to be a motor system disease and its diagnosis is based on the presence of a set of cardinal motor signs (e.g. rigidity, bradykinesia, rest tremor, and postural reflex disturbance). These symptoms of Parkinson's disease mainly result from the progressive degeneration of dopamine neurons of the *substantia nigra pars compacta* that project predominantly to the striatum. Today there is considerable evidence showing that deficits in olfactory and cognitive functions precede the classical motor symptoms seen in Parkinson's disease. The beneficial effects of the drugs currently available for the treatment of Parkinson's disease (such as levodopa) on improving the cognitive function affected in this disease is controversial. Thus, the management of non-motor symptoms of Parkinson's disease remains a challenge. Over the last decade, regular physical exercise has been implicated to an increased plasticity in the adult brain (such as increase in neurogenesis and cognitive processes and neurotrophic factors production). Research is now emerging on a possible influence of physical exercise in the neurodegenerative process associated to Parkinson's disease. The present chapter attempts to review results reported in different clinical studies and animal models to provide a comprehensive picture of the role of physical exercise in Parkinson's disease. Although many of the

* Corresponding author: Aderbal S. Aguiar Jr, PhD, Laboratório Experimental de Doenças Neurodegenerativas, Departamento de Farmacologia, Universidade Federal de Santa Catarina, Campus Trindade, 88049-900, Florianópolis, SC, Brazil., Phone (55) 48 3721 9764 ext 223 – Fax (55) 48 3337 5479., E-mail address: aderbalaguiar@gmail.com

training programs investigated were accompanied by some degree of oxidative stress, which should be taken into account in physical training programs for this population, it is important to emphasize that this response did not promote any negative impact on the rehabilitation aspects of Parkinson's disease patients. Taken together, the current literature suggests that regular physical exercise can present beneficial effects in Parkinson's disease patients evaluated through different tests. It might also afford protection against dopaminergic neurons death and motor dysfunction elicited in experimental models. Finally, this chapter shows recent findings from our laboratory indicating that moderate physical exercise plays an important role into improvement cognitive deficits in an experimental model of Parkinson's disease, reinforcing the potential of physical exercise in the management of non-motor symptoms of Parkinson's disease.

Abbreviations

BDNF – brain-derived neurotrophic factor;
BBB – blood brain barrier;
BWSTT – body weight supported treadmill training;
CAT – catalase;
DA – dopamine;
DAT transporter;
DNA – deoxyribonucleic acid;
EMG – electromyographic;
GPX – glutathione peroxidase;
HR – heart rate;
H_2O_2 – hydrogen peroxide;
L-DOPA – levodopa;
MPTP – 1-methyl-4-phenyl-1,2,3,6-tetrahydroxypyridine;
MPP^+ – 1-methyl-4-phenylpyridinium;
PD – Parkinson's disease;
PT – physical therapy;
QoL – quality of life;
SNpc – substantia nigra pars compacta;
SOD – superoxide dismutase;
TH – tyrosine hydroxylase;
6-OHDA – 6-hydroxydopamine

Introduction

Ever since James Parkinson described shaking palsy in 1817, scientists and clinicians have been searching for effective treatment options to Parkinson's disease (PD). Before the introduction of levodopa (L-DOPA) in the late 1960s, physical therapy was widely considered to be a critical component in the management of PD. By the early 1970s, L-DOPA had become widely available and many believed it to be a cure for PD. This led to a decreased interest in alternative treatments, such as physical therapy and physical exercise – main issues of this chapter. Within a few years, however, it became apparent that L-DOPA's efficacy does not last indefinitely, and that with long term use can cause side effects that may even surpasses the original parkinsonian symptoms, such as the 'on off' effect, dyskinesias and neuropsychiatric manifestations [1-3]. As science continues to search for a lasting "cure" for PD, there has been a renewed interest in non-pharmacological treatment options as adjuncts to drug therapy. In this way, several scientists changed the focus of exercise and PD from clinics and rehabilitation centers to experimental interventions in research centers and laboratory utilizing animal models of PD. Today, in addition to the standard drug regime, physical therapy is often prescribed by itself or with other treatment options, such as occupational therapy and speech therapy. In addition, several studies are pointing to physical exercise such as promise neuroprotective strategy in the PD.

A possible explanation to it begins in 1890, when William James first recognized that one of the most important features of animal behavior is the ability to carry out meaningful change [4]: the 'behavioral plasticity'. Since then, this concept of plasticity has been further developed to include structural change in the brain at the cellular, molecular, and system levels. Maintaining brain health and plasticity throughout life is an important public health goal, and it is increasingly clear that behavioral stimulation and exercise can help us to achieve it. The decline of neurological functions is an inevitable aged-related process derived from distinct factors since brain shrink and neurotrophic failure until tissue oxidation, among several others [5-8]. It stimulated the search for approaches to maintain or improve the biology of aged brain, such as the physical exercise and free leisure time (see Figure 6-1) (6, 9, 10). Physical exercise induces central and periphery allostatic changes leading to differential upstream of vascular and neurotrophic support, increasing newborn of synapses and neurons, and alleviating excessive oxidative stress in old-aged subjects [4, 9, 11]. Such intervention is particularly crucial from middle age onwards, when the brain faces a series of challenges that can include the pathogenesis of neurodegenerative diseases like Alzheimer's disease (AD) and PD[4, 12].

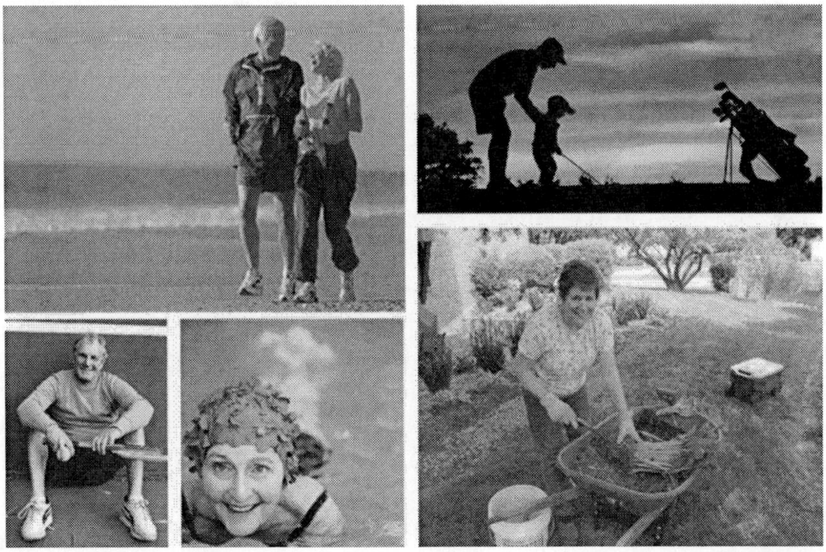

Figure 6.1. Be physically active protects against the aging-related cognitive decline and risk rate of several neurological diseases.

Over the past 20 years, an increasing number of studies on humans have shown the benefits of exercise on brain health and function, particularly in aging populations. Of high importance, physical exercise has been identified with one therapeutic alternative to minimize motor and non-motor symptoms of PD and it might also afford protection against dopaminergic neurons death and motor dysfunction elicited in rodent models of PD [13-18].

However, despite strong evidences regarding physical therapy and exercise benefits in the PD, the role of these environmental approaches remains controversial. They are safety and feasible to PD patients. But what is the main role of physical therapy and exercise in the PD: palliative, curative, or neuroprotective? The present chapter attempts to review evidences reported in different clinical studies and animal models to provide a comprehensive picture of the role of physical therapy and exercise in PD.

Physical Therapy and Exercise in Parkinson's Disease: The Current Palliative Approach

A wide variety of health professionals – physical therapists, occupational therapists, gerontologists, neurologists, psychologists, and others – may be involved in the rehabilitation of PD patients. Often physical therapy focuses on the impairments (e.g., neurological symptoms), functional limitations (e.g., walking, stair climbing, reaching, grasping), and disabilities (e.g., hobbies, sport, and social activities) and is comprised of mobility exercises, gait training (with and without the application of external cues), training of daily activities, relaxation therapy, and breathing exercises, among others [15]. Another goal is to educate the individual (as well as partner and family) about the disease process and the benefits of exercise therapy [15]. Goals of occupational therapy include maximizing fine motor coordination, especially of the upper extremities, reducing energy expenditure, increasing safety and independence, and improving quality of life and efficiency of activities of daily living [19]. Moreover, it has been suggested that physical therapy is an important adjunct to anti-PD drugs [15].

Physical therapy may serve as an important adjunct to the available pharmacological and neurosurgical treatment regimes with regard to neurologic symptoms (e.g., tremor, bradykinesia, and rigidity), walking ability, ADLs (activities of daily living), and quality of life (QoL) [15]. It should be noticed, however, that physical therapy is mainly focused on mobility strategies rather than neurologic symptoms, such as rigidity and tremor [15]. In this way, there are numerous intervention studies evaluating the effects of physical therapy in addition to the anti-PD pharmacological treatment, which seems to be an interesting approach to the problems of mobility that accompany the motor symptoms of the disease. They are summarized on Table 6-1. Generally, the approach is palliative and the main aim of physical therapy is to maximize functional ability and minimize secondary complications through movement rehabilitation within a context of education and support for the whole person.The rehabilitation management in patients with PD should preferably be a multidisciplinary effort with a wide variety of health professionals – physical therapists, occupational therapists, speech-language pathologists, gerontologists, neurologists, psychologists, and others, in which professionals work together as a team to address physical, behavioral and cognitive presentations resulting from PD.

Table 1. Overview of clinical outcomes in patients with Parkinson's disease submitted to physical exercise

Reference	HandY	Intervention	Significative outcomes
(22, 23)	1-3	Muscle strengthening	↑ 1RM, ↑ fat-free mass, ↑ bone mineral density
(24, 25)		Lower body resistance training and balance training	↑ equilibrium composite score
(26, 27)		Physical therapy	↓ UPDRS scores after follow-up
(28)	2-3	Cycling and treadmill	↑ VO_2max, ↑ movement initiation
(13)		Exercises to improve ROM, endurance, balance, gait and fine motor dexterity	↓ UPDRS score
(29)		Exercise to improve axial rotation, functional reach, time supine and stand, 360° turn, 6-min walking distance and 10-min walking time	↑ functional axial rotation, ↑ functional reach, ↓ time to complete 360° return
(30, 31)		Gait and step training	↑ gait speed, cadence and step test
(16, 32, 33)		BWSTT	↑ gait
(34, 35)	2-4	Training program involving sitting, standing and gait activities in relation to bed	↑ turning in bed, ↑ rising from a chair, ↓ falling.
(36)	3 or higher	Exercise	↓ mortality

Abbreviations – ↑: improvement; ↓: decrease; BWSTT: Body Weight-Supported Treadmill Training; HandY: Hoehn and Yahr; ROM: Range of Motion; UPDRS: Unified Parkinson's Disease Rating Scale; 1RM: maximal muscle contraction.

In addition, several strategies should be developed in order to ensure the adherence of patients to rehabilitation programs. For example, there are interesting evidences on the implementation of physical therapy in groups of patients with PD [15]. Gauthier et al. (1987) [20]and Palmer et al. (1986) [21] reported improvement of psychological well-being. Gauthier et al. (1987) [20] also reported facilitation of several positive behavioral changes as additional effects of group treatment.

Generally, both individual and group physical therapy treatment focuses on the impairments (e.g., neurologic symptoms), functional limitations (e.g., walking, stair climbing, reaching, and grasping), and disabilities (e.g., hobbies, sport, and social activities) and comprises of range of motion (ROM) and flexibility exercises [15, 29], gait and equilibrium training (with and without the application of external cues) [15, 37], exercises of mobility and coordination [15, 38], training of daily activities [15, 39], relaxation therapy [15], and breathing exercises [15, 29]. These studies reported positive results for the groups that received the intervention, such as improvement in gait [16, 33], increased spinal flexibility [29], better functional reach [36, 40] improved axial mobility [29, 40], improved motor ability [40], increased muscle strength, and reduction in number of falls [17]. These improvements are important for daily activities such as turning over, moving in bed, standing from a sitting position, reaching forward while sitting or standing, turning while standing, and walking. Another goal is to educate the individual (as well as caregivers, partners and the family) about the disease process and the benefits of exercise therapy. Moreover, it has been suggested that physical therapy is an important adjunct to the anti-parkinsonian medication (15), more forward we will address this issue.

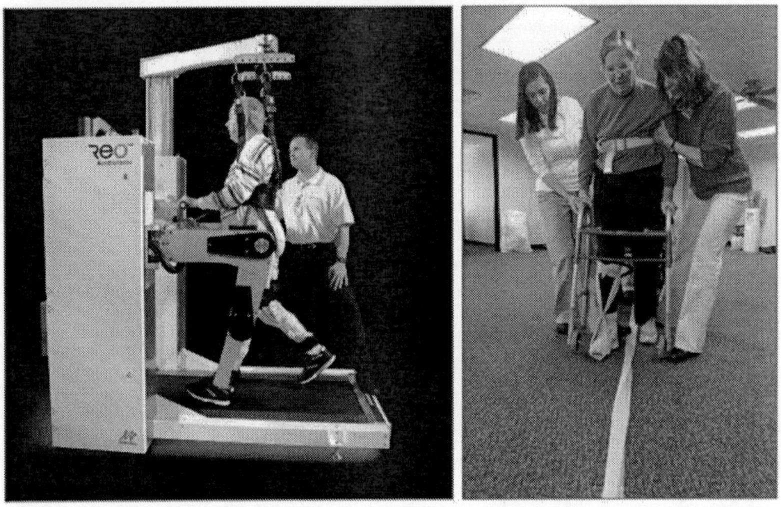

Figure 6.2. The physical rehabilitation of Parkinson's disease patients has been improved with the use of more efficient strategies for these patients, as BWSTT and the use of sensory cues. BWSTT - body weight-supported treadmill training.

In addition to the conventional physiotherapy regimes, a number of experimental physical therapy programs have been evaluated, such as body weight supported treadmill training (BWSTT) and sensory cueing for the treatment of gait (see Figure 6-2).

Animal research in the 1960s suggested that cats with transected spinal cords could produce stepping patterns after several weeks of BWSTT, in which the cat was partially supported in a sling and its hind limbs were manually assisted on a treadmill. This ability was attributed to a so-called central pattern generator, said to be produced in the lumbosacral spinal cord below the injury in response to sensory information associated with locomotion. This research into spinal cord "learning" has led to investigations of a possible central pattern generator in humans. The BWSTT was found to be superior to regular physiotherapy, especially as far as short step gait is concerned [16, 33, 38].

A central pattern generator mechanism is postulated. In parkinsonism, electromyographic (EMG) studies revealed that reduced leg extensor activation might contribute to gait disorder [41]. The absolute EMG amplitude of gastrocnemius muscles during the stance phase of stepping with normal body loading was significantly smaller in persons with PD than in age-matched healthy controls [42]. This contraction during stepping was reduced by body weight support, but the load sensitivity was less in persons with PD than in healthy subjects [43]. Body weight support might compensate for the diminished push-off of the leg experienced by Parkinson's patients in the latter half of stance phase of the gait. Improvement in postural reflex might be also involved in the mechanism since patients had better postural reflex outcomes after BWSTT than physical therapy. Moreover, reorganization especially in the supplementary cortical motor area might also be a possible mechanism underlying the improvement [16, 33].

Some researchers are interested in the phenomenon of sensory cueing [44]. One of the most interesting features of PD is that, despite severe motor symptoms, patients are sometimes still able to perform complex movements almost normally under certain conditions [44, 45]. For example, some patients will inexplicably freeze while walking through a doorway, but will have no trouble at all climbing a flight of stairs [46]. It appears that the underlying problem has more to do with motor control than with actual motor function. The challenge lies in enabling patients to access this ability at will and to use it in normal, daily function. This occurs because the basal ganglia, the focal point of impairment in PD, have been shown to be involved in the execution of automatic and repetitive movement [44, 47]. The basal ganglia are neural structures within the motor and cognitive control circuits in the mammalian forebrain and are interconnected with the neocortex by multiple loops [48]. Dysfunction in these parallel loops caused by damage to the striatum results in major defects in voluntary movement [48]. It is probably involved in two separate elements of motor control [49]. First, the basal ganglia prove phasic cues to the supplementary motor area, which is responsible for activating and deactivating submovements within the complete movement sequence. Submovements are hypothesized building blocks of human movement, discrete ballistic movements of which more complex movements are composed. Second, the basal ganglia are relate in the transmission of motor set information, i.e., they are responsible for accurate execution of each submovement element [44]. With this hypothesis, it is possible to explain two primary gait deficiencies seen in PD [44]. The movement execution is not smooth because internal rhythmic cues are not being properly supplied [47, 50]. Two of the hallmark features of PD gait: freezing [46, 51] and festination [52], may both be manifestations of a problem with the maintenance of an internal gait rhythm [46]. Second, because of the deficient motor set, some abnormalities are observed in the movement elements [44, 49]. Thus, for example, PD gait is characterized by short, shuffling steps and decreased or absent arm swing. Other interesting hypothesis is that basal ganglia mediate a form of learning and memory in which stimulus-response (S-R) associations or habits are incrementally acquired [53], and cueing techniques may induces neuroplasticity responses in this region. Different cueing techniques have been used [44]. To enhance basal ganglia function, some authors provide external rhythmic auditory cues to supplement the absent or deficient internal rhythm [54, 55]. Other utilized visual cues to set the proper stride length, thus providing external information to help augment the defective motor set [56, 57]. To reroute the movement through a non automatic pathway, attentional cues have been used to focus attention on walking and thus remove it from the automatic basal ganglia pathway. Alternatively, visual cues may be employed to activate the visual motor pathway instead of the automatic motor pathway.

In relation to physical exercise itself, the number of evidences is fewer than PT in patients with PD. But this is an interesting issue due to two mains aspects of exercise in middle-aged and older populate. First, the safety recommendations to exercise practice in this population due their greatest proportion of chronic disease burden, disability, and health care attention [58, 59]. Aging is a complex process involving many variables (e.g., genetics, lifestyle factors, and chronic diseases) that interact with one another, greatly influencing the manner in which we age [60, 61].

For example, approximately 88% of those over age 65 have at least one chronic health condition, and large numbers of older adults suffer from impaired functioning and well-being [58, 59]. In general, the evidences support a protective effect of regular physical activity (both aerobic and strength exercises) on functional limitation among older adults and extend this protective effect to middle-aged men and women [59-61]. The second aspect regarding physical exercise in aging is the well knowledge beneficial neurobiological effects of physical exercise in clinical [59-62] and experimental studies (these will be discussed later). For example, the peak cardiovascular (peak heart rate [HR]) and maximal oxygen uptake (VO_2max) responses to graded exercise achieved by subjects with PD were similar to controls at lower levels of exercise [63, 64], while half the subjects with PD displayed abnormal cardiovascular responses at higher exercise intensities [64]. Autonomic dysfunction [65, 66], rigidity, bradykinesia and the secondary disability and immobility that occur with PD can contribute to this cardiovascular de-conditioning, so that evidences of impaired cardiovascular response to postural changes on laboratory testing [67, 68], decreased latency to achieve exercise-induced fatigue [69-71], increased HR response and blood lactate level [7], and decrease maximal ventilatory levels during the exercise [73, 74]. The general muscle inactivity per se, secondary to the neurological disorder, are the most common secondary complaints of PD patients and is associated with reduced activity and poorer QoL. However, all of these variables showed to be modifiable by physical training in PD patients [16, 17, 21, 33, 75-77].Despite some inconsistencies in the literature, the current evidence suggests slightly that physical therapy is beneficial for PD patients. Various methodological considerations might explain the small benefit, including the outcomes measured, the stage of the patients when therapy was initiated, its duration and the type of therapy used [78]. The same may be applied to physical exercise. Overall, while it is clear that further studies will be needed, exercise-induced neuroprotection appears to be a potential protective strategy for PD.

Back to the Bench: Running as Neuroprotective Strategy in Experimental Models of Parkinson's Disease

Increased prevalence of PD in modern societies has been classically related to an increasingly aging population [79-81]. But the striatal dopamine (DA) pattern loss in normal aging differs substantially from that typically observed in idiopathic PD; therefore, the cause of PD cannot be primarily an age-dependent neurodegenerative process.

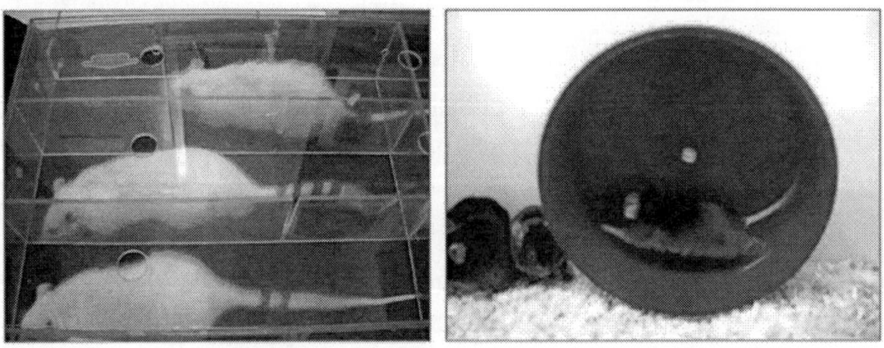

Figure 6.3. Physical exercise also can be experimentally modeled using muridae-adapted treadmill and running wheels.

In addition, we propose in this chapter that sedentary life may be an additional risk factor for PD development due to several evidences showing exercise-induced neuroprotection. For example, non-exercised rats displayed age-dependent decreases in vascularization and growth factor expression [82] and were more sensible to DA loss [83], which were reversed by physical exercise. These changes may enhance the vulnerability of dopaminergic neurons and the risk of developing PD, and may be reduced by exercise [82, 83]. Furthermore, several studies demonstrated positive effects of physical exercise in animal models of PD (see Figure 6-3) [14, 83-85].

Tillerson et al. (2003) [14] reported behavioral improvement after treadmill exercise in two rodent models of basal ganglia injury [the 6-OHDA (6-hydroxydopamine)[1] rat and MPTP (1-methyl-4-phenyl-1,2,3,6-tetrahydroxypyridine)[2]-lesioned mouse] and concluded that exercise might act largely through neuroprotective mechanisms because exercise was started within 12 hours of lesioning, and MPTP and 6-OHDA may take several days to complete neuronal death [86, 87]. Exercise resulted also in decreased DA transporter (DAT, a membrane-spanning protein that binds to DA and provides the primary mechanism of DA clearance from synapses) expression compared to non-trained mice exposed to MPTP via intraperitoneal (i.p.) injection [88]. Several mechanisms have been shown to regulate DAT activity including: [1] gene and protein expression of transporter number; [2] phosphorylation activated through glutamate receptors such as the mGluR5 metabotropic receptor; and [3] internalization within endosomes mediated by DA (89). Alterations in DAT activity can influence the synaptic occupancy of DA. An intervention (such as exercise) that down-regulates DAT expression may therefore results in increased DA occupancy in the synaptic cleft. The DAT down-regulation in exercised animals could also account for the superior running capabilities of intoxicated and control groups compared to the untrained groups [88]. These data deserve attention because DAT down-regulation may minimize symptoms by contributing to increased synaptic DA levels in early Parkinson disease, but at the expense of leading to increased extracellular DA catabolism and oscillating levels of DA that are associated to appearance of dyskinesias [90]. For example, DAT knockout mice display biochemical and behavioral dopaminergic hyperactivity despite decreases in the striatal levels of enzyme tyrosine hydroxylase (TH, L-tyrosine → dihydroxyphenylalanine [DOPA], the precursor of DA) and DA and these observations were not due to loss of either DA neurons or projections [91, 92]. An interesting contrast can be drawn between knockout mice, in which as little as 5% of normal DA leads to hyperactivity, and patients with PD in whom similarly low levels of DA cause debilitating impairment in locomotion. A similar down-regulation of DAT can be induced in rodents exposed to environmental enrichment[93, 94] and proven neuroprotection against MPTP toxicity [94]. Protection could be due to a reduced amount of MPP^+ taken up into DA terminals via DAT. Probably this event is associated to signaling of cellular toxicity.

[1] 6-hydroxydopamine (6-OHDA) is a neurotoxin used to selectively kill dopaminergic and noradrenergic neurons. 6-OHDA enters the neurons via the dopamine and noradrenaline reuptake transporters. The main use for 6-OHDA in scientific research is to induce Parkinsonism in laboratory animals such as mice, rats and monkeys, in order to develop and test new medicines for management of Parkinson's disease in humans.

[2] MPTP (1-methyl-4-phenyl-1,2,3,6-tetrahydropyridine) is a neurotoxin that causes permanent symptoms of Parkinson's disease by destroying dopaminergic neurons in the substantia nigra of the brain. It has been used in study disease models in various animal studies.

This chapter provides additional evidences that moderate physical exercise plays an important role in the improvement of motor and cognitive deficits verified in an experimental model of PD. Four consecutive weeks in running wheel or treadmill attenuated the motor disruption induced by 5 mg/kg subcutaneous injection of reserpine in rats (see Figure 6-4) [83]. The indole alkaloid reserpine (Figure 6-4), which is a catecholamine-depleting agent, has been used extensively to study DA neurotransmission. A single injection of reserpine (2.5 mg/kg, i.p.) reduces striatal DA concentrations by more than 90% within 2 h after administration [95].

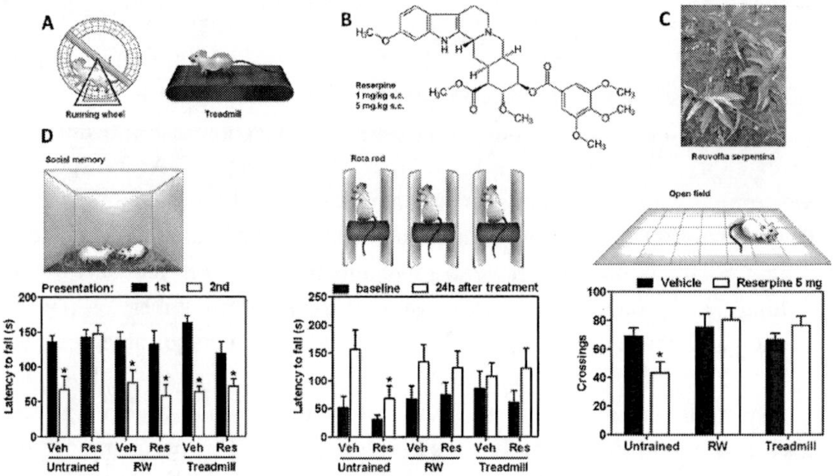

Figure 6.4. Four weeks of moderate physical training running wheel or treadmill reversed the cognitive (social memory test) and motor (open field and rota rod test) impairments induced by reserpine in rats. In the social memory test, sedentary reserpinized rats did not recognize the pup during the second exposition. In the rota rod and open field tests, reserpine administration induced, respectively, coordination and locomotion deficits in sedentary rats. In all tests, the running wheel and treadmill training reversed the impairments induced by reserpine. Reserpine is an indole alkaloid from the Rauvolfia serpentine (Indian snakeroot). Res – reserpine. RW – running wheel. Veh – vehicle.

The reserpine-induced DA depletion is long lasting and can be demonstrated for more than 60 days following a single injection in rats [96]. The reserpine-induced hypokinesia is also long lasting and persists for more than 30 days (96). The results presented in this chapter (Figure 6-4, 6-5, 6-6 and 6-7) corroborate previous observations that physical exercise ameliorates motor performance in neurointoxicant rodent models of PD, such as 6-OHDA [14, 88] and MPTP [14, 86, 88, 97] (see Table 6-2). Moreover, our findings demonstrate that physical exercise improve selectively social recognition memory deficits induced by 1 mg/kg subcutaneous injection of reserpine in rats (Figure 6-4), reinforcing the potential of physical exercise in the management of non-motor symptoms of PD.

Normally, when rodents are placed in a novel environment, they initially display a high level of exploratory activity, of which locomotion is an important, although not an exclusive component [98]. This class of spatial exploration is a complex cognitive process, modulated by the state of arousal, sensory processing, and a vast array of motivational factors (e.g. hunger, fear, curiosity, etc.) [98]. The systemic administration of reserpine to rodents is frequently used as a model of the motor disturbance of PD [99-101], and several clinically used anti-parkinsonian drugs have been shown to improve this motor impairment [102]. In accordance with these previous studies, the locomotion and exploratory activity are highly reduced in reserpine-treated (5 mg/kg) Wistar rats (Figure 6-4), probably due to the depletion of DA (and other monoamines) in the basal ganglia nuclei [99, 103]. Of high interest, both types – running wheel and treadmill – of exercise induced a full recovery of the locomotor performance of reserpinized animals in the open field and rota-rod tests (Figure 6-4).

Table 2. Overview of basic outcomes in experimental models of Parkinson's disease associating physical exercise

Reference	Animal model	Intervention	Outcomes
(104)	Intra-medial forebrain bundle 6-OHDA in Long Evan rats	Running wheel	↓ rotations following apomorphine challenge
(105, 106)	i.p. MPTP in C57BL/6 mice		Functional Subthreshold L-DOPA
(88)		Treadmill	↓ striatal DAT ↑ striatal DA D_2 receptors
(97, 107, 108)			↑ coordination ↑ striatal DA ↓ striatal TH and DAT
(109)			↑ striatal angiogenesis
(110)			↑ mitochondrial function
(111, 112)			↑ striatal D_2Receptor-like expression Change striatal AMPA receptor expression
(113)	i.c.v. 6-OHDA in Long Evan rats		↑ striatal DA No motor improvement
(14)	intra-striatal 6-OHDA in Fisher rats and i.p. MPTP in C57BL/6 mice		↑ striatal DA, DOPAC and HVA; ↑ TH in the SNpc; ↑ gait
(83)	i.p. reserpine in Wistar rats	Running wheel and treadmill	↓ motor and cognitive reserpine-induced impairments

Abbreviations: ↑: increase; ↓: decrease; 6-OHDA: 6-hydroxydopamine; MPTP: 1-methyl-4-phenyl-1,2,3,6 tetrahydropyridine; i.p.: intraperitoneal; i.c.v.: intracerebroventricular; DA: dopamine; DOPAC: 3,4-dihydroxyphenylacetic acid; HVA: homovallinic acid; SNpc: substantia nigra pars compacta; TH: tyrosine hydroxylase.

The efficacy of physical exercise in protecting DA neurons from degeneration *in vivo* was assessed qualitatively (rota-rod and rotation behavior) with the striatal 6-OHDA (Figure 6-5) progressive lesion C57BL6 mouse model of PD. As in reserpinized and exercised rats (Figure 6-4), trained 6-OHDA-mice revealed better rota-rod performance than sedentary 6-OHDA-mice (Figure 6-5).

Moreover, the progression of rotational behavior presented by apomorphine challenge (an agonist of D1 and D2 type DA receptors) was not observed in the exercised animals, and that the opposite occurred in sedentary animals with temporal increases in the number of rotations (Figure 6-5), which pharmacologically demonstrates the progressive death of striatal DA neurons.

These results reveal that physical exercise is a relevant intervention to several dopaminergic dysfunctions, since the depletion of monoamines (by reserpine, Figure 6-4) or death of neurons corresponding (by 6-OHDA, Figure 6-5). In this way, the problems of mobility that accompany the motor symptoms of PD generally minimized by PT and exercise interventions also demonstrate observable in animal models of PD. Thus, we can infer that these motor benefits observed in exercised PD patients [16, 17, 33, 75-77] can be associated with improvements in DA neurotransmission and a decreased DA neurons death. There are an extensive literature reporting it [14, 88, 97, 114] (see Table 6-2). The positive effects of exercise on motor function seem to be mediated, at least in part, by adaptive changes of DA system in basal ganglia and motor circuitry. For instance, Petzinger et al. (2007) [97] showed a highlight study demonstrating a partial return of striatal DA in MPTP-treated mice submitted to treadmill for 28 days.

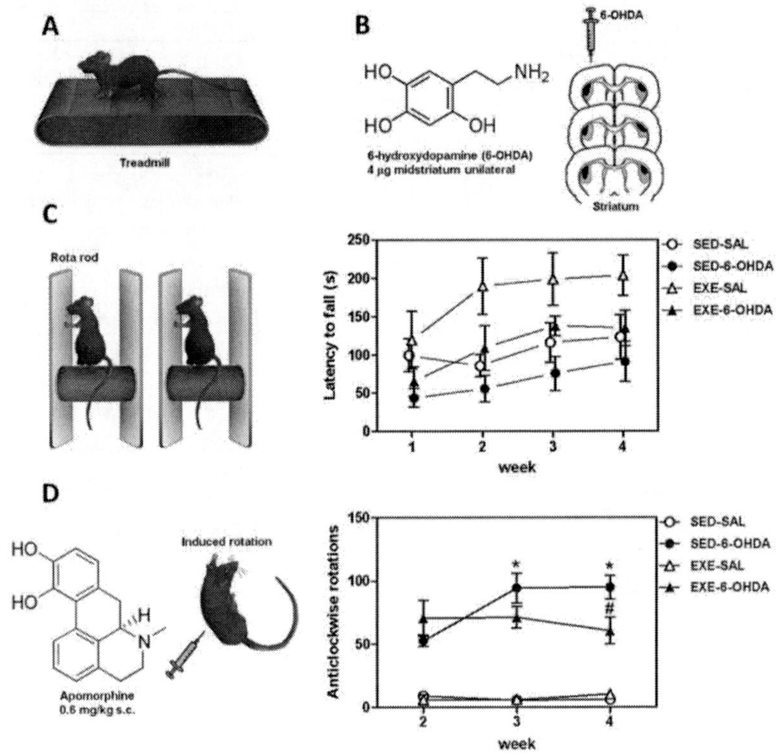

Figure 6.5. Mice with surgically 6-OHDA-lesioned right striatum had impaired motor coordination (rota rod task) and asymmetric movements (apomorphine challenge). These animals fall faster from a cylinder in motion and have rotational behavior after receiving a dopamine agonist. This rotational behavior occurs because the injured side of the dopamine receptors is more sensible than the non-injured side. Soon, the animals are turning after the administration of dopamine agonists. The figure illustrates that the exercised animals show higher coordination and lower sensitivity to agonists, indicating exercise-induced neuroprotection. Apomorphine is a non-selective dopamine agonist which activates both D1-like and D2-like receptors. It is a morphine decomposition product, hence the -morphine suffix. 6-OHDA – 6-hydroxydopamine. Exe – exercise. Sed – sedentary.

This effect was most pronounced within the dorsolateral striatum. In addition, the authors reported that exercise leads to the down-regulation of both DAT and TH expression in the striatum. A possible explanation for these regional specific effects may be because of use-dependent forms of synaptic plasticity. The high degree of engagement required from the dorsolateral striatum for forelimb and hind limb movement during treadmill exercise is supported by studies demonstrating that rats exposed to walking on a treadmill showed increases in cerebral blood flow and metabolic activity in motor circuits such as the primary motor cortex and the dorsolateral striatum [115-118].

To date, the majority of the studies performed with animal models of PD have focused upon their ability to induce nigrostriatal dopaminergic pathway damage and motor alterations associated with advanced phases of PD. Since PD is accompanied by alterations in a variety of functions including memory deficits [119, 120] and olfactory dysfunction [121-123], it seems important to evaluate whether the proposed animal models alter any of these functions. We therefore investigated the occurrence of cognitive alterations in rats after a single administration of a low dose of reserpine (1 mg/kg).

The data presented in Figure 6-4 demonstrates that the acute treatment with reserpine (1 mg/kg) induced pronounced deficits in the social recognition memory in rats. The social recognition memory is a particular model of olfactory memory mediated by olfactory cues [124] and may involve a non-procedural form of a short-term working memory based upon the olfactory discriminative ability of rats. The persistence with which an adult rat investigates a juvenile can be enhanced or decreased in a predictive manner by using inhibition and facilitation procedures [125]. It can be facilitated by memory-enhancing drugs and disrupted by pharmacological and pathophysiological models known to impair memory in rodents [126-128]. We found that rats treated with reserpine spent as much time investigating the familiar juvenile rat during the second presentation as they did on the first encounter, suggesting impairment in their ability to recognize the juvenile after a short period of time (30 min). Of high interest, the moderate physical training induced a full reversion of the short-term social memory deficits induced by reserpine in rats (Figure 6-4). Classically, exercise is knowledge to improve learning and memory in both humans and rodents [4, 129, 130]. In relation to basal ganglia, we found further exercise-induced basal ganglia benefits investigating implicit memory. The striatum in the basal ganglia-thalamocortical circuitry is a key neural substrate that is implicated in motor balance and procedural learning [53, 131]. We show that intranasal administration of MPTP (132) impairs procedural learning in the tone fear conditioning task (Figure 6-6), an indicative of basal ganglia cognitive dysfunction.

Classical fear conditioning occurs when initially innocuous conditioned stimuli (e.g., tone) are contingently paired with aversive unconditioned stimuli (e.g., foot shock) that reflexively activate unconditioned fear responses. We observed that 6 weeks of treadmill running exercise ameliorates the percentage freezing response of trained mice, showing better basal ganglia function than MPTP-treated sedentary animals (Figure 6-6).

However, the mechanisms are not yet completely understood. In line with this, regular physical exercise has been related to an increase in the number of new hippocampal cells [133, 134], an increase in brain plasticity [4], an increase in the production of neurotrophic factors [135-137], and an increase in learning and memory [88, 134, 137-139] In the past twenty years it has become clear that regular exercise beneficially affects brain function and could play an important preventive and therapeutic role in oxidative stress-associated diseases, such as the PD [140, 141].

The effects of exercise seem to be very complex and could include neurogenesis[4, 129, 133, 134] and synaptogenesis [142, 143] via neurotrophic factors [135, 136, 144] and stem cells [145], increased angiogenesis [146-148], decreased oxidative damage [12, 138, 149], and increased proteolytic degradation by proteasome [137, 138, 150] and neprilysin [151]. These structural changes are associated with enhanced performance on learning and memory and motor function tasks [145, 152, 153].

These exercise benefits are interesting to PD because studies in human post-mortem material indicate that free radicals are important in the pathogenesis of sporadic PD [154-156]. A selective 30–40% decrease in complex I activity of the mitochondrial respiratory chain has been found in the substantia nigra pars compacta (SNpc) of PD patients [157-159]. The cause of the decreased complex I activity in PD rem ains not clarified.

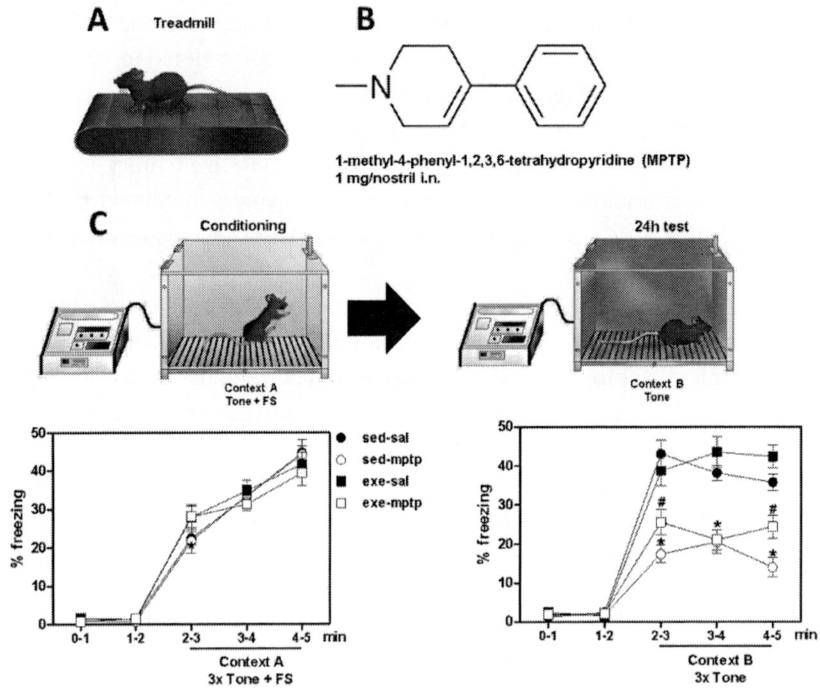

Figure 6.6. Mice had freezing responses after receiving a mild foot shock after a tone (graphics to the right). It's a basal-ganglia-dependent learning process. The MPTP-treatment affects the recall of these implicit memories, with partial protection of the exercise (graphics on the left). Exe – exercise. FS – foot shock. MPTP - 1-methyl-4-phenyl-1,2,3,6-tetrahydropyridine. Sed – sedentary.

A mitochondrial complex I defect could contribute to cell degeneration in PD through decreased ATP synthesis and a bioenergetic defect. Moreover, DA has a great potential to yield hydrogen peroxide (H_2O_2) and other free radicals [66, 140, 155, 160]. There are several studies reporting the effects of exercise on the brain antioxidant system. For example, physical exercise resulted in increased activities of the main antioxidant enzymes superoxide dismutase (SOD), catalase (CAT), and glutathione peroxidase (GPX) in the striatum of rodents [161-163]. The laboratory of professor Radak in (local) showed that regular exercise training attenuated the age-related accumulation of protein oxidative damage in the brain of rats, increased the activity of the proteasome complex, and improved brain function [138, 139, 150, 164]. Recently, we found that low-moderate intensity physical training induces increased in the activity of mitochondrial complex I of mice brain (Figure 6-7). Moreover, when we isolated mitochondrias from brain of trained mice and treated it with 1-methyl-4-phenylpyridinium (MPP^+) – the MPTP metabolite, the complex I inhibition was lower in the brain mitochondrias of trained mice when compared to sedentary controls (Figure 6-7). This is very interesting due to characteristic complex I inhibition in the substantia nigra of PD patients (157, 165, 166). These data supports the physical exercise such as useful tool in the oxidative stress etiology of PD.

Moreover, the pathological hallmarks of PD are the neurodegeneration of specific subnuclei of the SNpc, with severe obliteration of their neuromelanin-laden projection neurons – frequently is considered to be the most important hallmark of PD – and the presence specific α-synuclein-immunoreactive inclusion bodies, which develop as spindle- or thread-like Lewy neurites in cellular processes, and in the form of globular Lewy bodies in neuronal perikarya [167-169]. Many studies suggest that the death of DA cells in PD is linked to protein aggregation [170-172] and dysfunction of the ubiquitin proteasome pathway [166, 173, 174]. There are increasing evidences demonstrated that physical exercise may engage proteasome function [175-177] in the brain of rats associated to decreased oxidative damaged to lipids, proteins and DNA [137, 138, 176, 177]. These alterations could mean faster protein turnover, resulting in a smaller amount of physiologically inactive oxidatively modified 'junk'.

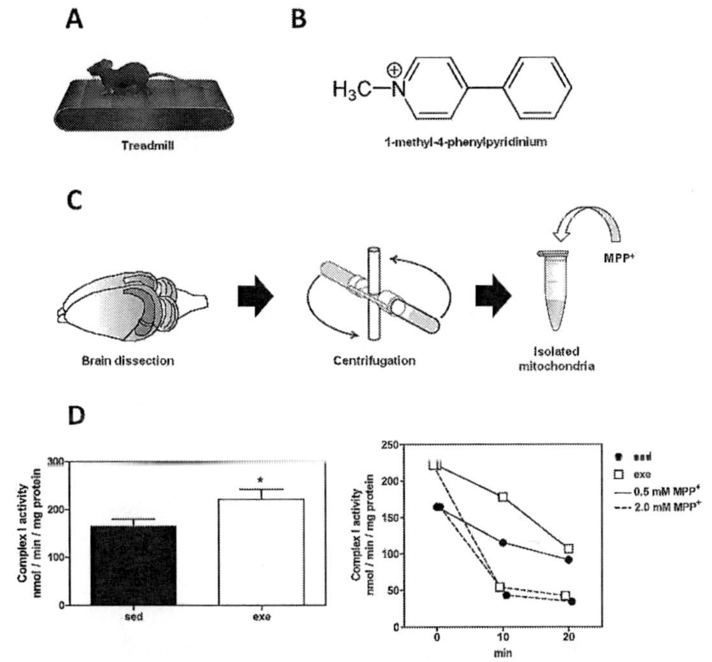

Figure 6.7. Mitochondria isolated from the brain of physically trained animals show higher mitochondrial complex I activity in relation to sedentary controls. In addition, these mitochondria of exercised animals are also more resistant to pharmacological inhibition of the mitochondrial complex I activity. This may explain the neuroprotective effects of physical exercise in experimental models of Parkinson's disease. Exe – exercise. MPP+ - 1-methyl-4-phenylpyridinium. Sed – sedentary.

In this way the oxidatively modified proteins would not hamper cell function, which otherwise might occur because of a massive accumulation of oxidized biomolecules dysfunctional brains. However, the effect of exercise over the main protein aggregation in the PD α-synuclein and Lewy body formation remains unstudied.

Other relevant aspect of exercise is your potential to increase neurotrophins. The neurotrophins are signaling molecules and have been proposed to play central roles in a variety of forms of synaptic plasticity [178, 179].

The expression and protein content of neurotrophins have been shown to be up-regulated by exercise mainly in the hippocampus (180). On the other hand, the striatum evidences are less inconsistent, with some authors demonstrating no changes [181, 182], increases [136, 183] or even decreased [181]levels.

Recent data from our laboratory showed that level running exercise induces no changes in the striatal levels of brain derived neurotrophic factors while an eccentric running program increased it in mice [135].

This result supports preliminary clinical findings demonstrating that eccentric physical training increased muscle strength and reduced PD-related bradykinesia in PD patients [75, 76].

Physical Therapy, Exercise and L-Dopa

The treatment of PD is very complex due to the progressive nature of the disease and the array of motor and non-motor features combined with early and late side effects associated with therapeutic interventions. While no treatments have yet been shown to slow the progression of the disease, some palliative pharmacologic therapies are available, as well as several forms of surgery and numerous non-pharmacological approaches, for example physical exercise and physical therapy. Since the own neurotransmitter DA does not cross the blood-brain barrier (BBB), it is replaced by giving its precursor L-DOPA, which does it [184-187]. The introduction of L-DOPA in the PD pharmacological therapy date from 1960s, and still remains the most effective therapy for motor symptoms where alleviates all the cardinal motor symptoms of PD [185-187]. Carbidopa (in the United States) or Benserazide (not available in the United States) are included in the standard L-DOPA oral formulation to inhibit dopa decarboxylase in the periphery. These drugs did not cross the BBB [185-187] and avoid intolerable side effects due to DA conversion in gastrointestinal tract. In this way, L-DOPA and physical therapy or exercise interactions are important due to involvement of exercise in the intrinsic regulation of central DA neurotransmission. For example, it is well established increases in the DA synthesis and release [188]. Moreover, D2 mRNA levels grew and D2 inhibition decreased in DA neurons of the SNpc after exercise [188]. These changes may be involved in the mechanisms by which habitually physically active animals are better able to delay fatigue compared to sedentary controls [188]. In addition, the striatal DA receptor's content of endurance trained rats was higher than untrained controls [188, 189]. However, no D1 changes were identified until now.

l-dopa is a large neutral amino acid that is absorbed in the gut and transported across the BBB by the large neutral amino acid transporter[185-187]. So far, the effects of exercise on l-dopa absorption from the gastrointestinal tract remains not enlightened [190], only a trend for a better l-dopa absorption under physical exercise [191]. However, several evidences showed unchanged plasma l-dopa levels [192] and similar [192, 193] or higher [194] motor scores of PD patients after exercise in relation to rest subjects. Perhaps, the increase of blood pressure and HR in response to exercise may contribute to a better l-dopa transport over the BBB and reduced l-dopa storage in peripheral tissues [194, 195]. While the effects of exercise on l-dopa gut absorption and BBB transport remains unclear, hemiparetic stroke patients are benefited by l-dopa medication [196]. In this case, brain L-DOPA is metabolized in noradrenaline and increase the efficacy of PT [196], having a probable relationship with physical therapy and exercise in PD patients.

On the other hand, the most problematic adverse effects of L-DOPA are the motor fluctuations and dyskinesia that constitute the long-term L-DOPA syndrome [197-200] and neuropsychiatric symptoms [1, 201-203]. In this aspect, there seems to be no influence of physical exercise, at levels ordinarily experienced by PD patients, in the pathogenesis of these motor fluctuations [192]. Actually, L-DOPA treated PD patients experimented less dyskinesias occurrence during exercise than in rest conditions with unchanged number of involuntary movements [191]. However, L-DOPA treated PD patients sometimes report a reduced exercise

capacity and onset of fatigue [197, 204]. Because DA is hypothesized to be critically involved in movement, a decreased DA neurotransmission and indirect L-DOPA efficacy during physical activity would hasten the onset of fatigue [188]

While an increase in DA neurotransmission would be sufficient to delay the onset of fatigue [188]. So, a putative association between reduced exercise capacities as possible consequence of altered L-DOPA pharmacokinetics was investigated in several clinical studies in PD patients. Again, no significant differences between rest/exercise L-DOPA pharmaco-kinetic behavior appeared [191, 193].

Only a trend for a better L-DOPA absorption under physical exercise and an increase of the L-DOPA EC_{50} that implies a right shift of the concentration effect curve under exercise [191].

Conclusion

The findings reviewed in this chapter indicate that physical exercise improves the motor and non motor impairments of PD patients. Data obtained in basic research has indicated the potential neuroprotective of physical exercise in neurointoxicant models of PD.

In particular, our new findings indicate that moderate physical exercise might afford protection against memory dysfunction in two rodent models (reserpine and MPTP), reinforcing it cognitive enhancing properties that may be of interest in the management of cognitive declines associated to PD. Finally, a better evaluation of the potential of combining physical exercise and the current drugs available in PD therapy is also indicated.

References

[1] Moskovitz, C; Moses, H, 3rd; Klawans, HL. Levodopa-induced psychosis: a kindling phenomenon. *Am. J. Psychiatry*. 1978 (135), 669-75.

[2] Ambani, LM; Van Woert, MH. Start hesitation--a side effect of long-term levodopa therapy. *N. Engl. J. Med*. 1973 (288), 1113-5.

[3] Marsden, CD; Parkes, JD. "On-off" effects in patients with Parkinson's disease on chronic levodopa therapy. *Lancet*. 1976 (1), 292-6.

[4] Cotman, CW; Berchtold, NC. Exercise: a behavioral intervention to enhance brain health and plasticity. *Trends. Neurosci.* 2002 (25), 295-301.

[5] Anderton, BH. Ageing of the brain. *Mech. Ageing. Dev.* 2002 (123), 811-7.

[6] Farooqui, T; Farooqui, AA. Aging: an important factor for the pathogenesis of neurodegenerative diseases. *Mech. Ageing. Dev.* 2009 (130), 203-15.

[7] Ames, BN; Shigenaga, MK; Hagen, TM. Oxidants, antioxidants, and the degenerative diseases of aging. *Proc. Natl. Acad. Sci. USA*. 1993 (90), 7915-22.

[8] Rovio, S; Spulber, G; Nieminen, LJ; Niskanen, E; Winblad, B; Tuomilehto, J; Nissinen, A; Soininen, H; Kivipelto, M. The effect of midlife physical activity on structural brain changes in the elderly. *Neurobiol. Aging*. 2010 (31), 1927-36.

[9] Colcombe, SJ; Kramer, AF; Erickson, KI; Scalf, P; McAuley, E; Cohen, NJ; Webb, A; Jerome, GJ; Marquez, DX; Elavsky, S. Cardiovascular fitness, cortical plasticity, and aging. *Proc. Natl. Acad. Sci. USA*. 2004 (101), 3316-21.

[10] Aguiar, AS, Jr.; Tuon, T; Albuquerque, MM; Rocha, GS; Speck, AE; Araujo, JC; Dafre, AL; Prediger, RD; Pinho, RA. The exercise redox paradigm in the Down's syndrome: improvements in motor function and increases in blood oxidative status in young adults. *J. Neural. Transm.* 2008 (115), 1643-50.

[11] Knaepen, K; Goekint, M; Heyman, EM; Meeusen, R. Neuroplasticity - exercise-induced response of peripheral brain-derived neurotrophic factor: a systematic review of experimental studies in human subjects. *Sports Med.* 2010 (40), 765-801.

[12] Mattson, MP. Neuroprotective signaling and the aging brain: take away my food and let me run. *Brain. Res.* 2000 (886), 47-53.

[13] Comella, CL; Stebbins, GT; Brown-Toms, N; Goetz, CG. Physical therapy and Parkinson's disease: a controlled clinical trial. *Neurology*. 1994 (44), 376-8.

[14] Tillerson, JL; Caudle, WM; Reveron, ME; Miller, GW. Exercise induces behavioral recovery and attenuates neurochemical deficits in rodent models of Parkinson's disease. *Neuroscience*. 2003 (119), 899-911.

[15] de Goede, CJ; Keus, SH; Kwakkel, G; Wagenaar, RC. The effects of physical therapy in Parkinson's disease: a research synthesis. *Arch. Phys. Med. Rehabil.* 2001 (82), 509-15.

[16] Miyai, I; Fujimoto, Y; Ueda, Y; Yamamoto, H; Nozaki, S; Saito, T; Kang, J. Treadmill training with body weight support: its effect on Parkinson's disease. *Arch. Phys. Med. Rehabil.* 2000 (81), 849-52.

[17] Hirsch, MA; Toole, T; Maitland, CG; Rider, RA. The effects of balance training and high-intensity resistance training on persons with idiopathic Parkinson's disease. *Arch. Phys. Med. Rehabil.* 2003 (84), 1109-17.

[18] Cohen, AD; Tillerson, JL; Smith, AD; Schallert, T; Zigmond, MJ. Neuroprotective effects of prior limb use in 6-hydroxydopamine-treated rats: possible role of GDNF. *J. Neurochem.* 2003 (85), 299-305.

[19] Mutch, WJ; Strudwick, A; Roy, SK; Downie, AW. Parkinson's disease: disability, review, and management. *Br. Med. J. (Clin Res Ed)*, 1986 (293), 675-7.

[20] Gauthier, L; Dalziel, S; Gauthier, S. The benefits of group occupational therapy for patients with Parkinson's disease. *Am. J. Occup. Ther.* 1987 (41), 360-5.

[21] Palmer, SS; Mortimer, JA; Webster, DD; Bistevins, R; Dickinson, GL. Exercise therapy for Parkinson's disease. *Arch. Phys. Med. Rehabil.* 1986 (67), 741-5.

[22] Hass, CJ; Collins, MA; Juncos, JL. Resistance training with creatine monohydrate improves upper-body strength in patients with Parkinson disease: a randomized trial. *Neurorehabil. Neural. Repair*. 2007 (21), 107-15.

[23] Pang, MY; Mak, MK. Trunk muscle strength, but not trunk rigidity, is independently associated with bone mineral density of the lumbar spine in patients with Parkinson's disease. *Mov. Disord*. 2009 (24), 1176-82.

[24] Toole, T; Hirsch, MA; Forkink, A; Lehman, DA; Maitland, CG. The effects of a balance and strength training program on equilibrium in Parkinsonism: A preliminary study. *NeuroRehabilitation*. 2000 (14), 165-74.

[25] Falvo, MJ; Schilling, BK; Earhart, GM. Parkinson's disease and resistive exercise: rationale, review, and recommendations. *Mov. Disord*. 2008 (23), 1-11.

[26] Marchese, R; Diverio, M; Zucchi, F; Lentino, C; Abbruzzese, G. The role of sensory cues in the rehabilitation of parkinsonian patients: a comparison of two physical therapy protocols. *Mov. Disord*. 2000 (15), 879-83.

[27] Dixon, L; Duncan, D; Johnson, P; Kirkby, L; O'Connell, H; Taylor, H; Deane, KH. Occupational therapy for patients with Parkinson's disease. *Cochrane. Database Syst. Rev*. 2007 CD002813.

[28] Bergen, JL; Toole, T; Elliott, RG, 3rd; Wallace, B; Robinson, K; Maitland, CG. Aerobic exercise intervention improves aerobic capacity and movement initiation in Parkinson's disease patients. *NeuroRehabilitation*. 2002 (17), 161-8.

[29] Schenkman, M; Cutson, TM; Kuchibhatla, M; Chandler, J; Pieper, CF; Ray, L; Laub, KC. Exercise to improve spinal flexibility and function for people with Parkinson's disease: a randomized, controlled trial. *J. Am. Geriatr. Soc*. 1998 (46), 1207-16.

[30] Protas, EJ; Mitchell, K; Williams, A; Qureshy, H; Caroline, K; Lai, EC. Gait and step training to reduce falls in Parkinson's disease. *NeuroRehabilitation*. 2005 (20), 183-90.

[31] Mirelman, A; Maidan, I; Herman, T; Deutsch, JE; Giladi, N; Hausdorff, JM. Virtual reality for gait training: can it induce motor learning to enhance complex walking and reduce fall risk in patients with Parkinson's disease? *J. Geronto.l A Biol. Sci. Med. Sci*. 2011 (66), 234-40.

[32] Fisher, BE; Wu, AD; Salem, GJ; Song, J; Lin, CH; Yip, J; Cen, S; Gordon, J; Jakowec, M; Petzinger, G. The effect of exercise training in improving motor performance and corticomotor excitability in people with early Parkinson's disease. *Arch. Phys. Med. Rehabil*. 2008 (89), 1221-9.

[33] Miyai, I; Fujimoto, Y; Yamamoto, H; Ueda, Y; Saito, T; Nozaki, S; Kang, J. Long-term effect of body weight-supported treadmill training in Parkinson's disease: a randomized controlled trial. *Arch. Phys. Med. Rehabil*. 2002 (83), 1370-3.

[34] Allen, NE; Canning, CG; Sherrington, C; Lord, SR; Latt, MD; Close, JC; O'Rourke, SD; Murray, SM; Fung, VS. The effects of an exercise program on fall risk factors in people with Parkinson's disease: a randomized controlled trial. *Mov. Disord*. 2010 (25), 1217-25.

[35] Nieuwboer, A; De Weerdt, W; Dom, R; Truyen, M; Janssens, L; Kamsma, Y. The effect of a home physiotherapy program for persons with Parkinson's disease. *J. Rehabil. Med*. 2001 (33), 266-72.

[36] Kuroda, K; Tatara, K; Takatorige, T; Shinsho, F. Effect of physical exercise on mortality in patients with Parkinson's disease. *Acta. Neurol. Scand*. 1992 (86), 55-9.

[37] Thaut, MH; McIntosh, GC; Rice, RR; Miller, RA; Rathbun, J; Brault, JM. Rhythmic auditory stimulation in gait training for Parkinson's disease patients. *Mov. Disord.* 1996 (11), 193-200.

[38] Crizzle, AM; Newhouse, IJ. Is physical exercise beneficial for persons with Parkinson's disease? *Clin. J. Sport. Med.* 2006 (16), 422-5.

[39] Lun, V; Pullan, N; Labelle, N; Adams, C; Suchowersky, O. Comparison of the effects of a self-supervised home exercise program with a physiotherapist-supervised exercise program on the motor symptoms of Parkinson's disease. *Mov. Disord.* 2005 (20), 971-5.

[40] Baatile, J; Langbein, WE; Weaver, F; Maloney, C; Jost, MB. Effect of exercise on perceived quality of life of individuals with Parkinson's disease. *J. Rehabil. Res. Dev.* 2000 (37), 529-34.

[41] Dietz, V; Zijlstra, W; Prokop, T; Berger, W. Leg muscle activation during gait in Parkinson's disease: adaptation and interlimb coordination. *Electroencephalogr. Clin. Neurophysiol.* 1995 (97), 408-15.

[42] Dietz, V; Leenders, KL; Colombo, G. Leg muscle activation during gait in Parkinson's disease: influence of body unloading. *Electroencephalogr. Clin. Neurophysiol.* 1997 (105), 400-5.

[43] Dietz, V; Colombo, G. Influence of body load on the gait pattern in Parkinson's disease. *Mov. Disord.* 1998 (13), 255-61.

[44] Rubinstein, TC; Giladi, N; Hausdorff, JM. The power of cueing to circumvent dopamine deficits: a review of physical therapy treatment of gait disturbances in Parkinson's disease. *Mov. Disord.* 2002 (17), 1148-60.

[45] Glickstein, M; Stein, J. Paradoxical movement in Parkinson's disease. *Trends Neurosci.*1991 (14), 480-2.

[46] Giladi, N; Treves, TA; Simon, ES; Shabtai, H; Orlov, Y; Kandinov, B; Paleacu, D; Korczyn, AD. Freezing of gait in patients with advanced Parkinson's disease. *J. Neural. Transm.* 2001 (108), 53-61.

[47] Cunnington, R; Iansek, R; Bradshaw, JL; Phillips, JG. Movement-related potentials in Parkinson's disease. Presence and predictability of temporal and spatial cues. *Brain.* 1995 (118 (Pt 4)), 935-50.

[48] Graybiel, AM; Aosaki, T; Flaherty, AW; Kimura, M. The basal ganglia and adaptive motor control. *Science.* 1994 (265), 1826-31.

[49] Morris, ME; Iansek, R; Matyas, TA; Summers, JJ. Stride length regulation in Parkinson's disease. Normalization strategies and underlying mechanisms. *Brain.* 1996 (119 (Pt 2)), 551-68.

[50] Hausdorff, JM; Cudkowicz, ME; Firtion, R; Wei, JY; Goldberger, AL. Gait variability and basal ganglia disorders: stride-to-stride variations of gait cycle timing in Parkinson's disease and Huntington's disease. *Mov. Disord.* 1998 (13), 428-37.

[51] Giladi, N; McMahon, D; Przedborski, S; Flaster, E; Guillory, S; Kostic, V; Fahn, S. Motor blocks in Parkinson's disease. *Neurology.* 1992 (42), 333-9.

[52] Giladi, N; Shabtai, H; Rozenberg, E; Shabtai, E. Gait festination in Parkinson's disease. *Parkinsonism Relat. Disord.* 2001 (7), 135-8.

[53] Packard, MG; Knowlton, BJ. Learning and memory functions of the Basal Ganglia. *Annu. Rev. Neurosci.* 2002 (25), 563-93.

[54] Cubo, E; Leurgans, S; Goetz, CG. Short-term and practice effects of metronome pacing in Parkinson's disease patients with gait freezing while in the 'on' state: randomized single blind evaluation. *Parkinsonism Relat. Disord.* 2004 (10), 507-10.

[55] Enzensberger, W; Fischer, PA. Metronome in Parkinson's disease. *Lancet.* 1996 (347), 1337.

[56] Morris, ME; Iansek, R; Matyas, TA; Summers, JJ. The pathogenesis of gait hypokinesia in Parkinson's disease. *Brain.* 1994 (117 (Pt 5)), 1169-81.

[57] Azulay, JP; Van Den Brand, C; Mestre, D; Blin, O; Sangla, I; Pouget, J; Serratrice, G. [Automatic motion analysis of gait in patients with Parkinson disease: effects of levodopa and visual stimulations]. *Rev. Neurol. (Paris).* 1996 (152), 128-34.

[58] Lonergan, ET; Krevans, JR. A national agenda for research on aging. *N. Eng.l J. Med.* 1991 (324), 1825-8.

[59] Huang, Y; Macera, CA; Blair, SN; Brill, PA; Kohl, HW, 3rd; Kronenfeld, JJ. Physical fitness, physical activity, and functional limitation in adults aged 40 and older. *Med. Sci. Sports Exerc.* 1998 (30), 1430-5.

[60] American College of Sports Medicine Position Stand. Exercise and physical activity for older adults. *Med .Sci Sports Exerc.* 1998 (30), 992-1008.

[61] Chodzko-Zajko, WJ; Proctor, DN; Fiatarone Singh, MA; Minson, CT; Nigg, CR; Salem, GJ; Skinner, JS. American College of Sports Medicine position stand. Exercise and physical activity for older adults. *Med. Sci. Sports Exerc.* 2009 (41), 1510-30.

[62] Colcombe, S; Kramer, AF. Fitness effects on the cognitive function of older adults: a meta-analytic study. *Psychol. Sci.* 2003 (14), 125-30.

[63] Protas, EJ; Stanley, RK; Jankovic, J; MacNeill, B. Cardiovascular and metabolic responses to upper- and lower-extremity exercise in men with idiopathic Parkinson's disease. *Phys. Ther.* 1996 (76), 34-40.

[64] Werner, WG; DiFrancisco-Donoghue, J; Lamberg, EM. Cardiovascular response to treadmill testing in Parkinson disease. *J. Neurol. Phys. Ther.* 2006 (30), 68-73.

[65] Gelb, DJ; Oliver, E; Gilman, S. Diagnostic criteria for Parkinson disease. *Arch. Neurol.* 1999 (56), 33-9.

[66] Olanow, CW; Tatton, WG. Etiology and pathogenesis of Parkinson's disease. *Annu. Rev. Neurosci.* 1999 (22), 123-44.

[67] Hughes, AJ; Daniel, SE; Lees, AJ. The clinical features of Parkinson's disease in 100 histologically proven cases. *Adv. Neurol.* 1993 (60), 595-9.

[68] Takahashi, A. Autonomic nervous system disorders in Parkinson's disease. *Eur. Neurol.* 1991 (31 Suppl 1), 41-7.

[69] Canning, CG; Alison, JA; Allen, NE; Groeller, H. Parkinson's disease: an investigation of exercise capacity, respiratory function, and gait. *Arch. Phys. Med. Rehabil.* 1997 (78), 199-207.

[70] Stanley, RK; Protas, EJ; Jankovic, J. Exercise performance in those having Parkinson's disease and healthy normals. *Med. Sci. Sports. Exerc*, 1999 (31), 761-6.

[71] Lou, JS. Physical and mental fatigue in Parkinson's disease: epidemiology, pathophysiology and treatment. *Drugs. Aging.*2009 (26), 195-208.

[72] Reuter, I; Engelhardt, M; Stecker, K; Baas, H. Therapeutic value of exercise training in Parkinson's disease. *Med. Sci. Sports Exerc.* 1999 (31), 1544-9.

[73] Koseoglu, F; Inan, L; Ozel, S; Deviren, SD; Karabiyikoglu, G; Yorgancioglu, R; Atasoy, T; Ozturk, A. The effects of a pulmonary rehabilitation program on pulmonary

function tests and exercise tolerance in patients with Parkinson's disease. *Funct. Neurol.* 1997 (12), 319-25.

[74] Haas, BM; Trew, M; Castle, PC. Effects of respiratory muscle weakness on daily living function, quality of life, activity levels, and exercise capacity in mild to moderate Parkinson's disease. *Am. J. Phys. Med.Rehabil.* 2004 (83), 601-7.

[75] Dibble, LE; Hale, T; Marcus, RL; Gerber, JP; Lastayo, PC. The safety and feasibility of high-force eccentric resistance exercise in persons with Parkinson's disease. *Arch. Phys. Med. Rehabil.* 2006 (87), 1280-2.

[76] Dibble, LE; Hale, TF; Marcus, RL; Gerber, JP; Lastayo, PC. High intensity eccentric resistance training decreases bradykinesia and improves quality of life in persons with Parkinson's disease: A preliminary study. *Parkinsonism Relat. Disord.* 2009.

[77] Goodwin, VA; Richards, SH; Taylor, RS; Taylor, AH; Campbell, JL. The effectiveness of exercise interventions for people with Parkinson's disease: a systematic review and meta-analysis. *Mov. Disord.*2008 (23), 631-40.

[78] Toulouse, A; Sullivan, AM. Progress in Parkinson's disease-where do we stand? *Prog. Neurobiol.* 2008 (85), 376-92.

[79] Mayeux, R. Epidemiology of neurodegeneration. *Annu. Rev. Neurosci.* 2003 (26), 81-104.

[80] Mayeux, R; Marder, K; Cote, LJ; Denaro, J; Hemenegildo, N; Mejia, H; Tang, MX; Lantigua, R; Wilder, D; Gurland, B; et al. The frequency of idiopathic Parkinson's disease by age, ethnic group, and sex in northern Manhattan, 1988-1993. *Am. J. Epidemiol.* 1995 (142), 820-7.

[81] Kish, SJ; Shannak, K; Rajput, A; Deck, JH; Hornykiewicz, O. Aging produces a specific pattern of striatal dopamine loss: implications for the etiology of idiopathic Parkinson's disease. *J. Neurochem.* 1992 (58), 642-8.

[82] Villar-Cheda, B; Sousa-Ribeiro, D; Rodriguez-Pallares, J; Rodriguez-Perez, AI; Guerra, MJ; Labandeira-Garcia, JL. Aging and sedentarism decrease vascularization and VEGF levels in the rat substantia nigra. Implications for Parkinson's disease. *J. Cereb. Blood Flow Metab.* 2009 (29), 230-4.

[83] Aguiar, AS, Jr.; Araujo, AL; da-Cunha, TR; Speck, AE; Ignacio, ZM; De-Mello, N; Prediger, RD. Physical exercise improves motor and short-term social memory deficits in reserpinized rats. *Brain Res. Bull.* 2009 (79), 452-7.

[84] Jones, TA; Schallert, T. Use-dependent growth of pyramidal neurons after neocortical damage. *J. Neurosci.* 1994 (14), 2140-52.

[85] Stroemer, RP; Kent, TA; Hulsebosch, CE. Neocortical neural sprouting, synaptogenesis, and behavioral recovery after neocortical infarction in rats. *Stroke.* 1995 (26), 2135-44.

[86] Jackson-Lewis, V; Jakowec, M; Burke, RE; Przedborski, S. Time course and morphology of dopaminergic neuronal death caused by the neurotoxin 1-methyl-4-phenyl-1, 2, 3 ,6- tetrahydropyridine. *Neurodegeneration.* 1995 (4), 257-69.

[87] Jackson-Lewis, V; Smeyne, RJ. MPTP and SNpc DA neuronal vulnerability: role of dopamine, superoxide and nitric oxide in neurotoxicity. Minireview. *Neurotox Res.* 2005 (7), 193-202.

[88] Fisher, BE; Petzinger, GM; Nixon, K; Hogg, E; Bremmer, S; Meshul, CK; Jakowec, MW. Exercise-induced behavioral recovery and neuroplasticity in the 1-methyl-4-

phenyl-1,2,3,6-tetrahydropyridine-lesioned mouse basal ganglia. *J. Neurosci. Res.* 2004 (77), 378-90.

[89] Page, G; Peeters, M; Najimi, M; Maloteaux, JM; Hermans, E. Modulation of the neuronal dopamine transporter activity by the metabotropic glutamate receptor mGluR5 in rat striatal synaptosomes through phosphorylation mediated processes. *J. Neurochem.* 2001 (76), 1282-90.

[90] Troiano, AR; de la Fuente-Fernandez, R; Sossi, V; Schulzer, M; Mak, E; Ruth, TJ; Stoessl, AJ. PET demonstrates reduced dopamine transporter expression in PD with dyskinesias. *Neurology.* 2009 (72), 1211-6.

[91] Jaber, M; Dumartin, B; Sagne, C; Haycock, JW; Roubert, C; Giros, B; Bloch, B; Caron, MG. Differential regulation of tyrosine hydroxylase in the basal ganglia of mice lacking the dopamine transporter. *Eur. J. Neurosci.* 1999 (11), 3499-511.

[92] Fauchey, V; Jaber, M; Caron, MG; Bloch, B; Le Moine, C. Differential regulation of the dopamine D1, D2 and D3 receptor gene expression and changes in the phenotype of the striatal neurons in mice lacking the dopamine transporter. *Eur. J. Neurosci.* 2000 (12), 19-26.

[93] Zhu, J; Apparsundaram, S; Bardo, MT; Dwoskin, LP. Environmental enrichment decreases cell surface expression of the dopamine transporter in rat medial prefrontal cortex. *J. Neurochem.* 2005 (93), 1434-43.

[94] Bezard, E; Jaber, M; Gonon, F; Boireau, A; Bloch, B; Gross, CE. Adaptive changes in the nigrostriatal pathway in response to increased 1-methyl-4-phenyl-1,2,3,6-tetrahydropyridine-induced neurodegeneration in the mouse. *Eur. J. Neurosci.* 2000 (12), 2892-900.

[95] Kuczenski, R. Differential effects of reserpine and tetrabenazine on rat striatal synaptosomal dopamine biosynthesis and synaptosomal dopamine pools. *J. Pharmacol. Exp. Ther.* 1977 (201), 357-67.

[96] Naudon, L; Leroux-Nicollet, I; Raisman-Vozari, R; Botton, D; Costentin, J. Time-course of modifications elicited by reserpine on the density and mRNA synthesis of the vesicular monoamine transporter, and on the density of the membrane dopamine uptake complex. *Synapse.* 1995 (21), 29-36.

[97] Petzinger, GM; Walsh, JP; Akopian, G; Hogg, E; Abernathy, A; Arevalo, P; Turnquist, P; Vuckovic, M; Fisher, BE; Togasaki, DM; Jakowec, MW. Effects of treadmill exercise on dopaminergic transmission in the 1-methyl-4-phenyl-1,2,3,6-tetrahydropyridine-lesioned mouse model of basal ganglia injury. *J. Neurosci.* 2007 (27), 5291-300.

[98] Kelley, AE; Cador, M; Stinus, L. Behavioral analysis of the effect of substance P injected into the ventral mesencephalon on investigatory and spontaneous motor behavior in the rat. *Psychopharmacology. (Berl)*, 1985 (85), 37-46.

[99] Carlsson, A. Monoamine-depleting drugs. *Pharmacol Ther [B]*, 1975 (1), 393-400.

[100] Colpaert, FC. Pharmacological characteristics of tremor, rigidity and hypokinesia induced by reserpine in rat. *Neuropharmacology.* 1987 (26), 1431-40.

[101] Kaur, S; Starr, MS. Antiparkinsonian action of dextromethorphan in the reserpine-treated mouse. *Eur. J. Pharmacol.* 1995 (280), 159-66.

[102] Menzaghi, F; Whelan, KT; Risbrough, VB; Rao, TS; Lloyd, GK. Interactions between a novel cholinergic ion channel agonist, SIB-1765F and L-DOPA in the reserpine model of Parkinson's disease in rats. *J. Pharmacol. Exp. Ther.* 1997 (280), 393-401.

[103] Elverfors, A; Nissbrandt, H. Reserpine-insensitive dopamine release in the substantia nigra? *Brain Res*. 1991 (557), 5-12.

[104] Mabandla, M; Kellaway, L; St Clair Gibson, A; Russell, VA. Voluntary running provides neuroprotection in rats after 6-hydroxydopamine injection into the medial forebrain bundle. *Metab. Brain Dis*. 2004 (19), 43-50.

[105] Archer, T; Fredriksson, A. Physical exercise attenuates MPTP-induced deficits in mice. *Neurotox. Res*. 2010 (18), 313-27.

[106] Fredriksson, A; Stigsdotter, IM; Hurtig, A; Ewalds-Kvist, B; Archer, T. Running wheel activity restores MPTP-induced functional deficits. *J. Neural Transm*. 2010.

[107] Gorton, LM; Vuckovic, MG; Vertelkina, N; Petzinger, GM; Jakowec, MW; Wood, RI. Exercise effects on motor and affective behavior and catecholamine neurochemistry in the MPTP-lesioned mouse. *Behav. Brain Res*. 2010 (213), 253-62.

[108] Smith, BA; Goldberg, NR; Meshul, CK. Effects of treadmill exercise on behavioral recovery and neural changes in the substantia nigra and striatum of the 1-methyl-4-phenyl-1,2,3,6-tetrahydropyridine-lesioned mouse. *Brain Res*. 2011.

[109] Al-Jarrah, M; Jamous, M; Al Zailaey, K; Bweir, SO. Endurance exercise training promotes angiogenesis in the brain of chronic/progressive mouse model of Parkinson's Disease. *NeuroRehabilitation*. (26), 369-73.

[110] Lau, YS; Patki, G; Das-Panja, K; Le, WD; Ahmad, SO. Neuroprotective effects and mechanisms of exercise in a chronic mouse model of Parkinson's disease with moderate neurodegeneration. *Eur. J. Neurosci*.2011.

[111] VanLeeuwen, JE; Petzinger, GM; Walsh, JP; Akopian, GK; Vuckovic, M; Jakowec, MW. Altered AMPA receptor expression with treadmill exercise in the 1-methyl-4-phenyl-1,2,3,6-tetrahydropyridine-lesioned mouse model of basal ganglia injury. *J. Neurosci. Res*. 2010 (88), 650-68.

[112] Vucckovic, MG; Li, Q; Fisher, B; Nacca, A; Leahy, RM; Walsh, JP; Mukherjee, J; Williams, C; Jakowec, MW; Petzinger, GM. Exercise elevates dopamine D2 receptor in a mouse model of Parkinson's disease: in vivo imaging with [(1)F]fallypride. *Mov. Disord*. 2010 (25), 2777-84.

[113] Poulton, NP; Muir, GD. Treadmill training ameliorates dopamine loss but not behavioral deficits in hemi-parkinsonian rats. *Exp. Neurol*. 2005 (193), 181-97.

[114] Zhang, WQ; Tilson, HA; Nanry, KP; Hudson, PM; Hong, JS; Stachowiak, MK. Increased dopamine release from striata of rats after unilateral nigrostriatal bundle damage. *Brain Res*.1988 (461), 335-42.

[115] Brown, LL; Sharp, FR. Metabolic mapping of rat striatum: somatotopic organization of sensorimotor activity. *Brain Res*. 1995 (686), 207-22.

[116] Cospito, JA; Kultas-Ilinsky, K. Synaptic organization of motor corticostriatal projections in the rat. *Exp. Neurol*. 1981 (72), 257-66.

[117] Ebrahimi, A; Pochet, R; Roger, M. Topographical organization of the projections from physiologically identified areas of the motor cortex to the striatum in the rat. *Neurosci. Res*. 1992 (14), 39-60.

[118] Holschneider, DP; Maarek, JM; Yang, J; Harimoto, J; Scremin, OU. Functional brain mapping in freely moving rats during treadmill walking. *J. Cereb. Blood Flow Metab*. 2003 (23), 925-32.

[119] Bosboom, JL; Stoffers, D; Wolters, E. Cognitive dysfunction and dementia in Parkinson's disease. *J. Neural Transm*. 2004 (111), 1303-15.

[120] Dubois, B; Pillon, B. Cognitive deficits in Parkinson's disease. *J. Neurol.* 1997 (244), 2-8.
[121] Doty, RL. The olfactory vector hypothesis of neurodegenerative disease: is it viable? *Ann. Neurol*, 2008 (63), 7-15.
[122] Hawkes, CH; Shephard, BC; Daniel, SE. Olfactory dysfunction in Parkinson's disease. *J. Neurol. Neurosurg. Psychiatry*. 1997 (62), 436-46.
[123] Hawkes, CH; Shephard, BC; Daniel, SE. Is Parkinson's disease a primary olfactory disorder? *QJM*, 1999 (92), 473-80.
[124] Sawyer, TF; Hengehold, AK; Perez, WA. Chemosensory and hormonal mediation of social memory in male rats. *Behav. Neurosci.* 1984 (98), 908-13.
[125] Dantzer, R; Bluthe, RM; Koob, GF; Le Moal, M. Modulation of social memory in male rats by neurohypophyseal peptides. *Psychopharmacology. (Berl)*, 1987 (91), 363-8.
[126] Perio, A; Terranova, JP; Worms, P; Bluthe, RM; Dantzer, R; Biziere, K. Specific modulation of social memory in rats by cholinomimetic and nootropic drugs, by benzodiazepine inverse agonists, but not by psychostimulants. *Psychopharmacology (Berl)*, 1989 (97), 262-8.
[127] Prediger, RD; Takahashi, RN. Ethanol improves short-term social memory in rats. Involvement of opioid and muscarinic receptors. *Eur. J. Pharmacol.* 2003 (462), 115-23.
[128] Terranova, JP; Perio, A; Worms, P; Le Fur, G; Soubrie, P. Social olfactory recognition in rodents: deterioration with age, cerebral ischaemia and septal lesion. *Behav. Pharmacol.* 1994 (5), 90-8.
[129] Cotman, CW; Berchtold, NC; Christie, LA. Exercise builds brain health: key roles of growth factor cascades and inflammation. *Trends. Neurosci.* 2007 (30), 464-72.
[130] Cotman, CW; Engesser-Cesar, C. Exercise enhances and protects brain function. *Exerc. Sport. Sci. Rev.* 2002 (30), 75-9.
[131] Kitabatake, Y; Hikida, T; Watanabe, D; Pastan, I; Nakanishi, S. Impairment of reward-related learning by cholinergic cell ablation in the striatum. *Proc. Natl. Acad. Sci. USA.* 2003 (100), 7965-70.
[132] Prediger, RD; Aguiar, AS, Jr.; Rojas-Mayorquin, AE; Figueiredo, CP; Matheus, FC; Ginestet, L; Chevarin, C; Bel, ED; Mongeau, R; Hamon, M; Lanfumey, L; Raisman-Vozari, R. Single intranasal administration of 1-methyl-4-phenyl-1,2,3,6-tetrahydropyridine in C57BL/6 mice models early preclinical phase of Parkinson's disease. *Neurotox Res.* (17), 114-29.
[133] van Praag, H; Christie, BR; Sejnowski, TJ; Gage, FH. Running enhances neurogenesis, learning, and long-term potentiation in mice. *Proc. Natl. Acad. Sci. USA.* 1999 (96), 13427-31.
[134] van Praag, H; Kempermann, G; Gage, FH. Running increases cell proliferation and neurogenesis in the adult mouse dentate gyrus. *Nat. Neurosci.* 1999 (2), 266-70.
[135] Aguiar, AS, Jr.; Speck, AE; Prediger, RD; Kapczinski, F; Pinho, RA. Downhill training upregulates mice hippocampal and striatal brain-derived neurotrophic factor levels. *J. Neural. Transm.* 2008 (115), 1251-5.
[136] Neeper, SA; Gomez-Pinilla, F; Choi, J; Cotman, CW. Physical activity increases mRNA for brain-derived neurotrophic factor and nerve growth factor in rat brain. *Brain Res.* 1996 (726), 49-56.

[137] Ogonovszky, H; Berkes, I; Kumagai, S; Kaneko, T; Tahara, S; Goto, S; Radak, Z. The effects of moderate-, strenuous- and over-training on oxidative stress markers, DNA repair, and memory, in rat brain. *Neurochem. Int.* 2005 (46), 635-40.

[138] Radak, Z; Kaneko, T; Tahara, S; Nakamoto, H; Pucsok, J; Sasvari, M; Nyakas, C; Goto, S. Regular exercise improves cognitive function and decreases oxidative damage in rat brain. *Neurochem. Int.* 2001 (38), 17-23.

[139] Radak, Z; Toldy, A; Szabo, Z; Siamilis, S; Nyakas, C; Silye, G; Jakus, J; Goto, S. The effects of training and detraining on memory, neurotrophins and oxidative stress markers in rat brain. *Neurochem. Int.* 2006 (49), 387-92.

[140] Halliwell, B. Oxidants and the central nervous system: some fundamental questions. Is oxidant damage relevant to Parkinson's disease, Alzheimer's disease, traumatic injury or stroke? *Acta. Neurol. Scand. Suppl.* 1989 (126), 23-33.

[141] Halliwell, B. Reactive oxygen species and the central nervous system. *J. Neurochem.* 1992 (59), 1609-23.

[142] Black, JE; Isaacs, KR; Anderson, BJ; Alcantara, AA; Greenough, WT. Learning causes synaptogenesis, whereas motor activity causes angiogenesis, in cerebellar cortex of adult rats. *Proc. Natl. Acad. Sci. U SA.* 1990 (87), 5568-72.

[143] Chen, YC; Chen, QS; Lei, JL; Wang, SL. Physical training modifies the age-related decrease of GAP-43 and synaptophysin in the hippocampal formation in C57BL/6J mouse. *Brain Res.* 1998 (806), 238-45.

[144] Gomez-Pinilla, F; Ying, Z; Roy, RR; Molteni, R; Edgerton, VR. Voluntary exercise induces a BDNF-mediated mechanism that promotes neuroplasticity. *J. Neurophysiol.* 2002 (88), 2187-95.

[145] Schmidt-Hieber, C; Jonas, P; Bischofberger, J. Enhanced synaptic plasticity in newly generated granule cells of the adult hippocampus. *Nature.* 2004 (429), 184-7.

[146] Isaacs, KR; Anderson, BJ; Alcantara, AA; Black, JE; Greenough, WT. Exercise and the brain: angiogenesis in the adult rat cerebellum after vigorous physical activity and motor skill learning. *J. Cereb. Blood Flow Metab.* 1992 (12), 110-9.

[147] Ide, K; Secher, NH. Cerebral blood flow and metabolism during exercise. *Prog. Neurobiol.* 2000 (61), 397-414.

[148] Secher, NH; Seifert, T; Van Lieshout, JJ. Cerebral blood flow and metabolism during exercise: implications for fatigue. *J. Appl. Physiol.* 2008 (104), 306-14.

[149] Liu, J; Yeo, HC; Overvik-Douki, E; Hagen, T; Doniger, SJ; Chyu, DW; Brooks, GA; Ames, BN. Chronically and acutely exercised rats: biomarkers of oxidative stress and endogenous antioxidants. *J. Appl. Physiol.* 2000 (89), 21-8.

[150] Radak, Z; Sasvari, M; Nyakas, C; Kaneko, T; Tahara, S; Ohno, H; Goto, S. Single bout of exercise eliminates the immobilization-induced oxidative stress in rat brain. *Neurochem. Int.* 2001 (39), 33-8.

[151] Adlard, PA; Perreau, VM; Pop, V; Cotman, CW. Voluntary exercise decreases amyloid load in a transgenic model of Alzheimer's disease. *J. Neurosci.* 2005 (25), 4217-21.

[152] Russo-Neustadt, A; Ha, T; Ramirez, R; Kesslak, JP. Physical activity-antidepressant treatment combination: impact on brain-derived neurotrophic factor and behavior in an animal model. *Behav. Brain. Res.* 2001 (120), 87-95.

[153] Vaynman, S; Ying, Z; Gomez-Pinilla, F. Exercise induces BDNF and synapsin I to specific hippocampal subfields. *J. Neurosci. Res.* 2004 (76), 356-62.

[154] Jenner, P; Olanow, CW. Understanding cell death in Parkinson's disease. *Ann. Neurol.*1998 (44), S72-84.

[155] Jenner, P; Olanow, CW. Oxidative stress and the pathogenesis of Parkinson's disease. *Neurology*. 1996 (47), S161-70.

[156] Hunot, S; Brugg, B; Ricard, D; Michel, PP; Muriel, MP; Ruberg, M; Faucheux, BA; Agid, Y; Hirsch, EC. Nuclear translocation of NF-kappaB is increased in dopaminergic neurons of patients with parkinson disease. *Proc. Natl. Acad. Sci. USA*. 1997 (94), 7531-6.

[157] Schapira, AH. Mitochondrial complex I deficiency in Parkinson's disease. *Adv. Neurol.*1993 (60), 288-91.

[158] Cooper, JM; Mann, VM; Krige, D; Schapira, AH. Human mitochondrial complex I dysfunction. *Biochim. Biophys. Acta*. 1992 (1101), 198-203.

[159] Parker, WD, Jr.; Boyson, SJ; Parks, JK. Abnormalities of the electron transport chain in idiopathic Parkinson's disease. *Ann. Neurol*. 1989 (26), 719-23.

[160] Dauer, W; Przedborski, S. Parkinson's disease: mechanisms and models. *Neuron*. 2003 (39), 889-909.

[161] Aguiar, AS, Jr.; Tuon, T; Soares, FS; da Rocha, LG; Silveira, PC; Pinho, RA. The effect of n-acetylcysteine and deferoxamine on exercise-induced oxidative damage in striatum and hippocampus of mice. *Neurochem. Res*. 2008 (33), 729-36.

[162] Somani, SM; Husain, K. Exercise training alters kinetics of antioxidant enzymes in rat tissues. *Biochem. Mol. Biol. Int*. 1996 (38), 587-95.

[163] Devi, SA; Kiran, TR. Regional responses in antioxidant system to exercise training and dietary vitamin E in aging rat brain. *Neurobiol. Aging*. 2004 (25), 501-8.

[164] Radak, Z; Chung, HY; Goto, S. Systemic adaptation to oxidative challenge induced by regular exercise. *Free Radic. Biol. Med*. 2008 (44), 153-9.

[165] Fahn, S; Cohen, G. The oxidant stress hypothesis in Parkinson's disease: evidence supporting it. *Ann. Neurol*. 1992 (32), 804-12.

[166] Betarbet, R; Sherer, TB; MacKenzie, G; Garcia-Osuna, M; Panov, AV; Greenamyre, JT. Chronic systemic pesticide exposure reproduces features of Parkinson's disease. *Nat. Neurosci*. 2000 (3), 1301-6.

[167] Braak, H; Del Tredici, K; Rub, U; de Vos, RA; Jansen Steur, EN; Braak, E. Staging of brain pathology related to sporadic Parkinson's disease. *Neurobiol. Aging*. 2003 (24), 197-211.

[168] Braak, H; Ghebremedhin, E; Rub, U; Bratzke, H; Del Tredici, K. Stages in the development of Parkinson's disease-related pathology. *Cell Tissue. Res*. 2004 (318), 121-34.

[169] Schulz, JB. Neuronal pathology in Parkinson's disease. *Cell Tissue. Res*. 2005 (320), 211.

[170] Polymeropoulos, MH; Lavedan, C; Leroy, E; Ide, SE; Dehejia, A; Dutra, A; Pike, B; Root, H; Rubenstein, J; Boyer, R; Stenroos, ES; Chandrasekharappa, S; Athanassiadou, A; Papapetropoulos, T; Johnson, WG; Lazzarini, AM; Duvoisin, RC; Di Iorio, G; Golbe, LI; Nussbaum, RL. Mutation in the alpha-synuclein gene identified in families with Parkinson's disease. *Science*. 1997 (276), 2045-7.

[171] Baba, M; Nakajo, S; Tu, PH; Tomita, T; Nakaya, K; Lee, VM; Trojanowski, JQ; Iwatsubo, T. Aggregation of alpha-synuclein in Lewy bodies of sporadic Parkinson's disease and dementia with Lewy bodies. *Am. J. Pathol*. 1998 (152), 879-84.

[172] Dawson, TM; Dawson, VL. Molecular pathways of neurodegeneration in Parkinson's disease. *Science*. 2003 (302), 819-22.

[173] Kitada, T; Asakawa, S; Hattori, N; Matsumine, H; Yamamura, Y; Minoshima, S; Yokochi, M; Mizuno, Y; Shimizu, N. Mutations in the parkin gene cause autosomal recessive juvenile parkinsonism. *Nature*. 1998 (392), 605-8.

[174] Leroy, E; Boyer, R; Auburger, G; Leube, B; Ulm, G; Mezey, E; Harta, G; Brownstein, MJ; Jonnalagada, S; Chernova, T; Dehejia, A; Lavedan, C; Gasser, T; Steinbach, PJ; Wilkinson, KD; Polymeropoulos, MH. The ubiquitin pathway in Parkinson's disease. *Nature*, 1998 (395), 451-2.

[175] Szabo, Z; Ying, Z; Radak, Z; Gomez-Pinilla, F. Voluntary exercise may engage proteasome function to benefit the brain after trauma. *Brain Res*. 2009

[176] Goto, S; Naito, H; Kaneko, T; Chung, HY; Radak, Z. Hormetic effects of regular exercise in aging: correlation with oxidative stress. *Appl. Physiol. Nutr. Metab*. 2007 (32), 948-53.

[177] Radak, Z; Kumagai, S; Taylor, AW; Naito, H; Goto, S. Effects of exercise on brain function: role of free radicals. *Appl. Physiol. Nutr. Metab*. 2007 (32), 942-6.

[178] Barbacid, M. The Trk family of neurotrophin receptors. *J. Neurobiol*. 1994 (25), 1386-403.

[179] McAllister, AK; Katz, LC; Lo, DC. Neurotrophins and synaptic plasticity. *Annu. Rev. Neurosci*. 1999 (22), 295-318.

[180] Mattson, MP; Magnus, T. Ageing and neuronal vulnerability. *Nat. Rev. Neurosci*. 2006 (7), 278-94.

[181] Dobrossy, MD; Dunnett, SB. Environmental enrichment affects striatal graft morphology and functional recovery. *Eur. J. Neurosci*. 2004 (19), 159-68.

[182] Dobrossy, MD; Dunnett, SB. Morphological and cellular changes within embryonic striatal grafts associated with enriched environment and involuntary exercise. *Eur. J. Neurosci*. 2006 (24), 3223-33.

[183] Cechetti, F; Fochesatto, C; Scopel, D; Nardin, P; Goncalves, CA; Netto, CA; Siqueira, IR. Effect of a neuroprotective exercise protocol on oxidative state and BDNF levels in the rat hippocampus. *Brain Res*. 2008 (1188), 182-8.

[184] Calne, DB. Treatment of Parkinson's disease. *N. Engl. J. Med*. 1993 (329), 1021-7.

[185] Horstink, M; Tolosa, E; Bonuccelli, U; Deuschl, G; Friedman, A; Kanovsky, P; Larsen, JP; Lees, A; Oertel, W; Poewe, W; Rascol, O; Sampaio, C. Review of the therapeutic management of Parkinson's disease. Report of a joint task force of the European Federation of Neurological Societies and the Movement Disorder Society-European Section. Part I: early (uncomplicated) Parkinson's disease. *Eur. J. Neurol*. 2006 (13), 1170-85.

[186] Kieburtz, K. Issues in neuroprotection clinical trials in Parkinson's disease. *Neurology*. 2006 (66), S50-7.

[187] Rascol, O; Goetz, C; Koller, W; Poewe, W; Sampaio, C. Treatment interventions for Parkinson's disease: an evidence based assessment. *Lancet*. 2002 (359), 1589-98.

[188] Foley, TE; Fleshner, M. Neuroplasticity of dopamine circuits after exercise: implications for central fatigue. *Neuromolecular Med*. 2008 (10), 67-80.

[189] Gilliam, PE; Spirduso, WW; Martin, TP; Walters, TJ; Wilcox, RE; Farrar, RP. The effects of exercise training on [3H]-spiperone binding in rat striatum. *Pharmacol Biochem. Behav*. 1984 (20), 863-7.

[190] Carter, JH; Nutt, JG; Woodward, WR. The effect of exercise on levodopa absorption. *Neurology*. 1992 (42), 2042-5.

[191] Reuter, I; Harder, S; Engelhardt, M; Baas, H. The effect of exercise on pharmacokinetics and pharmacodynamics of levodopa. *Mov. Disord*. 2000 (15), 862-8.

[192] Mouradian, MM; Juncos, JL; Serrati, C; Fabbrini, G; Palmeri, S; Chase, TN. Exercise and the antiparkinsonian response to levodopa. *Clin. Neuropharmacol*. 1987 (10), 351-5.

[193] Goetz, CG; Thelen, JA; MacLeod, CM; Carvey, PM; Bartley, EA; Stebbins, GT. Blood levodopa levels and unified Parkinson's disease rating scale function: with and without exercise. *Neurology*. 1993 (43), 1040-2.

[194] Muhlack, S; Welnic, J; Woitalla, D; Muller, T. Exercise improves efficacy of levodopa in patients with Parkinson's disease. *Mov. Disord*. 2007 (22), 427-30.

[195] Muller, T; Erdmann, C; Bremen, D; Schmidt, WE; Muhlack, S; Woitalla, D; Goetze, O. Impact of gastric emptying on levodopa pharmacokinetics in Parkinson disease patients. *Clin. Neuropharmacol*. 2006 (29), 61-7.

[196] Scheidtmann, K. Advances in adjuvant pharmacotherapy for motor rehabilitation: effects of levodopa. *Restor. Neurol. Neurosci*. 2004 (22), 393-8.

[197] Fahn, S; Oakes, D; Shoulson, I; Kieburtz, K; Rudolph, A; Lang, A; Olanow, CW; Tanner, C; Marek, K. Levodopa and the progression of Parkinson's disease. *N. Engl. J. Med*. 2004 (351), 2498-508.

[198] Ahlskog, JE; Muenter, MD. Frequency of levodopa-related dyskinesias and motor fluctuations as estimated from the cumulative literature. *Mov. Disord*. 2001 (16), 448-58.

[199] Bhidayasiri, R; Truong, DD. Motor complications in Parkinson disease: clinical manifestations and management. *J. Neurol. Sci*. 2008 (266), 204-15.

[200] Jankovic, J. Motor fluctuations and dyskinesias in Parkinson's disease: clinical manifestations. *Mov. Disord*. 2005 (20 Suppl 11), S11-6.

[201] Factor, SA; Molho, ES; Podskalny, GD; Brown, D. Parkinson's disease: drug-induced psychiatric states. *Adv. Neurol*. 1995 (65), 115-38.

[202] Friedman, JH; Factor, SA. Atypical antipsychotics in the treatment of drug-induced psychosis in Parkinson's disease. *Mov. Disord*. 2000 (15), 201-11.

[203] Nausieda, PA; Weiner, WJ; Kaplan, LR; Weber, S; Klawans, HL. Sleep disruption in the course of chronic levodopa therapy: an early feature of the levodopa psychosis. *Clin. Neuropharmacol*. 1982 (5), 183-94.

[204] van Hilten, JJ; Weggeman, M; van der Velde, EA; Kerkhof, GA; van Dijk, JG; Roos, RA. Sleep, excessive daytime sleepiness and fatigue in Parkinson's disease. *J. Neural Transm. Park Dis. Dement. Sect*. 1993 (5), 235-44.

In: Striatum: Anatomy, Functions and Role in Disease
Editors: Hugo T. Maldonado and Ignacio M. Ortega
ISBN 978-1-61942-384-8

Chapter III

Impaired Nigrostriatal Dopaminergic Neurotransmission in Huntington's Disease: Insights from the R6/1 Transgenic Mouse Model

Joana Gil-Mohapel[1], *Patricia S. Brocardo*[1], *Ruben Smith*[2], *Sören Lagerkvist*[3], *Jia-Yi Li*[4] *and Åsa Petersén*[5]

[1] Division of Medical Sciences, Island Medical Program, University of Victoria, Victoria, BC, Canada
[2] Department of Neurology, Lund University Hospital, Lund, Sweden
[3] NeuroSearch Sweden AB, Göteborg, Sweden
[4] Wallenberg Neuroscience Center, Department of Experimental Medical Science, Lund University, Lund, Sweden
[5] Translational Neuroendocrine Research Unit, Lund University, Lund, Sweden

Abstract

Background: Huntington's disease (HD) is the most common polyglutamine neurodegenerative disorder. The mutation consists of an unstable expansion of CAG repeats within the coding region of the *HD* gene, which expresses the protein huntingtin. Although the abnormal protein is ubiquitously expressed throughout the organism, cell degeneration occurs mainly in the brain, particularly in the striatum. Motor disturbances, associated with the loss of voluntary movement coordination, are the classical symptoms of HD. Previous studies have shown that the nigrostriatal dopaminergic system is impaired in transgenic mouse models of HD. In this study, we have further characterized deficits in the regulation of the nigrostriatal dopaminergic pathway in R6/1 transgenic HD mice.

Results: We examined R6/1 mice at 18-19 weeks of age using *in vivo* microdialysis. Specifically, we analyzed the maximum capacity of the nigrostriatal neurons to release dopamine (DA) in the striatum following KCl-induced depolarization of the plasma membrane and after administration of amphetamine. We used high-performance liquid chromatography (HPLC) to measure the levels of DA and its metabolites 3,4-dihydroxyphenylacetic acid (DOPAC) and homovanillic acid (HVA) in the dialysis perfusates. Intrastriatal infusion of both KCl and amphetamine rapidly increased the extracellular levels of DA in the dialysates in both R6/1 and wild-type mice, but the increase was significantly greater in the wild-type animals. In addition, we assessed the total DA tissue levels in the striatum contralateral to the side where we had performed intracerebral dialysis. The striatal tissue levels of DA were significantly decreased in R6/1 mice as compared with their wild-type littermate controls. We also observed a significant and progressive reduction in the mRNA and protein levels of tyrosine hydroxylase (TH) in R6/1 mice compared to their wild-type littermates. This may be the underlying cause for the reduced levels of DA release and tissue content.

Conclusions: Our results support earlier observations indicating that the dopaminergic nigrostriatal pathway is severely affected in R6/1 transgenic HD mice. Based on the present study and previous literature that we review here, we suggest that a dysfunctional nigrostriatal dopaminergic pathway is likely to contribute to some of the symptoms associated with HD.

Keywords: Amphetamine; Dopamine; Dopamine transporter; Exocytosis; Huntington's disease; *in vivo* microdialysis; Nigrostriatal pathway; R6/1 transgenic mice; Striatum; Tyrosine hydroxylase

List of Abbreviations

ANOVA	analysis of variance
CAG	cytosine-adenine-guanine
DA	dopamine
DARPP-32	DA and cyclic-AMP regulated phosphoprotein of a molecular weight of 32 kDa
DAT	dopamine transporter
DOPAC	3,4-dihydroxyphenylacetic acid
ECL	enhanced chemical luminescence
GAPDH	glyceraldehyde-3-phosphate dehydrogenase
HD	Huntington's disease
HPLC	high-performance liquid chromatography
HRP	horseradish peroxidase
HVA	homovanillic acid
$HO^{\bullet}$	hydroxyl radical
H_2O_2	hydrogen peroxide
IEG	immediate early gene
JNK	c-Jun N-terminal kinase
NIIs	neuronal intranuclear inclusions
n.s.	non-significant difference
$O_2^{\bullet}$	superoxide
PBS	phosphate buffered saline

PCR	polymerase chain reaction
PFA	paraformaldehyde
PVDF	polyvinylidene difluoride
ROS	reactive oxygen species
RT-PCR	real-time polymerase chain reaction
SDS-PAGE	sodium dodecyl sulfate-polyacrylamide gel electrophoresis
SEM	standard error of the mean
SNAP-25	synaptosome-associated protein 25
TH	tyrosine hydroxylase
TPH	tryptophan hydroxylase
YAC	yeast artificial chromosome

1. Introduction

1.1. Huntington's Disease

Huntington's disease (HD) is the most common polyglutamine neurodegenerative disorder with a prevalence of 3 to 10 affected subjects per 100,000 individuals in Western Europe and North America (for review see Vonsattel and DiFiglia, 1998). The disease is caused by an unstable expansion of cytosine-adenine-guanine (CAG) repeats within the coding region of the *HD* gene, which encodes the protein huntingtin. This mutation results in a stretch of glutamine residues located in the NH_2-terminal of huntingtin (1993).

In most cases the onset of the disease occurs in midlife, between the ages of 35 and 50 years. The disease progresses over time and is invariably fatal 15 to 20 years after the onset of the first symptoms. Motor disturbances, associated with the loss of voluntary movement coordination, are the classical symptoms of HD, with bradykinesia and rigidity appearing in later stages of the disease. Cognitive capacities are also severely affected during the course of the disease with the slowing of intellectual processes being the first sign of cognitive impairment in HD patients (for review see Gil and Rego, 2008). In fact, deficits in some cognitive functions can in some cases be detected decades before the onset of motor symptoms. These cognitive impairments deteriorate over time and late-stage HD patients show profound dementia (Folstein and Folstein, 1983). Moreover, psychiatric symptoms including personality changes, irritability, apathy, depression, and anxiety are common (Dewhurst et al., 1970; Folstein et al., 1983; Jensen et al., 1993; Duff et al., 2007; van Duijn et al., 2007, 2010; Vaccarino et al., 2011).

Mutant huntingtin is ubiquitously expressed throughout the body. However, cell degeneration occurs mainly in the brain, particularly in the striatum and certain layers of the cortex (for review see Vonsattel and DiFiglia, 1998; Gil and Rego, 2008). Nevertheless, cell loss can also be detected in other brain regions, including the hippocampus and the lateral hypothalamus (Spargo et al., 1993; Rosas et al., 2003; Petersen et al., 2005; for review see Vonsattel and DiFiglia, 1998). One of the neuropathological hallmarks of the disease is the intracellular accumulation of the mutant protein, leading to the formation of insoluble ubiquitinated neuronal intranuclear inclusions (NIIs) and protein aggregates in dystrophic neurites (DiFiglia et al., 1997).

The genetic predictability of HD gives it the potential to take advantage of early intervention therapies aimed at retarding or halting its progression. Unfortunately, while a great deal has been learned about this disorder since the discovery of the *HD* gene in 1993 (1993), there is still no cure or even a satisfactory treatment for this devastating disorder. Nevertheless, various mechanisms have now been implicated in the pathogenesis of HD (for review see Gil and Rego, 2008). At the neuronal level, both a loss of function of normal huntingtin and a toxic gain of function conferred by the polyglutamine expansion are thought to contribute to HD pathology, promoting the activation of proteases, protein misfolding and inhibition of protein degradation, transcription deregulation, synaptic dysfunction, metabolic and mitochondrial dysfunction, and oxidative stress, which over the years culminate in neurodegeneration and cell loss (for review see Gil and Rego, 2008). On the other hand, at the level of neuronal circuits, the decrease in striatal neuroprotection and the massive release of glutamate from the corticostriatal terminals, leading to striatal excitotoxicity, highly suggest that initial cortical dysfunction underlies striatal neurodegeneration in HD. However, a dysfunction of the nigrostriatal dopaminergic pathway has also been suggested to affect the striatum. Thus, the neuronal dysfunction induced by mutant huntingtin in non-striatal brain regions (namely the cortex and the substantia nigra) might be a crucial initial step in HD (for review see Gil and Rego, 2008; Andre et al., 2010) (Figure 1).

In this chapter, we will focus on the role of the nigrostriatal pathway in HD neuropathology. We will review the studies that have shown alterations in dopamine (DA) neurotransmission in HD and present previously unpublished results obtained with the R6/1 HD transgenic mouse model that support this hypothesis.

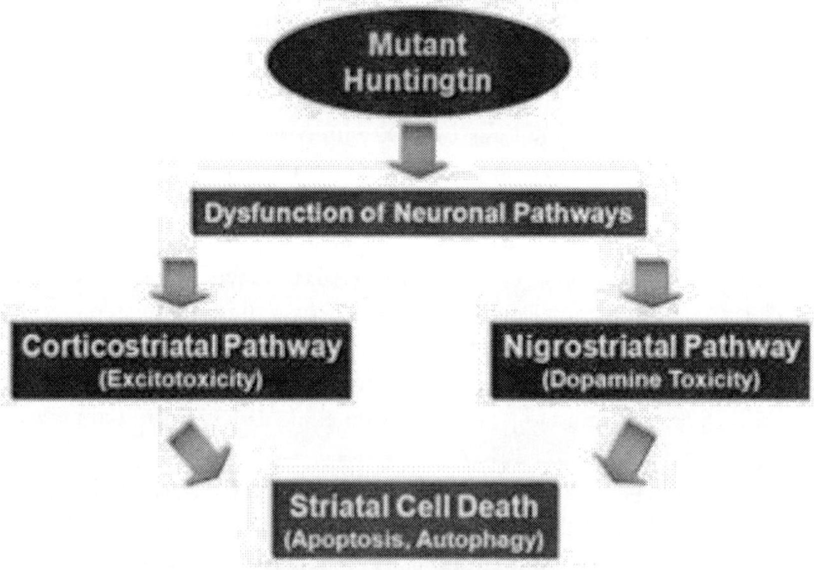

Figure 1. Intracellular dysfunction induced by mutant huntingtin progressively causes the degeneration of relevant neuronal pathways. A dysfunction of corticostriatal and nigrostriatal pathways can have deleterious consequences in the striatum. In particular, excitotoxicity (caused by an increased glutamatergic neurotransmittion) and dysregulation of dopaminergic neurotransmittion can promote a cascade of events that ultimately contributes to the loss of striatal neurons by either apoptosis and/or autophagy in the HD brain.

1.2. The R6 Transgenic Mice for Huntington's Disease

The most commonly used HD transgenic mouse models are the R6 lines (R6/1 and R6/2), which express exon 1 of the human *HD* gene (corresponding to approximately 3% of the entire gene) with 115 and 150 CAG repeats respectively (Mangiarini et al., 1996). Since their generation in 1996, the R6 mice have also been widely used in the screening of therapeutic strategies for HD (for review see Li et al., 2005; Gil and Rego 2009).

The phenotype and neuropathology observed in these mice replicate several features of the human condition, including a progressive and biphasic motor deterioration characterized by an initial hyperactive phase followed by a hypoactive phase (Carter et al., 1999; Luesse et al., 2001; Bolivar et al., 2003, 2004). R6 mice also show cognitive impairment, which can be detected at an early stage of the disease progression (Lione et al., 1999; Murphy et al., 2000) and appears to be correlated with deficits in synaptic plasticity (Murphy et al., 2000).

At the neuropathological level, R6 mice display a marked reduction in brain size that is accompanied by severe striatal atrophy (Mangiarini et al., 1996). Furthermore, R6 mice also show accumulation of ubiquitinated nuclear and cytoplasmic inclusions of the mutant protein (Davies et al., 1997; Li et al., 1999), altered levels of neurotransmitters and their receptors (Young et al., 1998), and compromised gene expression (Olson et al., 2000; Zucker et al., 2005). However, R6 mice show reduced neuronal loss in the striatum, with only one study reporting a 25% decrease in the total number of striatal cells present in 12-week-old transgenic mice (Stack et al., 2005). On the other hand, "dark cell degeneration" has been described in a small number of neurons at a very late stage in the development of the disease (Iannicola et al., 2000; Turmaine et al., 2000; Yu et al., 2003; Stack et al., 2005). Nevertheless, loss of hypothalamic neurons has been reported in end-stage R6/2 mice (Petersen et al., 2005; van der Burg et al., 2008). Importantly, this phenomenon might underlie not only the sleep disturbances (Petersen et al., 2005) and alterations in the circadian rhythm (Morton et al., 2005), but also the metabolic changes and weight loss (van der Burg et al., 2008) that are observed in these HD mice. Moreover, loss of retinal ganglion neurons has also been found in these transgenic animals (Helmlinger et al., 2002).

At the peripheral level, R6 mice show a decrease in body weight (Mangiarini et al., 1996), diabetes (Hurlbert et al., 1999; Luesse et al., 2001; Bjorkqvist et al., 2005) and other neuroendocrine abnormalities (Bjorkqvist et al., 2006; for review see Petersen and Bjorkqvist, 2006), as well as premature death (Mangiarini et al., 1996).

1.3. Nigrostriatal Dysfunction in Huntington's Disease

DA is a major neuromodulator in the striatum as well as other neural areas and is involved in numerous functions, including motor activity, cognition, motivation, emotion, and food intake, to name a few (Wise, 2004; Volkow et al., 2011). The DA pathways responsible for these functions have received much attention because their dysfunction is involved in the etiology of numerous pathological conditions. In particular, several lines of evidence have implicated a dysregulation of the nigrostriatal dopaminergic pathway in the selective striatal degeneration observed in HD (for review see Gil and Rego, 2008), which may account for some of the motor and non-motor manifestations of the disease.

Indeed, several studies have shown degeneration of nigrostriatal projections (Ferrante and Kowall, 1987; Ginovart et al., 1997; Bohnen et al., 2000; Suzuki et al., 2001), atrophy of dopaminergic neurons in the substantia nigra (Oyanagi et al., 1989; Yohrling et al., 2003), as well as a striking reduction of the dopaminergic striatal neuronal population in post-mortem brain tissue from HD patients (Huot et al., 2007). Aggregates of mutant huntingtin were also found in the substantia nigra pars compacta (Gutekunst et al., 1999). Furthermore, a marked loss of tyrosine hydroxylase (TH; the rate-limiting enzyme for DA biosynthesis) (Yohrling et al., 2003) and a down-regulation of the DA transporter (DAT) are known to occur in HD brains (Augood et al., 1997; Ginovart et al., 1997). Although these studies strongly suggest that a pre-synaptic deficit can contribute to the dysfunction of the nigrostriatal pathway in HD, others have found that DA levels and TH activity were actually increased in the striatum of post-mortem HD brains (Spokes, 1981). It is possible however that an initial increase of DA release or abnormal extracellular levels of DA (along with elevated extracellular glutamate levels) will induce excitotoxicity, loss of cortical and striatal neurons, and loss of DA terminals, ultimately leading to a later decrease in DA neurotransmission in the striatum.

At the post-synaptic level, a reduction in DA receptors (i.e., D1 and D2 receptors) and DA uptake sites have also been shown not only in symptomatic HD patients (Cross and Rossor, 1983; Lawrence et al., 1998), but also in pre-symptomatic HD carriers (van Oostrom et al., 2005) suggesting an early dysfunctional DA signalling in HD. In agreement, in both pre-symptomatic and symptomatic patients, positron emission tomography for D1 and D2 ligands found that both striatal D1 and D2 receptor levels were reduced by 45–50% and that this loss progressed by 3–5% per year (Andrews et al., 1999; van Oostrom et al., 2009). Interestingly, loss of D2 DA receptors was previously suggested to be a sensitive indicator of early neuronal impairment in preclinical carriers of the *HD* mutation (van Oostrom et al., 2005). Importantly, this reduction in the expression of DA receptors appears to be a consequence of mutant huntingtin-induced transcriptional dysregulation (Runne et al., 2008), which has been shown to play an important role in the pathophysiology of HD. Overall, these results suggest that both a pre-synaptic and a post-synaptic impairment may contribute to a dysfunctional nigrostriatal pathway (Table I).

Importantly, this nigrostriatal dysfunction may be one of the underlying causes of the motor (e.g., akinesia and dystonia) and cognitive deficits that are characteristic of HD. Indeed, the loss of both pre- and post-synaptic markers of DA neurotransmission is positively correlated with cognitive performance in asymptomatic and symptomatic HD patients (for review see Backman and Farde, 2001). Furthermore, late stages of the disease are normally characterized by bradykinesia and rigidity, symptoms that may be directly caused by the progressive loss of DA receptors in the striatum.

In vitro and *in vivo* studies have also shown that DA itself can enhance polyglutamine toxicity. Indeed, we have previously shown that postnatal cultures of R6/2 striatal neurons display increased sensitivity to exposure to DA with induction of autophagy when compared to cultures derived from wild-type littermate mice (Petersen et al 2001). Using primary cultures of striatal neurons transiently expressing exon 1 of mutant huntingtin, Charvin et al. (2005) have also shown that low doses of DA act synergistically with mutant huntingtin to activate the pro-apoptotic transcription factor c-Jun through a mechanism that is thought to involve the production of reactive oxygen species (ROS) and the activation of the c-Jun N-terminal kinase (JNK) pathway. Importantly, DA also increased aggregate formation in this *in vitro* model, which could be reversed by a selective D2 receptor antagonist (Charvin et al.,

2005). In another study, double mutant mice (generated by crossing a DAT knock-out mouse with a knock-in HD mouse model expressing huntingtin with 92 CAG repeats) exhibited increased stereotypic activity at 6 months of age, followed by a progressive decline of their locomotor hyperactivity. In this hyperdopaminergic mouse model of HD the appearance of NIIs and neuropil aggregates was shown to occur much earlier and to a greater extent in the striatum and other dopaminergic brain regions as compared to control HD mice (Cyr et al., 2006). Thus, based on the results from these studies, it is reasonable to conclude that DA exacerbates mutant huntingtin aggregation both *in vitro* and *in vivo*, although the relationship between DA-mediated aggregation and striatal neurodegeneration needs to be clarified.

Table I. Evidence for nigrostriatal dopaminergic dysfunction in the HD brain

Nigrostriatal Dopaminergic Dysfunction in HD Patients	
Pre-synaptic Dysfunction	**References**
Atrophy of DA neurons in substantia nigra	Oyanagi et al., 1989 Yohrling et al., 2003
NIIs of mutant huntingtin in substantia nigra	Gutekunst et al., 1999
TH reduction in substantia nigra	Yohrling et al., 2003
DAT reduction in substantia nigra	Augood et al., 1997 Ginovart et al., 1997
Degeneration of nigrostriatal projections	Ferrante and Kowall, 1987 Ginovart et al., 1997 Bohnen et al., 2000 Suzuki et al., 2001
Reduction in the number of DA neurons in striatum	Huot et al., 2007
Post-synaptic Dysfunction	**References**
Reduction in DA D1 and D2 receptors in striatum	Cross and Rossor, 1983 Lawrence et al., 1998 van Oostrom et al., 2005
Decrease in DA binding sites in striatum	Andrews et al., 1999 van Oostrom et al., 2009

DA, dopamine; DAT, dopamine transporter; NIIs, neuronal intranuclear inclusions; TH, tyrosine hydroxylase.

Deficits in DA neurotransmission are also thought to exacerbate the dysregulation of the corticostriatal pathway. Indeed, Tang et al. (2007) have shown that DA in the presence of glutamate induced apoptosis in primary striatal cell cultures derived from yeast artificial chromosome (YAC) 128 HD transgenic mice [which express the full-length human HD gene with 128 CAG repeats (Slow et al 2003)]. These results indicate that glutamate and DA signaling pathways may act synergistically to induce an increase in intracellular Ca^{2+} concentration in the HD brain (Tang et al., 2007). Furthermore, a decrease in DA D2 receptor modulation of the pre-synaptic terminal was shown to parallel the age-dependent alterations in corticostriatal activity that are observed in YAC128 HD transgenic mice (Joshi et al., 2009).

Importantly, DA itself can be a source of ROS and a trigger of oxidative stress. Under normal conditions, the enzyme monoamino oxidase converts DA into 3,4-dihydrophenyl-acetic acid (DOPAC) and hydrogen peroxide (H_2O_2). However, DA can also undergo a nonenzymatic process of auto-oxidation producing DA quinones and H_2O_2, and a DA semiquinone and superoxide ($O_2^{\bullet-}$). H_2O_2 and $O_2^{\bullet-}$ can be further oxidized, respectively, through the Fenton (in the presence of transition metal ions) and the Haber-Weiss reactions, producing the extremely reactive hydroxyl radical ($HO^{\bullet}$) (Sulzer and Zecca, 2000, for review). Another possibility is that DA can increase neuronal vulnerability through interactions with the mitochondria. Indeed, primary cultures of striatal neurons expressing mutant huntingtin were shown to be vulnerable to DA, and this vulnerability could be correlated with a reduction in the activity of mitochondrial complex II (Benchoua et al., 2008). Thus, by promoting an increase in the production of ROS and a dysregulation of mitochondrial function, DA might actively contribute to the degeneration of striatal medium-sized spiny neurons in HD.

1.4. Nigrostriatal Dysfunction in R6 HD Transgenic Mice

In R6 mice, abnormalities of the nigrostriatal system have been reported both pre- and post-synaptically. At the post-synaptic level, i.e. in striatal neurons, the reduced expression of DA D1 and D2 receptors can be detected as early as 4 weeks in R6/2 mice (Cha et al., 1998). A reduced expression of the DA receptor signaling protein DARPP-32 (DA and cyclic-AMP regulated phosphoprotein of a molecular weight of 32 kDa) is apparent at the same time (Bibb et al., 2000; Luthi-Carter et al., 2000; van Dellen et al., 2000). Moreover, these mice exhibit defects in DA-regulated ion channels and in the D1/DARPP-32 signaling cascade (Bibb et al., 2000). Importantly, basal immediate early gene (IEG) expression, an index of dopaminergic signal transduction, was found to be altered in the R6/2 striatum at 12 weeks (Spektor et al., 2002). Indeed, while D2-antagonist-induced IEG mRNA levels were found to be reduced in the R6/2 striatum, D1-agonist-induced IEG mRNA levels were shown to be increased (Spektor et al., 2002). Possibly, the increased IEG response after D1 receptor agonist stimulation may be due to D1 receptor supersensitization, which in turn is caused by a diminished dopaminergic input.

Furthermore, at the pre-synaptic level, the nigrostriatal terminals of 16-week-old R6/1 mice were found to release reduced amounts of DA, both at baseline and after malonate stimulation, as measured by *in vivo* microdialysis (Petersen et al., 2002). This may account for the reported D1 receptor super-sensitization. Moreover, 9-week-old R6/2 mice also display attenuated motor activation in response to cocaine (a DAT inhibitor that potentiates the action of physiologically released DA) (Hickey et al., 2002), further supporting the notion of an impaired capacity to release DA.

1.5. Objectives

The goal of the present study was to further characterize the dysfunction of the dopaminergic nigrostriatal pathway at the pre-synaptic level (i.e., at the level of DA synthesis and release) in a transgenic mouse model of HD. Thus, we performed *in vivo* microdialysis in

18- to 19-week-old R6/1 mice by infusing KCl (which depolarizes plasma membranes inducing the release of DA from the vesicular pool), and amphetamine (which leads to a DAT-mediated efflux of DA) through the dialysis probe. This technique allowed us to evaluate the contribution of the two major DA releasing routes for the reduced release of DA that was previously reported (Petersen et al., 2002). Furthermore, we also investigated whether alterations in the expression of TH, the rate-limiting enzyme for the biosynthesis of DA, could contribute for the dysfunction of the dopaminergic nigrostriatal pathway in these HD transgenic mice.

2. Materials and Methods

2.1. Transgenic Animals

Heterozygous male R6/1 mice were purchased from Jackson Laboratories (Bar Harbor, ME, USA) and bred with CBA x C57BL/6J wild-type females. Tails of the offspring were used to obtain DNA for determination of the genotype using a polymerase chain reaction (PCR) assay as previously described (Mangiarini et al., 1996). The animals were housed under a 12-hour light-dark cycle with food and water *ad libitum.* All the work involving animals was approved by the Ethical Committee for the use of laboratory animals at Lund University, Sweden.

2.2. *In Vivo* Microdialysis

R6/1 (n = 7) and wild-type littermates (n = 8) at 18-19 weeks of age were anesthetized with a mixture of 1% halothane and O_2/N_2O. The anesthesia was maintained during microdialysis by free-breathing into a mask fitted over the nose of the mouse. Body temperature was maintained at 37°C using a temperature-regulating heating pad throughout the entire surgical procedure. A microdialysis probe of concentric design (CMA/11, Carnegie Medicin AB, Stockholm, Sweden; length = 2 mm; outer diameter = 0.24 mm) was inserted into the right striatum through a hole drilled in the skull, at the following stereotactic coordinates: 0.8 mm rostral to bregma; 2.2 mm lateral to the midline; 2.8 mm ventral from the dural surface; with the tooth-bar set at zero. The probes were perfused at a rate of 2 μl/min with sterile Ringer solution (145 mM NaCl, 3 mM KCl, 1.3 mM $CaCl_2$, 1 mM $MgCl_2$, pH = 6.0; Apoteksbolaget, Täby, Sweden) through the dialysis session. Perfusate samples were collected every 20 min, starting 60 min after probe implantation (i.e., the first 120 μl were discarded). Subsequently, three basal values (60 min) were obtained, after which the perfusion fluid was switched to one containing KCl (60 mM) for 20 min. The perfusion medium was then switched back to normal Ringer solution and an additional three 20 min dialysate samples were collected. Amphetamine (10 μM) was then perfused through the microdialysis probe for 20 min, after which three more 20 min samples were collected in Ringer solution, yielding a total of 11 samples collected per mouse. Each 40 μl sample was divided into 2 aliquots of 20 μl each, immediately frozen in liquid nitrogen and stored at –80°C until processed.

2.3. Determination of the Dialysate DA, DOPAC and HVA Levels

The quantification of the levels of the monoamine neurotransmitter DA and its acidic metabolites DOPAC and homovanillic acid (HVA) present in the dialysate samples was performed at Carlsson Research AB, Göteborg, Sweden, by high performance liquid chromatography (HPLC) separation and electrochemical detection, according to a method developed by Lagerkvist et al. (unpublished results). Briefly, the analytical method is based on two chromatographic separations dedicated for amines or acids, respectively. The two chromatographic systems share a common auto injector with a 10-port valve and two sample loops for simultaneous injection on the two systems. The acids are separated by reverse phase chromatography while the amines are separated by reverse phase ion pairing preceded by a reverse phase separation in a column switching configuration.

2.4. Analysis of Whole Tissue Striatal DA Levels

Immediately after microdialysis, R6/1 and wild-type mice were killed by cervical dislocation and the brains were rapidly removed on ice. The two hemispheres were separated and the left hemisphere was used to dissect the left striatum, which was immediately frozen on dry ice and stored at –80°C until being processed. The determination of the whole tissue striatal DA levels was then carried out at Carlsson Research AB, Göteborg, Sweden. Briefly, the striata were thawed and homogenized in 1 ml of 0.1 N perchloric acid containing 5% EDTA. After centrifugation at 14,000 *g* for 30 minutes, 200 μl of the supernatant was filtered through a 0.22 μm glass filter and 20 μl were then injected into the HPLC equipment and the DA levels were determined as described above (Section 2.3).

2.5. Evaluation of Correct Microdialysis Probe Placement

After separation of the two brain hemispheres, the right hemisphere (i.e., the one where the microdialysis probe was inserted) was fixed for 24 hours in 4% paraformaldehyde (PFA) and dehydrated in 20% sucrose/0.1 M phosphate buffered saline (PBS). Serial coronal sections were cut on a freezing sliding microtome at 30 μm thickness. Tissue from wild-type and transgenic mice were processed in parallel to control for staining intensity. In order to evaluate the correct placement of the microdialysis probes inside the striata, one series of brain sections was processed for the Nissl stain cresyl violet (ICN Biomedicals Inc., Aurora, OH, USA). Brain sections from each mouse were then observed under a 10x objective fitted onto a light microscope in order to evaluate the location of the lesion caused by the needle tract. In all R6/1 and wild-type mice used in this study the damage caused by the probe was located within the striatum, and therefore we concluded that all the microdialysis probes had been correctly placed.

2.6. Western-Blotting

The striatum and midbrain of R6/1 and wild-type control mice at 16 and 40 weeks of age (n = 4 mice/genotype/age) were dissected, snap-frozen in dry ice, and stored at -80°C until further processing. The brain samples were homogenized on ice in homogenization buffer containing 4 mM HEPES-NaOH (pH = 7.3), 2 mM EDTA, and 1 x of a cocktail of protease inhibitors (Sigma, Stockholm, Sweden) using a Vibra cell sonicator (Sonics and materials inc., Danbury, CT, USA). The homogenate was centrifuged at 1,000 *g* for 10 min. 1% SDS (final concentration) was added to the supernatant and the protein concentration was determined using the BioRad D_C protein assay kit (BioRad, Hercules, CA, USA). Samples were diluted to 1 mg/ml and Laemmli buffer containing beta-mercaptoethanol (3% final concentration) was added. 10 μg of protein were loaded per lane, separated by sodium dodecyl sulfate-polyacrylamide gel electrophoresis (SDS-PAGE), and transferred onto a polyvinylidene difluoride (PVDF) membrane (Amersham Pharmacia Biotech, Uppsala, Sweden). The primary antibodies used were mouse anti-TH (1:1000; Chemicon, Temecula, CA, USA - mAB318) and mouse anti-glyceraldehyde-3-phosphate dehydrogenase (GAPDH; 1:50000; Chemicon - mAB374). After rinsing, secondary antibodies (sheep anti-mouse IgG or donkey anti-rabbit IgG) conjugated with horseradish peroxidase (HRP) (Amersham Pharmacia Biotech) were used and the signals were detected with enhanced chemical luminescence (ECL) plus detection reagents (Amersham Pharmacia Biotech). The ECL exposed films were scanned and the intensity of the bands was measured. Incubations with antibodies were performed at least twice for every antibody and pair of animals (wild-type + R6/1). Levels of TH were calculated as a ratio to the levels of the loading control (GAPDH) and were expressed as percentage of the wild-type signal.

2.7. Real-Time PCR (RT-PCR)

Brains from R6/1 and wild-type animals at 16 and 40 weeks of age ($n \geq 4$ mice/ genotype/age) were dissected and immediately frozen in pulverized dry ice. The brains were kept at –80°C until being further processed. The brains were sectioned on ice into 2 mm sections and the ventral midbrain was quickly dissected out and homogenized in 500μl 1:1 PBS homogenization buffer (Applied Biosystems, Foster City, USA). RNA was purified from the homogenate using a HT6100 RNA preparation station (Applied Biosystems). RNA (0.3 μg) was reverse transcribed with the Advantage™ RT-for-PCR Kit (BD Biosciences, Palo Alto, USA) and random hexamer primers, according to the manufacturer's instructions. Quantitative PCR reactions were performed on the ABI PRISM® 7900 HT Sequence Detection System (Applied Biosystems) by mixing 2x TaqMan® Universal PCR Master Mix, 20x TaqMan® Gene Expression Assays (both from Applied Biosystems), nuclease free water and cDNA for a final reaction volume of 25 μl. TaqMan® Gene Expression Assays used were Mm00447546_m1 for TH and Mm00607939_s1 for beta-actin. Results for TH mRNA were standardized to the levels of beta-actin mRNA.

2.8. Statistical Analysis

The data were analyzed with unpaired Student's *t* tests or two-factor analysis of variance (ANOVA) with repeated measures when appropriate, using the Statview 5.4 package (Abacus Concepts, Berkeley, CA, USA). Data are presented as means ± standard error of the mean (SEM). A P value of < 0.05 was considered statistically significant.

3. Results

3.1. Whole Tissue Striatal DA Levels in R6/1 Mice

Our previous studies have shown no significant differences in the striatal concentration of DA between 16 week-old R6/1 mice and their wild-type littermate controls (Petersen et al., 2002). Interestingly, in the present study, the concentrations of DA in striatal tissue were 143 ± 11 nM for wild-type mice, and 68 ± 11 nM for R6/1 mice at 18-19 weeks of age (Student's *t* test, $P < 0.05$), hence revealing a significant reduction in DA tissue levels in the striatum of R6/1 mice at this stage.

3.2. Dialysate DA Striatal Levels in R6/1 Mice

For all sample collection time-points obtained during the microdialysis experiment the mean dialysate DA levels were significantly reduced in R6/1 as compared with their wild-type littermate controls [two-factor ANOVA with repeated measures, effect of genotype: $P < 0.001$; $F(1, 130) = 24.95$; interaction between time and genotype: $P < 0.0001$; $F(10, 130) = 20.68$)] (Figure 2).

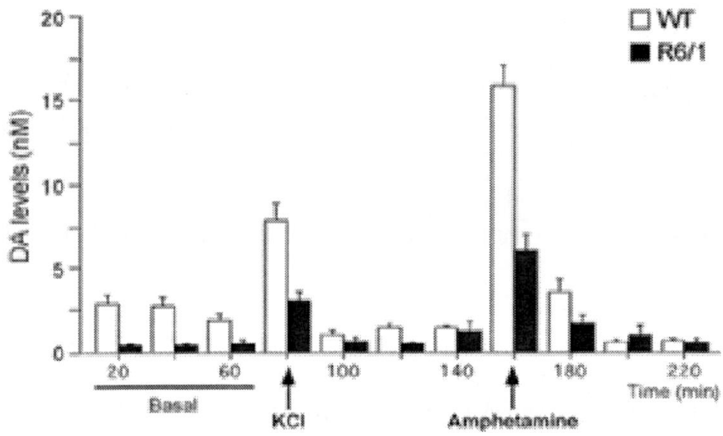

Figure 2. Measurement of DA dialysate striatal levels before and after local infusion of KCl and amphetamine. Dialysate samples were collected every 20 min, starting 60 min after the implantation of the microdialysis probe. Basal levels were obtained during the first three samples after which KCl (60 mM) was perfused through the microdialysis probe during 20 min. After a recovery period of 60 min, amphetamine (10 μM) was perfused for 20 min and three more subsequent 20 min samples were collected. There were significant reductions in DA dialysate levels at all time points in R6/1 mice as compared with their wild-type littermate controls (see text for details on statistical analysis). Data are presented as means ± SEM.

Stable basal striatal dialysate DA levels were achieved 1 hour after probe implantation. Three basal fractions of 20 minutes each were collected during that period. Basal striatal dialysate DA levels were reduced by approximately 76% in R6/1 mice as compared with their wild-type littermate controls (during 20 minutes of sample collection: R6/1 = 0.610 ± 0.10

nM; WT = 2.49 ± 0.41 nM; Student's *t* test, $P < 0.01$), which is in accordance with our previous observations (Petersen et al., 2002).

Intrastriatal KCl (60 mM) injection during 20 minutes rapidly raised the local dialysate DA levels in all animals (Figure 2). However, the release of DA induced by KCl was significantly greater in wild-type animals (7.87 ± 0.99 nM) than in R6/1 mice (2.90 ± 0.42 nM; Student t test, $P < 0.001$). After induction of DAT-mediated DA efflux by intrastriatal injection of amphetamine (10 μM) during 20 minutes the local dialysate DA levels were 15.81 ± 1.31 nM in wild-type and 5.82 ± 0.83 nM in R6/1 mice (Student's *t* test, $P < 0.0001$) (Figure 2). These results suggest that both pathways of DA release (KCl-induced exocytosis and amphetamine-mediated DA release) are impaired in R6/1 mice at 18-19 weeks of age.

3.3. Dialysate Basal Levels of DA Metabolites in R6/1 Mice

We also determined the basal dialysate striatal levels of the DA metabolites DOPAC and HVA (Figure 3). We found a 67% reduction in the basal dialysate DOPAC levels (WT: 162.84 ± 20.01 nM; R6/1: 53.39 ± 12.48 nM; Student's *t* test, $P < 0.001$), and a 69% decrease in the basal dialysate levels of HVA (WT: 179.70 ± 20.07 nM; R6/1: 56.35 ± 13.36 nM; Student's *t* test, $P < 0.001$). The significant reduction in the levels of both DA metabolites supports the concept that the dopaminergic nigrostriatal pathway is impaired in R6/1 mice at 18-19 weeks of age.

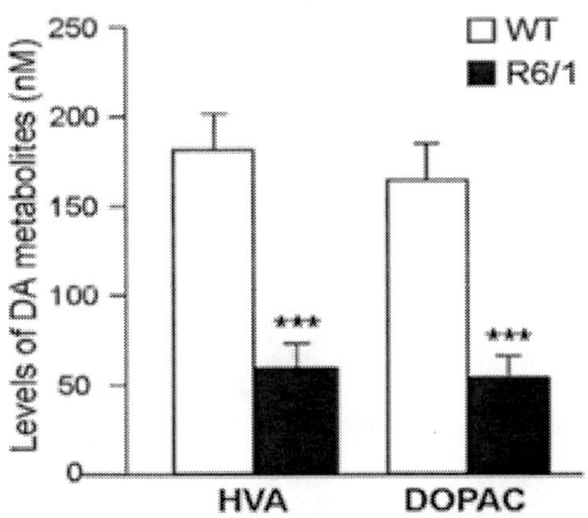

Figure 3. Basal dialysate striatal levels of the DA metabolites DOPAC and HVA. Dialysate samples were collected every 20 min, starting 60 min after the implantation of the microdialysis probe. Basal levels of DOPAC and HVA were obtained during the first three samples and the respective averages were determined. Both DOPAC and HVA striatal basal dialysate levels were significantly reduced in 18-19 week-old R6/1 mice as compared with their wild-type littermate controls (Student's t test, *** $P < 0.001$). Data are presented as means ± SEM.

3.4. TH Protein and mRNA Levels in the R6/1 Midbrain and Striatum

We analyzed the protein levels of TH in ventral midbrain and striatal homogenates using Western blots. At 16 weeks of age there was a decrease of protein TH levels, both in the midbrain and the striatum, to 82.4 ± 4% and 79.5 ± 1% of wild-type levels, respectively. At 40 weeks of age, the decrease was even further pronounced with midbrain and striatal TH protein levels being 54.9 ± 6% and 31.2 ± 10% of wild-type levels, respectively (Figures 4A and 4B). A two-factor ANOVA revealed significant changes with age [midbrain: $P = 0.01$, $F(1, 16) = 8.53$; striatum: $P < 0.01$, $F(1, 14) = 9.06$], genotype [midbrain: $P < 0.0001$, $F(1, 16) = 43.59$; striatum: $P < 0.0001$, $F(1, 14) = 31.27$], and a significant interaction between age and genotype [midbrain: $P = 0.01$, $F(1, 16) = 8.53$; striatum: $P < 0.01$, $F(1, 14) = 9.06$] for both brain regions analyzed.

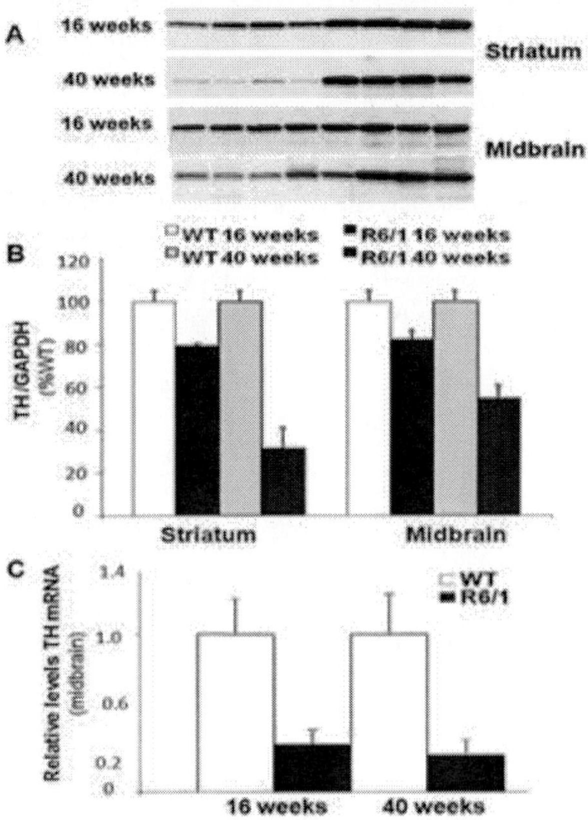

Figure 4. TH protein and mRNA levels. (A) TH protein levels in the striatum and the midbrain of 16- and 40- week-old R6/1 and wild-type mice. Two-factor ANOVA shows a decrease in TH protein levels with age for both the striatum and the midbrain ($P < 0.01$). Additionally, a significant decrease in TH protein levels was detected in R6/2 mice as compared with their wild-type littermate controls in the two brain regions analyzed ($P < 0.0001$). (B) mRNA levels for TH in the midbrain of R6/1 and wild-type mice with 16 and 40 weeks of age. Already at 16 weeks there is a decrease in TH mRNA levels. Two-factor ANOVA revealed no effect of age but a significant effect of genotype ($P < 0.01$) with TH mRNA levels being significantly reduced in R6/2 mice when compared with their wild-type littermate controls. Data are presented as means ± SEM.

To assess whether these reductions in protein levels corresponded to similar decreases in messenger levels, we prepared RNA from the ventral midbrain of 16- and 40-week-old animals and analyzed them using semi-quantitative RT-PCR. At 16 weeks of age TH mRNA levels were down to 30.5 ± 10 % of wild-type levels. At 40 weeks of age the mRNA levels were further decreased to 23.4 ± 10 % of wild-type levels (Figure 4C). A two-factor ANOVA revealed an effect of genotype [$P < 0.01$, F (1, 10) = 15.70], but no effect of age [*P* n.s., F (1, 10) = 0.03], nor an interaction between age and genotype [*P* n.s., F (1, 10) = 0.03].

4. Discussion

In this study we show that DA release due to membrane depolarization and reversal of the DAT is impaired in 18-19 week-old R6/1 mice. Furthermore, we demonstrate a significant decrease in tissue levels of DA in the R6/1 striatum, a result that is in agreement with previous studies showing that DA levels are significantly reduced in the striatum of 8- (Mochel et al., 2011), 9- (Hickey et al., 2002) and 12- week-old (Reynolds et al., 1999; Mochel et al., 2011) R6/2 mice.

Using intracerebral microdialysis, we also found a reduction in the basal extracellular levels of DA and two of its metabolites, DOPAC and HVA in the striatum of 18-19 week-old R6/1 mice. The observed decrease may reflect the reduced amount of DA that is available for catabolism in these mice. Interestingly, a reduction in whole tissue striatal DOPAC levels was also found in 9 week-old R6/2 mice (Hickey et al., 2002), while significant reductions in the DA metabolites HVA and 3-methoxytyramine have been detected in the striatum of 4 week-old pre-symptomatic R6/2 mice (Mochel et al., 2011). Together these results suggest that alterations in DA metabolism might occur early on in the course of the disease.

Finally, in the present study we also detected a progressive decrease in the mRNA and protein levels of TH, the rate-limiting enzyme in the biosynthesis of DA, which may contribute to the observed reduction in DA release and striatal DA levels. Taken together, these results and previous studies demonstrate that the function of the nigrostriatal dopaminergic pathway is severely impaired in R6/1 (Hickey et al., 2002; Petersen et al., 2002; present study) and R6/2 (Reynolds et al., 1999; Hickey et al., 2002; Mochel et al., 2011) HD transgenic mice.

4.1. R6 Mice Show Impaired DA Release

We have previously reported that DA release after malonate stimulation is reduced in 15-16 week-old R6/1 mice (Petersen et al., 2002), which is in agreement with the present findings of a reduction in extracellular DA after KCl-mediated exocytosis and amphetamine-induced efflux through DAT. Interestingly, we found that amphetamine evoked a greater release of DA than KCl in all mice. It has been demonstrated that amphetamine induces DA release via two distinct DAT-mediated mechanisms: (1) a slow process consistent with an exchange mechanism due to the reversal of the transporter; and (2) a rapid efflux through a channel-like mode of DAT that accounts for the release of a large quantity of DA molecules (Kahlig et al., 2005). Therefore, it is possible that these two mechanisms can account for the massive DA release we observed upon amphetamine infusion. Nevertheless, the amphetamine-induced DAT-mediated DA release was significantly decreased in R6/1 mice as compared to wild-type controls. However, the protein levels of DAT seem to be unchanged in R6/1 mice both at 16 (Petersen et al., 2002; Smith et al., unpublished data) and 40 weeks of age (Smith et al., unpublished data), suggesting that a decrease in DAT is unlikely to account for our results.

Further evidence for impaired DA release in HD mice comes from experiments showing that R6/2 exhibit an attenuated response to cocaine (Hickey et al., 2002; Johnson et al., 2006), and a reduced increase in activity in the open field when stimulated with a single dose of amphetamine (2.5 mg/kg) (Gil-Mohapel et al., unpublished observations). In addition, various *in vitro* studies also support this hypothesis. Johnson and colleagues (2006) demonstrated a progressive and significant reduction in DA release in brain slices from R6/2 mice starting at 6 weeks of age (Johnson et al 2006), whereas Ortiz et al. (2010) showed that brain slices from 12 week-old R6/2 mice released less DA than those from wild-type littermate controls. Moreover, the release of the reserve vesicular pool of DA, mobilized by treatment with cocaine, was shorter lived in R6/2 slices when compared with wild-type slices, even though the peak of DA release was identical between the two genotypes. This might be a consequence of the fact that the number of DA-containing vesicles that constitute the reserve pool was reduced by less than half in R6/2 mice (Ortiz et al., 2010). In a subsequent study, the same authors extended these results and showed that the peak of DA release was significantly diminished in R6/1 mice (52% of wild-type at 24 weeks of age). Moreover, the maximum rate of DA uptake was also shown to be decreased both at 16 and 24 weeks of age in R6/1 mice (51 and 48% of wild-type, respectively) (Ortiz et al., 2011).

4.2. Mechanisms Underlying the Reduced DA Release in R6 Mice

The mechanisms underlying the reduced release of DA that has been observed in both R6/1 and R6/2 HD transgenic mice are not yet fully understood. One possibility would be a loss of dopaminergic neurons or of their projections to the striatum. In our previous study, however, stereological analysis revealed no differences in the total number of dopaminergic neurons in the R6/1 substantia nigra at 16 weeks of age, even though there was a significant reduction in malonate-induced DA release already at that age (Petersen et al., 2002). Furthermore, the number of labeled substantia nigra neurons following intrastriatal injection of the retrograde tracer Fluorogold was normal in 16 week-old R6/1 mice, suggesting that the nigrostriatal projections were still intact at that age (Petersen et al., 2002).

Another possible explanation for the observed reduced DA release would be an impairment of the synthesis of this neurotransmitter. Although no differences in the protein levels of TH were detected in the earlier study (Petersen et al., 2002), here we report a significant 20% reduction of protein TH levels in 16 week-old R6/1 mice. This decrease was progressive and reached 70% in 40 week-old R6/1 mice. The reduction in TH protein levels corresponded to a similar decrease in the levels of TH mRNA at both ages. This suggests that the decreased TH protein levels are likely to be caused by a reduced *TH* gene transcription, which could be due to mutant huntingtin-mediated transcriptional dysregulation (for review see Sugars and Rubinsztein, 2003). Reduced TH protein levels have also been reported in end-stage 12 week-old R6/2 mice as assessed by fluorescence immunohistochemistry (Ariano et al., 2002) and western-blotting (Yohrling et al., 2003). Importantly, a decrease in TH has also been observed in human HD brains (Yohrling et al., 2003).

Although impaired DA synthesis is a likely cause of the reductions in extracellular DA levels, we cannot exclude that an impaired exocytosis contributes to the reduced DA release, at least in basal conditions and after KCl-induced depolarization. Indeed, mutant huntingtin is thought to abnormally interact with several different proteins involved in exocytosis and endocytosis (for review see Li et al., 2003; Smith et al., 2005a), such as rabphilin 3A (Smith et al 2007; Smith et al 2005b) and synaptosome-associated protein 25 (SNAP-25) (Smith et al 2007).

Results contradicting ours and showing no changes at the pre-synaptic level of the dopaminergic system in R6/2 mice have also been reported (Vetter et al., 2003). Vetter and colleagues performed *in vitro* release experiments and *in vivo* microdialysis in freely moving 12 week-old R6/2 mice, and did not detect any significant differences in electrically evoked DA release and/or changes in response to DA D2 receptor stimulation (Vetter et al., 2003). The reasons for this discrepancy are not clear and differences between the transgenic mouse lines (R6/1 and R6/2), colonies, and *in vivo* microdialysis techniques may provide an explanation. Within this scenario, it is interesting to point that in our laboratory R6/2 mice failed to survive during the long periods of anesthesia that were required to perform our particular microdialysis procedure.

Conclusion

In conclusion, we provide further evidence for an impaired release of DA and a consequent reduction in the striatal levels of this neurotransmitter and its metabolites in R6/1 mice.

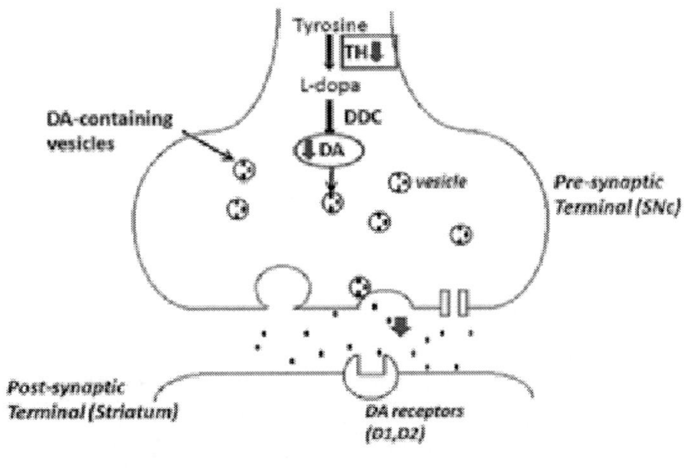

Figure 5. A pre-synaptic deficit contributes to a dysregulation of the dopaminergic nigrostriatal pathway in R6/1 HD transgenic mice. A decrease in the expression of TH (red arrow), the rate-limiting enzyme in the biosynthesis of DA, results in a reduction in the total levels of this neurotransmitter (red arrow). As a consequence, less DA is incorporated into vesicles, which results in a reduction of DA release (red arrow) through KCl-mediated depolarization of the plasma membrane and amphetamine-mediated DAT release. This deficit in pre-synaptic DA neurotransmission may contribute to some of the symptoms characteristic of this HD transgenic mouse model. Red arrows indicate the findings presented in this chapter. DA, dopamine; DAT, dopamine transporter; DDC, DOPA decarboxylase; SNc, substantia nigra pars compacta; TH, tyrosine hydroxylase.

We believe that this reduction is primarily due to a decrease in DA synthesis, which in turn is caused by a decreased TH expression. A dysfunctional nigrostriatal pathway is thus likely to contribute to some of the motor (such as bradykinesia and rigidity) and cognitive symptoms of the disease, which are observed in both late-stage R6 mice and HD patients (Figure 5).

Nevertheless, changes in other neurotransmitter signaling pathways (such as those regulated by the serotonergic system) might also contribute to some of the symptoms characteristic of this neurodegenerative disease. In agreement with this hypothesis, it has been shown that the activity of the rate-limiting enzyme for serotonin production, tryptophan hydroxylase (TPH), is also reduced in 4 week-old R6/2 mice (Yohrling et al., 2002) and there are significant decreases in serotonin and its metabolite 5-hydroxyindolacetic acid at the age of 12 weeks (Reynolds et al., 1999). Thus, it is clear that several neurotransmitter systems are affected in HD, and these changes appear to occur early in the disease process.

Acknowledgments

The work presented in this Book Chapter was performed in the Laboratory of Professor Patrik Brundin (Neuronal Survival Unit), at the Wallenberg Neuroscience Centre, Department of Experimental Medical Science, Lund University, Lund, Sweden. The authors are grateful to Birgit Haraldsson and Elsy Ling for excellent technical assistance with performing the in vivo microdialysis experiments and the genotyping of R6/1 mice respectively. JGM acknowledges the Portuguese Foundation for Science and Technology (FCT) for doctoral funding as well as the Natural Sciences and Engineering Research Council of Canada (NSERC) and the Michael Smith Foundation for Health Research (MSFH) for post-doctoral funding. ÅP is supported by the Swedish Research Council.

References

(1993). A novel gene containing a trinucleotide repeat that is expanded and unstable on Huntington's disease chromosomes. The Huntington's disease collaborative research group. *Cell,* 72, 971-983.

Andre, V. M., Cepeda, C. and Levine, M. S. (2010). Dopamine and glutamate in Huntington's disease: A balancing act. *CNS Neurosci. Ther.,* 16, 163-178.

Andrews, T. C., Weeks, R. A., Turjanski, N., Gunn, R. N., Watkins, L. H., Sahakian, B., Hodges, J. R., Rosser, A. E., Wood, N. W. and Brooks, D. J. (1999). Huntington's disease progression. PET and clinical observations. *Brain*, 122, 2353-2363.

Ariano, M. A., Aronin, N., Difiglia, M., Tagle, D. A., Sibley, D. R., Leavitt, B. R., Hayden, M. R. and Levine, M. S. (2002). Striatal neurochemical changes in transgenic models of Huntington's disease. *J. Neurosci. Res.,* 68, 716-729.

Augood, S. J., Faull, R. L. and Emson, P. C. (1997). Dopamine D1 and D2 receptor gene expression in the striatum in Huntington's disease. *Ann. Neurol.,* 42, 215-221.

Backman, L. and Farde, L. (2001). Dopamine and cognitive functioning: Brain imaging findings in Huntington's disease and normal aging. *Scand. J. Psychol.,* 42, 287-296.

Benchoua, A., Trioulier, Y., Diguet, E., Malgorn, C., Gaillard, M. C., Dufour, N., Elalouf, J. M., Krajewski, S., Hantraye, P., Deglon, N. and Brouillet, E. (2008). Dopamine determines the vulnerability of striatal neurons to the n-terminal fragment of mutant huntingtin through the regulation of mitochondrial complex II. *Hum. Mol. Genet.,* 17, 1446-1456.

Bibb, J. A., Yan, Z., Svenningsson, P., Snyder, G. L., Pieribone, V. A., Horiuchi, A., Nairn, A. C., Messer, A. and Greengard, P. (2000). Severe deficiencies in dopamine signaling in presymptomatic Huntington's disease mice. *Proc. Natl. Acad. Sci. U S A,* 97, 6809-6814.

Bjorkqvist, M., Fex, M., Renstrom, E., Wierup, N., Petersen, A., Gil, J., Bacos, K., Popovic, N., Li, J. Y., Sundler, F., Brundin, P. and Mulder, H. (2005). The R6/2 transgenic mouse model of Huntington's disease develops diabetes due to deficient beta-cell mass and exocytosis. *Hum. Mol. Genet.,* 14, 565-574.

Bjorkqvist, M., Petersen, A., Bacos, K., Isaacs, J., Norlen, P., Gil, J., Popovic, N., Sundler, F., Bates, G. P., Tabrizi, S. J., Brundin, P. and Mulder, H. (2006). Progressive alterations in the hypothalamic-pituitary-adrenal axis in the R6/2 transgenic mouse model of Huntington's disease. *Hum. Mol. Genet.,* 15, 1713-1721.

Bohnen, N. I., Koeppe, R. A., Meyer, P., Ficaro, E., Wernette, K., Kilbourn, M. R., Kuhl, D. E., Frey, K. A. and Albin, R. L. (2000). Decreased striatal monoaminergic terminals in Huntington disease. *Neurology*, 54, 1753-1759.

Bolivar, V. J., Manley, K. and Messer, A. (2003). Exploratory activity and fear conditioning abnormalities develop early in R6/2 Huntington's disease transgenic mice. *Behav. Neurosci.,* 117, 1233-1242.

Bolivar, V. J., Manley, K. and Messer, A. (2004). Early exploratory behavior abnormalities in R6/1 Huntington's disease transgenic mice. *Brain Res.,* 1005, 29-35.

Carter, R. J., Lione, L. A., Humby, T., Mangiarini, L., Mahal, A., Bates, G. P., Dunnett, S. B. and Morton, A. J. (1999). Characterization of progressive motor deficits in mice transgenic for the human Huntington's disease mutation. *J. Neurosci.,* 19, 3248-3257.

Cha, J. H., Kosinski, C. M., Kerner, J. A., Alsdorf, S. A., Mangiarini, L., Davies, S. W., Penney, J. B., Bates, G. P. and Young, A. B. (1998). Altered brain neurotransmitter receptors in transgenic mice expressing a portion of an abnormal human Huntington disease gene. *Proc. Natl. Acad. Sci. U S A,* 95, 6480-6485.

Charvin, D., Vanhoutte, P., Pages, C., Borrelli, E. and Caboche, J. (2005). Unraveling a role for dopamine in Huntington's disease: The dual role of reactive oxygen species and D2 receptor stimulation. *Proc. Natl. Acad. Sci. U S A,* 102, 12218-12223.

Cross, A. and Rossor, M. (1983). Dopamine D-1 and D-2 receptors in Huntington's disease. *Eur. J. Pharmacol.*, 88, 223-229.

Cyr, M., Sotnikova, T. D., Gainetdinov, R. R. and Caron, M. G. (2006). Dopamine enhances motor and neuropathological consequences of polyglutamine expanded huntingtin. *FASEB J.,* 20, 2541-2543.

Davies, S. W., Turmaine, M., Cozens, B. A., Difiglia, M., Sharp, A. H., Ross, C. A., Scherzinger, E., Wanker, E. E., Mangiarini, L. and Bates, G. P. (1997). Formation of neuronal intranuclear inclusions underlies the neurological dysfunction in mice transgenic for the HD mutation. *Cell,* 90, 537-548.

Dewhurst, K., Oliver, J. E. and Mcknight, A. L. (1970). Socio-psychiatric consequences of Huntington's disease. *Br. J. Psychiatry*, 116, 255-258.

Difiglia, M., Sapp, E., Chase, K. O., Davies, S. W., Bates, G. P., Vonsattel, J. P. and Aronin, N. (1997). Aggregation of huntingtin in neuronal intranuclear inclusions and dystrophic neurites in brain. *Science,* 277, 1990-1993.

Duff, K., Paulsen, J. S., Beglinger, L. J., Langbehn, D. R. and Stout, J. C. (2007). Psychiatric symptoms in Huntington's disease before diagnosis: The predict-HD study. *Biol. Psychiatry*, 62, 1341-1346.

Ferrante, R. J. and Kowall, N. W. (1987). Tyrosine hydroxylase-like immunoreactivity is distributed in the matrix compartment of normal human and Huntington's disease striatum. *Brain Res.*, 416, 141-146.

Folstein, S. E. and Folstein, M. F. (1983). Psychiatric features of Huntington's disease: Recent approaches and findings. *Psychiatr. Dev.*, 1, 193-205.

Folstein, S. E., Franz, M. L., Jensen, B. A., Chase, G. A. and Folstein, M. F. (1983). Conduct disorder and affective disorder among the offspring of patients with Huntington's disease. *Psychol. Med.*, 13, 45-52.

Gil, J. M. and Rego, A. C. (2008). Mechanisms of neurodegeneration in Huntington's disease. *Eur. J. Neurosci.*, 27, 2803-2820.

Gil, J. M. and Rego, A. C. (2009). The R6 lines of transgenic mice: A model for screening new therapies for Huntington's disease. *Brain Res. Rev.*, 59, 410-431.

Ginovart, N., Lundin, A., Farde, L., Halldin, C., Backman, L., Swahn, C. G., Pauli, S. and Sedvall, G. (1997). PET study of the pre- and post-synaptic dopaminergic markers for the neurodegenerative process in Huntington's disease. *Brain,* 120, 503-514.

Gutekunst, C. A., Li, S. H., Yi, H., Mulroy, J. S., Kuemmerle, S., Jones, R., Rye, D., Ferrante, R. J., Hersch, S. M. and Li, X. J. (1999). Nuclear and neuropil aggregates in Huntington's disease: Relationship to neuropathology. *J. Neurosci.*, 19, 2522-2534.

Helmlinger, D., Yvert, G., Picaud, S., Merienne, K., Sahel, J., Mandel, J. L. and Devys, D. (2002) Progressive retinal degeneration and dysfunction in R6 Huntington's disease mice. *Hum. Mol. Genet.*, 11, 3351-3359.

Hickey, M. A., Reynolds, G. P. and Morton, A. J. (2002). The role of dopamine in motor symptoms in the R6/2 transgenic mouse model of Huntington's disease. *J. Neurochem.,* 81, 46-59.

Huot, P., Levesque, M. and Parent, A. (2007). The fate of striatal dopaminergic neurons in Parkinson's disease and Huntington's chorea. *Brain*, 130, 222-232.

Hurlbert, M. S., Zhou, W., Wasmeier, C., Kaddis, F. G., Hutton, J. C. and Freed, C. R. (1999). Mice transgenic for an expanded CAG repeat in the Huntington's disease gene develop diabetes. *Diabetes,* 48, 649-651.

Iannicola, C., Moreno, S., Oliverio, S., Nardacci, R., Ciofi-Luzzatto, A. and Piacentini, M. (2000). Early alterations in gene expression and cell morphology in a mouse model of Huntington's disease. *J. Neurochem.*, 75, 830-839.

Jensen, P., Sorensen, S. A., Fenger, K. and Bolwig, T. G. (1993). A study of psychiatric morbidity in patients with Huntington's disease, their relatives, and controls. Admissions to psychiatric hospitals in Denmark from 1969 to 1991. *Br. J. Psychiatry*, 163,790-797.

Johnson, M. A., Rajan, V., Miller, C. E. and Wightman, R. M. (2006). Dopamine release is severely compromised in the R6/2 mouse model of Huntington's disease. *J. Neurochem.*, 97, 737-746.

Joshi, P. R., Wu, N. P., Andre, V. M., Cummings, D. M., Cepeda, C., Joyce, J. A., Carroll, J. B., Leavitt, B. R., Hayden, M. R., Levine, M. S. and Bamford, N. S. (2009). Age-dependent alterations of corticostriatal activity in the YAC128 mouse model of Huntington disease. *J. Neurosci.,* 29, 2414-2427.

Kahlig, K. M., Binda, F., Khoshbouei, H., Blakely, R. D., Mcmahon, D. G., Javitch, J. A. and Galli, A. (2005). Amphetamine induces dopamine efflux through a dopamine transporter channel. *Proc. Natl. Acad. Sci. U S A,* 102, 3495-3500.

Lawrence, A. D., Weeks, R. A., Brooks, D. J., Andrews, T. C., Watkins, L. H., Harding, A. E., Robbins, T. W. and Sahakian, B. J. (1998). The relationship between striatal dopamine receptor binding and cognitive performance in Huntington's disease. *Brain,* 121,1343-1355.

Li, J. Y., Popovic, N. and Brundin, P. (2005). The use of the R6 transgenic mouse models of Huntington's disease in attempts to develop novel therapeutic strategies. *NeuroRx,* 2, 447-464.

Li, J.-Y., Plomann, M. and Brundin, P. (2003). Huntington's disease: A synaptopathy? *Trends Mol. Med.,* 9, 414-420.

Li, X. J., Li, H., Li, S. H., Cheng, A. L., Mangiarini, L. and Bates, G. P. (1999). Ultrastructural localization and progressive formation of neuropil aggregates in Huntington's disease transgenic mice. *Hum. Mol. Genet.*, 8, 1227-1236.

Lione, L. A., Carter, R. J., Hunt, M. J., Bates, G. P., Morton, A. J. and Dunnett, S. B. (1999). Selective discrimination learning impairments in mice expressing the human Huntington's disease mutation. *J. Neurosci.,* 19, 10428-10437.

Luesse, H. G., Schiefer, J., Spruenken, A., Puls, C., Block, F. and Kosinski, C. M. (2001). Evaluation of R6/2 HD transgenic mice for therapeutic studies in Huntington's disease: Behavioral testing and impact of diabetes mellitus. *Behav. Brain Res.,* 126, 185-195.

Luthi-Carter, R., Strand, A., Peters, N. L., Solano, S. M., Hollingsworth, Z. R., Menon, A. S., Frey, A. S., Spektor, B. S., Penney, E. B., Schilling, G., Ross, C. A., Borchelt, D. R., Tapscott, S. J., Young, A. B., Cha, J. H. and Olson, J. M. (2000). Decreased expression of striatal signaling genes in a mouse model of Huntington's disease. *Hum. Mol. Genet.*, 9, 1259-1271.

Mangiarini, L., Sathasivam, K., Seller, M., Cozens, B., Harper, A., Hetherington, C., Lawton, M., Trottier, Y., Lehrach, H., Davies, S. W. and Bates, G. P. (1996). Exon 1 of the HD gene with an expanded CAG repeat is sufficient to cause a progressive neurological phenotype in transgenic mice. *Cell,* 87, 493-506.

Mochel, F., Durant, B., Durr, A. and Schiffmann, R. (2011). Altered dopamine and serotonin metabolism in motorically asymptomatic R6/2 mice. *Plos One,* 6, e18336.

Morton, A. J., Wood, N. I., Hastings, M. H., Hurelbrink, C., Barker, R. A. and Maywood, E. S. (2005). Disintegration of the sleep-wake cycle and circadian timing in Huntington's disease. *J. Neurosci.,* 25, 157-163.

Murphy, K. P., Carter, R. J., Lione, L. A., Mangiarini, L., Mahal, A., Bates, G. P., Dunnett, S. B. and Morton, A. J. (2000). Abnormal synaptic plasticity and impaired spatial cognition in mice transgenic for exon 1 of the human Huntington's disease mutation. *J. Neurosci.,* 20, 5115-5123.

Olson, J. M., Luthi-Carter, R., Strand, A., Peters, N. L., Solano, S. M., Hollingsworth, Z. R., Menon, A. S., Frey, A. S., Spektor, B. S., Penney, E. B., Schilling, G., Ross, C. A., Borchelt, D. R., Tapscott, S. J., Young, A. B. and Cha, J. H. J. (2000). Decreased expression of striatal signaling genes in a mouse model of Huntington's disease. *Hum. Mol. Genet.*, 9, 1259-1271.

Ortiz, A. N., Kurth, B. J., Osterhaus, G. L. and Johnson, M. A. (2010). Dysregulation of intracellular dopamine stores revealed in the R6/2 mouse striatum. *J. Neurochem.,* 112, 755-761.

Ortiz, A. N., Kurth, B. J., Osterhaus, G. L. and Johnson, M. A. (2011). Impaired dopamine release and uptake in R6/1 Huntington's disease model mice. *Neurosci. Lett.,* 492, 11-14.

Oyanagi, K., Takeda, S., Takahashi, H., Ohama, E. and Ikuta, F. (1989). A quantitative investigation of the substantia nigra in Huntington's disease. *Ann. Neurol.*, 26, 13-19.

Petersen, A. and Bjorkqvist, M. (2006). Hypothalamic-endocrine aspects in Huntington's disease. *Eur. J. Neurosci.,* 24, 961-967.

Petersen, A., Gil, J., Maat-Schieman, M. L., Bjorkqvist, M., Tanila, H., Araujo, I. M., Smith, R., Popovic, N., Wierup, N., Norlen, P., Li, J. Y., Roos, R. A., Sundler, F., Mulder, H. and Brundin, P. (2005). Orexin loss in Huntington's disease. *Hum. Mol. Genet.*, 14, 39-47.

Petersen, A., Larsen, K. E., Behr, G. G., Romero, N., Przedborski, S., Brundin, P. and Sulzer, D. (2001). Expanded CAG repeats in exon 1 of the Huntington's disease gene stimulate dopamine-mediated striatal neuron autophagy and degeneration. *Hum. Mol. Genet.*, 10, 1243-1254.

Petersen, A., Puschban, Z., Lotharius, J., Nicniocaill, B., Wiekop, P., O'connor, W. T. and Brundin, P. (2002). Evidence for dysfunction of the nigrostriatal pathway in the R6/1 line of transgenic Huntington's disease mice. *Neurobiol. Dis.,* 11, 134-146.

Reynolds, G. P., Dalton, C. F., Tillery, C. L., Mangiarini, L., Davies, S. W. and Bates, G. P. (1999). Brain neurotransmitter deficits in mice transgenic for the Huntington's disease mutation. *J. Neurochem.,* 72, 1773-1776.

Rosas, H. D., Koroshetz, W. J., Chen, Y. I., Skeuse, C., Vangel, M., Cudkowicz, M. E., Caplan, K., Marek, K., Seidman, L. J., Makris, N., Jenkins, B. G. and Goldstein, J. M. (2003). Evidence for more widespread cerebral pathology in early HD: An MRI-based morphometric analysis. *Neurology,* 60, 1615-1620.

Runne, H., Regulier, E., Kuhn, A., Zala, D., Gokce, O., Perrin, V., Sick, B., Aebischer, P., Deglon, N. and Luthi-Carter, R. (2008). Dysregulation of gene expression in primary neuron models of Huntington's disease shows that polyglutamine-related effects on the striatal transcriptome may not be dependent on brain circuitry. *J. Neurosci.,* 28, 9723-9731.

Slow, E. J., Van Raamsdonk, J., Rogers, D., Coleman, S. H., Graham, R. K., Deng, Y., Oh, R., Bissada, N., Hossain, S. M., Yang, Y. Z., Li, X. J., Simpson, E. M., Gutekunst, C. A., Leavitt, B. R. and Hayden, M. R. (2003). Selective striatal neuronal loss in a YAC128 mouse model of Huntington disease. *Hum. Mol. Genet.*, 12, 1555-1567.

Smith, R., Brundin, P. and Li, J. Y. (2005a). Synaptic dysfunction in Huntington's disease: A new perspective. *Cell Mol. Life Sci.,* 62, 1901-1912.

Smith, R., Klein, P., Koc-Schmitz, Y., Waldvogel, H. J., Faull, R. L., Brundin, P., Plomann, M. and Li, J. Y. (2007). Loss of SNAP-25 and rabphilin 3a in sensory-motor cortex in Huntington's disease. *J. Neurochem.*, 103, 115-123.

Smith, R., Petersen, A., Bates, G. P., Brundin, P. and Li, J. Y. (2005b). Depletion of rabphilin 3a in a transgenic mouse model (R6/1) of Huntington's disease, a possible culprit in synaptic dysfunction. *Neurobiol. Dis.,* 20, 673-684.

Spargo, E., Everall, I. P. and Lantos, P. L. (1993). Neuronal loss in the hippocampus in Huntington's disease: A comparison with HIV infection. *J. Neurol. Neurosurg. Psychiatry*, 56, 487-491.

Spektor, B. S., Miller, D. W., Hollingsworth, Z. R., Kaneko, Y. A., Solano, S. M., Johnson, J. M., Penney, J. B., Jr., Young, A. B. and Luthi-Carter, R. (2002). Differential D1 and D2 receptor-mediated effects on immediate early gene induction in a transgenic mouse model of Huntington's disease. *Brain Res. Mol. Brain Res.,* 102, 118-128.

Spokes, E. G. S. (1981). The neurochemistry of Huntingtons-chorea. *Trends Neurosci.,* 4, 115-118.

Stack, E. C., Kubilus, J. K., Smith, K., Cormier, K., Del Signore, S. J., Guelin, E., Ryu, H., Hersch, S. M. and Ferrante, R. J. (2005). Chronology of behavioral symptoms and neuropathological sequela in R6/2 Huntington's disease transgenic mice. *J. Comp. Neurol.*, 490, 354-370.

Sugars, K. L. and Rubinsztein, D. C. (2003). Transcriptional abnormalities in Huntington disease. *Trends Genet.*, 19, 233-238.

Sulzer, D. and Zecca, L. (2000). Intraneuronal dopamine-quinone synthesis: A review. *Neurotox. Res.*, 1, 181-195.

Suzuki, M., Desmond, T. J., Albin, R. L. and Frey, K. A. (2001). Vesicular neurotransmitter transporters in Huntington's disease: Initial observations and comparison with traditional synaptic markers. *Synapse,* 41, 329-336.

Tang, T. S., Chen, X., Liu, J. and Bezprozvanny, I. (2007). Dopaminergic signaling and striatal neurodegeneration in Huntington's disease. *J. Neurosci.,* 27, 7899-7910.

Turmaine, M., Raza, A., Mahal, A., Mangiarini, L., Bates, G. P. and Davies, S. W. (2000). Nonapoptotic neurodegeneration in a transgenic mouse model of Huntington's disease. *Proc. Natl. Acad. Sci. U S A*, 97, 8093-8097.

Vaccarino, A. L., Sills, T., Anderson, K. E., Bachoud-Levi, A. C., Borowsky, B., Craufurd, D., Duff, K., Giuliano, J., Groves, M., Guttman, M., Kupchak, P., Ho, A. K., Paulsen, J. S., Pedersen, K. F., Van Duijn, E., Van Kammen, D. P. and Evans, K. (2011). Assessment of depression, anxiety and apathy in prodromal and early Huntington disease. *PLoS Curr.,* 3, RRN1242.

Van Dellen, A., Welch, J., Dixon, R. M., Cordery, P., York, D., Styles, P., Blakemore, C. and Hannan, A. J. (2000). N-acetylaspartate and DARPP-32 levels decrease in the corpus striatum of Huntington's disease mice. *Neuroreport,* 11, 3751-3757.

Van Der Burg, J. M. M., Bacos, K., Wood, N. I., Lindqvist, A., Wierup, N., Woodman, B., Wamsteeker, J. I., Smith, R., Deierborg, T., Kuhar, M. J., Bates, G. P., Mulder, H., Erlanson-Albertsson, C., Morton, A. J., Brundin, P., Petersen, A. and Bjorkqvist, M. (2008). Increased metabolism in the R6/2 mouse model of Huntington's disease. *Neurobiol. Dis.*, 29, 41-51.

Van Duijn, E., Kingma, E. M. and Van Der Mast, R. C. (2007). Psychopathology in verified Huntington's disease gene carriers. *J. Neuropsychiatry Clin. Neurosci.*, 19, 441-448.

Van Duijn, E., Reedeker, N., Giltay, E. J., Roos, R. A. and Van Der Mast, R. C. (2010). Correlates of apathy in Huntington's disease. *J. Neuropsychiatry Clin. Neurosci.,* 22, 287-294.

Van Oostrom, J. C. H., Dekker, M., Willemsen, A. T. M., De Jong, B. M., Roos, R. A. C. and Leenders, K. L. (2009). Changes in striatal dopamine D2 receptor binding in pre-clinical Huntington's disease. *Eur. J. Neurol.,* 16, 226-231.

Van Oostrom, J. C. H., Maguire, R. P., Verschuuren-Bemelmans, C. C., Veenma-Van Der Duin, L., Pruim, J., Roos, R. A. C. and Leenders, K. L. (2005). Striatal dopamine D2 receptors, metabolism, and volume in preclinical Huntington disease. *Neurology,* 65, 941-943.

Vetter, J. M., Jehle, T., Heinemeyer, J., Franz, P., Behrens, P. F., Jackisch, R., Landwehrmeyer, G. B. and Feuerstein, T. J. (2003). Mice transgenic for exon 1 of Huntington's disease: Properties of cholinergic and dopaminergic pre-synaptic function in the striatum. *J. Neurochem.,* 85, 1054-1063.

Volkow, N.D., Wang, G.J., Baler, R.D. (2011). Reward, dopamine and the control of food intake: implications for obesity. *Trends Cogn. Sci.,* 15, 37-46.

Vonsattel, J. P. and Difiglia, M. (1998). Huntington disease. *J. Neuropathol. Exp. Neurol.,* 57, 369-384.

Wise, R.A. (2004). Dopamine, learning and motivation. *Nat. Rev. Neurosci.,* 5, 483-494.

Yohrling Iv, G. J., Jiang, G. C. T., Dejohn, M. M., Robertson, D. J., Vrana, K. E. and Cha, J.-H. J. (2002). Inhibition of tryptophan hydroxylase activity and decreased 5-HT1A receptor binding in a mouse model of Huntington's disease. *J. Neurochem.*, 82, 1416-1423.

Yohrling, G. J. T., Jiang, G. C., Dejohn, M. M., Miller, D. W., Young, A. B., Vrana, K. E. and Cha, J. H. (2003). Analysis of cellular, transgenic and human models of Huntington's disease reveals tyrosine hydroxylase alterations and substantia nigra neuropathology. *Brain Res. Mol. Brain Res., 119, 28-36.*

Young, A. B., Cha, J. H. J., Kosinski, C. M., Kerner, J. A., Alsdorf, S. A., Mangiarini, L., Davies, S. W., Penney, J. B. and Bates, G. P. (1998). Altered brain neurotransmitter receptors in transgenic mice expressing a portion of an abnormal human Huntington disease gene. *Proc. Natl. Acad. Sci. U S A,* 95, 6480-6485.

Yu, Z. X., Li, S. H., Evans, J., Pillarisetti, A., Li, H. and Li, X. J. (2003). Mutant huntingtin causes context-dependent neurodegeneration in mice with Huntington's disease. *J. Neurosci.,* 23, 2193-2202.

Zucker, B., Luthi-Carter, R., Kama, J. A., Dunah, A. W., Stern, E. A., Fox, J. H., Standaert, D. G., Young, A. B. and Augood, S. J. (2005). Transcriptional dysregulation in striatal projection- and interneurons in a mouse model of Huntington's disease: Neuronal selectivity and potential neuroprotective role of HAP1. *Hum. Mol. Genet.,* 14, 179-189.

In: Striatum: Anatomy, Functions and Role in Disease
Editors: Hugo T. Maldonado and Ignacio M. Ortega
ISBN 978-1-61942-384-8

Chapter IV

Behavioral and Neurochemical Interrelations between the Striatum and the Cerebellum

R. Lalonde[1] and C. Strazielle[2,*]
[1]University of Rouen, Faculty of Sciences, Department of Psychology, Mont-Saint-Aignan Cedex France
[2]University of Nancy, INSERM 954, Electron Microscopy Service, Faculty of Medicine, Vandoeuvre-les-Nancy France

Abstract

Deep cerebellar nuclei project directly to the susbantia nigra pars compacta and ventral tegmental area, source of dopamine input to the striatum, nucleus accumbens, and prefrontal cortex. Behavioral tests sensitive to lesions of either region in mutant mice include limb-clasping, changes in motor activity, and deficits in motor coordination and spatial orientation. The ascending anatomical projections from the cerebellum to the striatum may explain some of the behavioral similarities, as well as disynaptic projections from the subthalamic nucleus to cerebellar cortex. This hypothesis is supported by findings of neurochemical changes in basal ganglia as a consequence of cerebellar atrophy and neurochemical changes in cerebellum of mice with basal ganglia lesions.

Keywords: Striatum, Substantia nigra, Dopamine, *SNCA*, α-Synuclein, *Park2*, Parkin, UCHL1, Pitx3, *HD* gene, Huntington, Cerebellum, *Grid2*^{Lc} (*Lurcher*) mutant; *Girk2*^{Wv} (*Weaver*) mutant; *Rora*^{sg} (*staggerer*) mutant; Purkinje cells

* Corresponding author: Tel +33 02 35 14 61 08; Fax +33 02 35 14 63 49; Email: robert.lalonde@univ-rouen.fr

Introduction

The purpose of the present review is to describe the relation between the functions of the striatum and the cerebellum. We begin by describing anatomical pathways linking the cerebellum to the basal ganglia, followed by behavioral functions in which the two brain regions participate, based on studies in patients and mutant mice with degeneration of either region. Evidence showing neurochemical effects in basal ganglia in mice with cerebellar lesions, or, conversely, neurochemical effects in cerebellum of mice with basal ganglia lesions is summarized.

Cerebello-Striatal Pathways

The neostriatum (or dorsal striatum) receives direct excitatory input from the neocortex relating to motor, cognitive, and emotional functions, representing functionally distinct but parallel circuits [Graybiel, 1995; Parent and Hazrati, 1995a,b]. Topographic integration into specific subregions relays information in specific areas of pallidum and thalamus before being returned to the neocortex. Neostriatal activity is modulated by dopaminergic fibers originating from the substantia nigra pars compacta (SNc), while the ventral tegmental area (VTA) innervates the nucleus accumbens and prefrontal cortex.

In a similar manner, the cerebellum forms loops with the cerebral cortex, receiving inputs from widespread regions and returning information to the neocortex by relays in ventral thalamic nuclei. Although the basal ganglia and cerebellar loops function in isolation, different studies provide evidence of reciprocal influences between the two subcortical structures. In the ventrolateral thalamic nucleus, sites of projections are separate while convergence of nigral inhibition and cerebellar excitation has been reported in ventromedial cells of rats [Chenier and Deniau, 1982], though not in monkeys [Yamamoto et al, 1983].

Snider et al [1976] first described ascending cerebellar pathways to midbrain dopamine regions in cats. In rats, Perciavalle et al [1989] first provided evidence of a direct projection from the cerebellum to ventral midbrain tegmentum by using retrograde and anterograde horseradish peroxidase transport methods. Unilateral injections in the ventral midbrain tegmentum retrogradely labeled contralateral deep cerebellar nuclei (dentate and interpositus). Conversely, injection sites into deep cerebellar nuclei reached contralateral ventral midbrain tegmentum, including as expected, the red nucleus, but also the SNc and the VTA. Conversely, the subthalamic nucleus sends disynaptic efferents to the cerebellum [Bostan et al, 2010]. When rabies virus were injected into cerebellar cortex of monkeys, retrograde transneuronal transport were seen in the subthalamic nucleus via pontine nuclei. In particular, the subthalamic nucleus projects to the pontine reticular tegmental nucleus and the basal pontine nucleus in monkeys [Giolli et al, 2001] and the pedunculopontine tegmental nucleus in rats [Hammond et al, 1983; Kita and Kitai, 1987], all three precerebellar nuclei [Butcher and Wolf, 2004; Ruigbrok, 2004]. Moreover, high-frequency electric stimulation of the subthalamic nucleus in rats increased c-fos expression in cerebellar nuclei [Moers-Hornikx et al, 2011]. In addition, in rats and monkeys, the cerebellum, specifically the output fibers from deep cerebellar nuclei, project to the neostriatum via the thalamic nuclei [Ichinohe et al, 2000; Hoshi et al, 2005]. The cerebellar projections to basal ganglia and neocortex via thalamic and non-thalamic pathways and subthalamic efferents to the cerebellum via pontine nuclei are illustrated in Figure 1.

The question arises as to whether the cerebellum contributes to symptoms found in basal ganglia diseases. Conversely, the basal ganglia may contribute to symptoms found in cerebellar diseases. This question can be initiated by considering neurologic signs common to both, as well neurochemical changes seen in these diseases as determined by brain cartographies.

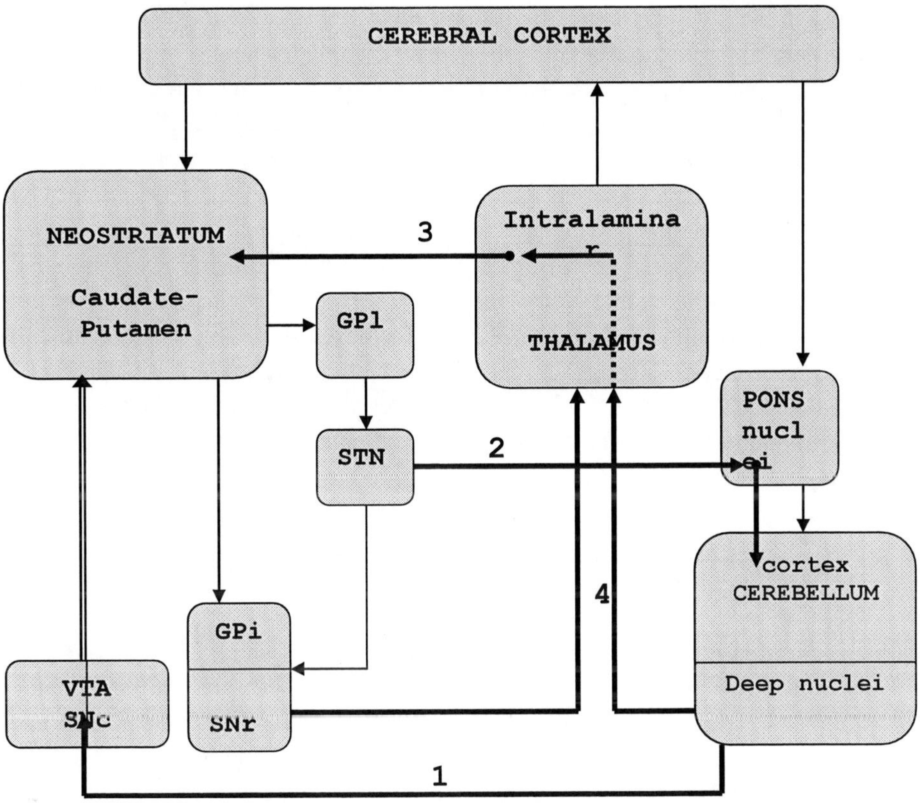

Figure 1. Reciprocal projections between the cerebellum and the basal ganglia (bold arrows - 1-4 pathways). Involved in the extrapyramidal control of movement, the cerebellum and basal ganglia have multisynaptic loops with the cerebral cortex. The thalamus is the efferent structure of the two regions before reaching the cortex: the caudal part of the ventrolateral nucleus (VLc) receives inputs from the cerebellum while its rostral part (VLr) receives inputs from the medial pallidum (GPi) and substantia nigra, pars reticulata (SNr).
1 = direct inputs from the cerebellar deep nuclei (dentate/interpositus nuclei) into the dopaminergic regions of the mesencephalon, the substantia nigra, pars compacta (SNc), and ventral tegmental area (VTA).
2 = disynaptic inputs from the subthalamic nucleus (STN) into the cerebellar cortex via pontic nuclei.
3 = disynpatic inputs from the deep cerebellar nuclei (mainly the dentate nucleus) into the striatum via the non-specific thalamic nuclei, particularly the intralaminar.
4 = convergence of inputs from the two subcortical structures in ventromedial nucleus (VM) of the thalamus.
The neostriatum is regulated by dopamine; the double-arrow illustrates the dopaminergic innervation from SNc and VTA.

Basal Ganglia Diseases and Animal Models

Parkinson's Disease: Neuropathology and Behavioral Dysfunctions

Parkinson's disease is mainly an age-related sporadic disorder, but of earlier onset when transmitted in autosomal dominant or recessive fashion [Marsden, 1982; Lee and Liu, 2008]. Primary symptoms are caused by degenerating neurons in SNc and VTA, resulting in decreased dopamine concentrations in striatum, nucleus accumbens, and prefrontal cortex. Dopamine loss in the putamen is mostly responsible for motor deficits such as akinesia (slow movement initiation), bradykinesia (slow movement completion), muscle rigidity, and resting tremor and dopamine loss in the caudate nucleus for cognitive and emotional disturbances, together with degeneration of ascending noradrenergic, serotoninergic, and cholinergic tracts [Dubois and Pillon, 1997]. Neuropsychological examination reveals a dysexecutive syndrome (deficient planning an organized sequence of events) [Meco et al, 1996; Saint-Cyr et al, 1988], with deficient memory [Hietanen et al, 1988] and visuospatial functions [Bowen et al, 1972; Hietanen et al, 1988].

Helmich et al [2011] and Mure et al [2011] presented evidence of a role for the cerebellum in resting tremor and Ni et al [2010] for postural tremor. The cerebellothalamic circuit appears to be driven into tremor generation at rest after receiving transient signals from dopamine-depleted basal ganglia. Functional magnetic resonance imaging (MRI) indicates increased recruitment of the cerebello-thalamocortical pathway over time by the hand shifted from non-symptomatic to symptomatic [Sen et al, 2010].

Genetic Murine Models of Parkinson's Disease

Parkinson-related genes include *SNCA*, *PARK2*, *UCHL1*, and *DJ1* [Lee and Liu, 2008] from which murine genetic models have been generated [Chesselet, 2008; Fleming et al, 2005; Kahle, 2008]. Transgenic mice with the disease-related $SNCA_{\mathrm{A53T}}$ mutation had lower dopamine transporter binding in dorsal striatum and nucleus accumbens than non-transgenic mice [Unger et al, 2006]. Deletion *SNCA* mice with the same mutation yielding truncated human α-synuclein had reduced SNc dopamine neuronal numbers [Wakamatsu et al, 2008]. Moreover, mice with the artificial (non-disease-related) $SNCA_{G88C+G209A}$ transgene [Richfield et al, 2002] and those with the artificial $SNCA_{120}$ one expressing human truncated α-synuclein [Tofaris et al, 2006] had reduced striatal dopamine concentrations. In addition, two transgenic models expressing non-mutated (wild-type) *SNCA* had fewer striatal dopaminergic terminals [Masliah et al, 2000] and lower TH-immunoreactivity in SNc and striatum [Shults et al, 2005].

In addition to *SNCA*, mice possessing the $UCHL1_{\mathrm{I93M}}$ transgene had reduced nigral TH^{+} neurons and striatal TH fiber terminals [Setsuie et al, 2007]. In view of disease-related loss-of-function *Park2* mutations [Lee and Liu, 2008], six parkin-deficient models have been developed with different exon deletions, though dopamine effects are minimal [Lalonde and Strazielle, 2007a]. In contrast, though not related to parkinsonian mutations, *Pitx3*-deficient aphakia (*ak*) mice, lacking a transcription factor selectively expressed in midbrain and retinal lens [Smidt et al, 2004], had reduced dopamine concentrations in striatum as a result of SNc degeneration [Hwang et al, 2003; Nunes et al, 2003; Smidt et al, 2004; van den Munckhof et al, 2003], but, unlike Parkinson patients, the mutants have severe dysfunction in visual acuity.

Huntington's Disease: Neuropathology and Behavioral Dysfunctions

Huntington's dementia is caused by an autosomal dominant gain-of-malfunction mutation of the *HDH* (*huntingtin*) gene and characterized by degenerating neurons in the caudate and the putamen, particularly medium spiny neurons containing GABA, to a lesser degree in prefrontal cortex, substantia nigra, thalamus, subthalamic nuclei, and cerebellum [Bates et al, 2002; Browne, 1997; Harper, 1996; Roos, 1986; Rosas et al, 2003]. The cerebellar damage may be important, insomuch as the presenting symptom of some Huntington cases, though rarely, is cerebellar ataxia [Kageyama et al, 2003]. The mutated protein is expressed in cerebellum, though at a lower level than neocortex [Aronin et al, 1995]. Motor dysfunction in patients with Huntington's disease include chorea, dystonia, tremor, gait disturbances, and rigidity. The patients are marked at an early age by hyperactivity followed by hypoactivity and apathy. Anterograde amnesia is one of the cardinal symptoms as well as the dysexecutive syndrome [Butters et al, 1978, 1985] and visuospatial disorientation [Boll et al, 1974; Mohr et al, 1991].

Genetic Murine Models of Huntington's Disease

Transgenic mice expressing mutant human *HDH* mimic Huntington's disease, characterized by multiple cytosine-adenine-guanine (CAG) repeats [Heng et al, 2008]. R6/1 and R6/2 transgenic mice express exon 1 of mutated *HDH* with CAG repeats, larger in the latter [Mangiarini et al, 1996]. Other transgenic models include mice expressing *HDH* with 16, 48, and 89 CAG repeats [Reddy et al, 1998]. Knock-ins comprise Hdh_{Q71}, Hdh_{Q92}, Hdh_{Q94}, Hdh_{Q111}, Hdh_{Q140}, and Hdh_{Q150} [Menalled et al, 2000, 2002, 2003] or Hdh_{Q92} and Hdh_{Q111} [Wheeler et al, 1999, 2000, 2002] mutants, where the number corresponds to CAG repeats added to human/murine chimeric exon 1, while another Hdh_{Q150} knock-in contains murine exon 1 with 150 CAG repeats [Heng et al, 2007; Lin et al, 2001].

Mouse Behavior

We compare behavioral tests sensitive to lesions of the basal ganglia with those sensitive to lesions of the cerebellum, namely in mutant mice modeling spinocerebellar ataxias (SCAs). For example, human SCA type 1 is transmitted in an autosomal dominant manner and caused by CAG repeat expansions of the *SCA1* gene, encoding ataxin-1, expressed in the nuclei of Purkinje cells [Clark and Orr, 2000; Skinner et al, 1997]. There is an adult-onset degeneration of the cerebellum and brainstem, leading to ataxia, dysarthria, and bulbar symptoms. Neuropsychological testing in SCA patients reveals deficits in specific visuospatial and executive functions without dementia, of subtler nature than in Huntington's disease [Botez-Marquard and Botez, 1993; Garrard et al, 2008].

Table 1. Mutant mice with cerebellar or basal ganglia lesions with the abnormal paw-clasping reflex

Mutant (name)	Mutation (type)	Pathology	References
Girk2^{Wv}	natural	cerebellum, susbstantia nigra	[*Lalonde, 1987a*]
Rora^{sg}	natural	cerebellum	[*Lalonde, 1987b*]
Cacna1a$^{tg\text{-}rol}$	natural	cerebellum	[*Takahashi et al, 2009, 2010*]
Cacna1a$^{tg\text{-}la}$	natural	cerebellum	[*Alonso et al, 2008*]
ATXN3/Q79	transgenic	cerebellum	[*Chou et al, 2008*]
ATXN3/Q84	transgenic	cerebellum	[*Cemal et al, 2002*]
ATXN7/Q52	transgenic	cerebellum	[*Chou et al, 2010*]
ATXN7/Q92	transgenic	cerebellum	[*Garden et al, 2002*]
R6/1, R6/2	transgenic	striatum	[*Mangiarini et al, 1996*]
HD/Q89, *HD*/Q48	transgenic	striatum	[*Reddy et al, 1998*]
Hd150	transgenic	striatum	[*Heng et al, 2007*] [*Lin et al, 2001*]

Limb-Clasping

When adult rodents are picked up by the tail and slowly lowered towards a horizontal surface, they extend all four paws in anticipation of ground contact, a response triggered by either visual or tactile stimuli [Lalonde and Strazielle, 2011]. In addition to sensory pathways, this placing reflex depends on spinal motor pathways responsible for moving fore- and hindlimbs. Under pathological conditions, limb-flexion and clasping occur instead of extension. The role of the dorsal striatum in triggering limb-clasping is supported by findings in murine models of Huntington's disease with striatal anomalies (Table 1). Indeed, R6/1 and R6/2 transgenic mice display hindlimb clasping, of earlier onset in the latter, probably due to a greater number of polyglutamatine repeats [Mangiarini et al, 1996]. Limb-clasping was also noted in *HDH* transgenic mice with 48 and 89 CAG repeats, though not in those with only 16 [Reddy et al, 1998]. The same response was observed in Hdh_{Q150} knock-in mice with 150 CAG repeats [Heng et al, 2007; Lin et al, 2001]. However, to our knowledge, limb-clasping has not been reported among parkinsonian models. The contribution of the striatum to limb-clasping and its modulation by dopamine is indicated by data showing hindlimb clasping in mice after systemic administration of the neurotoxin, 3-nitropropionic acid (3-NP), causing damage to dorsal striatum, the clasping being potentiated by systemic administration of methyl-phenyl-tetrahydro-pyridine (MPTP), causing damage to the SNc [Fernagut et al, 2004]. However, it is uncertain whether MPTP alone can cause limb-clasping.

The contribution of the cerebellum in pathologic reflexes is indicated by limb-clasping and the bat-like posture (all four limbs bound tightly together) in spontaneous mutant mice with cerebellar atrophy, notably *Girk2*^{Wv} (*Weaver*) [Lalonde, 1987a]. This autosomal semi-dominant mutation comprises a base pair substitution of an inward rectifying K^+ channel strongly expressed in cerebellum and ventral midbrain [Patil et al, 1995]. In cerebellum, the main depleted cell type is the granule cell [Hirano and Dembitzer, 1973]. Unlike the loss of post-migratory granule cells found in *Grid2*^{Lc} (*Lurcher*) mutants [Wetts and Herrup, 1982], the *Girk2*^{Wv} granule cell decrement is mostly pre-migratory, pyknotic cells observed in the external granule cell layer as early as the day of birth, prior to their migration to the internal granule cell layer [Smeyne and Goldowitz, 1989]. There is a more limited Purkinje cell loss [Blatt and Eisenman, 1985; Herrup and Trenkner, 1987]. Unlike cerebellar mutants with more severe Purkinje cell atrophy such as *Grid2*^{Lc} [Caddy and Biscoe, 1979], the number of inferior olive neurons was not reduced in *Girk2*^{Wv} mutants [Blatt and Eisenman, 1985].

In addition to the cerebellum, *Girk2*^{Wv} mutants have degeneration in SNc [Triarhou et al, 1988], leading to reduced dopamine innervation [Strazielle et al, 1998] and concentrations in dorsal striatum [Roffler-Tarlov and Graybiel, 1986; Roffler-Tarlov et al., 1996; Triarhou et al., 1988]. Thus, limb-clasping in this mutant may be due to basal ganglia pathology. However, the spontaneous *Rora*^{sg} (*staggerer*) mutant, whose gene encodes retinoid-like orphan nuclei receptor α (RORA), also characterized by massive granule and Purkinje cell depletion [Herrup, 1983; Herrup and Mullen, 1979] but with normal dopamine concentrations in dorsal striatum [Roffler-Tarlov and Graybiel, 1986], shows the same limb-clasping phenotype [Lalonde, 1987b], supporting the hypothesis that cerebellar damage alone can initiate the pathologic reflex. However, cerebellar damage may induce neural changes in basal ganglia that trigger the response.

Another worthy observation is that the presence of ataxia in a cerebellar mutant does not guarantee observations of the paw-clasping response, as revealed in the *Grid2*^{Lc} mutant [Zuo et al, 1997]. This autosomal semi-dominant mutation comprises a gain-in-malfunction of the *Grid2* gene encoding the GluRδ2 ionotropic glutamate receptor [Zuo et al, 1997], functionally related with the amino-methyl-isoxazoleproprionate (AMPA) receptor [Landsend et al, 1997]. The chronically depolarized membrane potential of *Grid2*^{Lc} Purkinje cells [Zuo et al, 1997] is likely responsible for their nearly complete disappearance [Caddy and Biscoe, 1979], whereas the massive degeneration of granule cells is secondary to this [Wetts and Herrup, 1982], together with the lighter loss in inferior olive neurons through retrograde degeneration [Caddy and Biscoe, 1979] and in deep cerebellar nuclei through anterograde degeneration [Heckroth et al, 1994]. Like the ataxic *Rora*^{sg} mutant [Herrup, 1983; Herrup and Mullen, 1979], the ataxic *Grid2*^{Lc} mutant has massive degeneration of cerebellar cortex [Caddy and Biscoe, 1979], and yet only the former clasps [Lalonde, 1987b; personal observations]. One possible reason for this dissociation is the degree of atrophy between the two mutants in the only output cell out of the cerebellar cortex, the Purkinje cell. Indeed, the Purkinje cell loss is nearly complete in *Grid2*^{Lc} [Caddy and Biscoe, 1979], but represents 75% in *Rora*^{sg} [Herrup, 1983; Herrup and Mullen, 1979]. Total Purkinje cell loss may be better compensated by other brain regions than subtotal loss.

Because of combined cerebellar and SNc damage, it is not surprising to note neurochemical changes in the neostriatum of *Girk2*^{Wv} mutants, particularly reduced dopamine innervation [Strazielle et al, 1998] and concentrations [Roffler-Tarlov and Graybiel, 1986; Roffler-Tarlov et al, 1996; Triarhou et al., 1988], along with changes in basal ganglia pathways, such as augmented regional brain metabolism determined by cytochrome oxidase histochemistry (COX) in the subthalamic nucleus [Table 2; Strazielle et al, 2006], augmented neural activity in this structure being a feature of Parkinson's disease [Lozano et al, 2002].

Table 2. Cytochrome oxidase variations between mutants and controls (expressed in differences of percentage) in brain regions of 3 ataxic mutants, *Lurcher, Weaver and staggerer*

Regions (name)	*Grid2*^{Lc} *Lurcher*	*Girk2*^{Wv} *Weaver*	*Rora*^{sg} *staggerer*
Cerebellum			
-cortex	-	+ 25 **	-
-nuclei			
dentate	+ 47 **	+ 18 *	+ 20 **
interpositus	+ 45 **	-	+ 18 **
fastigial	+ 42 **	-	+ 35 **
Mesencephalon			
-substantia nigra	-	+ 200 **	-
-ventral tegmental area	-	+ 40 *	+ 17 *
-red nucleus	+ 14 *	-	+ 14 *
-reticular pontis	-	-16 *	-
-subthalamic nucleus	-	+ 13 *	-

* P<0.01; ** P<0.001 (- : non significant).

The contribution of the cerebellum to the paw-clasping phenotype is further demonstrated by observing other ataxic mice with cerebellar atrophy, such as the spontaneous *Cacna1a*$^{tg\text{-}rol}$ (*rolling Nagoya*) mutation of a calcium channel [Takahashi et al., 2009, 2010], corresponding to the gene responsible for SCA6, as well as two SCA3 transgenic models *ATXN3*/Q79 [Chou et al, 2008] and *ATXN3*/Q84 [Cemal et al, 2002] and two SCA7 transgenic models *ATXN7*/Q52 [Chou et al, 2010] and *ATXN7*/Q92 [Garden et al, 2002]. Paw-clasping is even observed in mutants with cerebellar dysfunction without overt ataxia, notably in heterozygotes with the *leaner* mutation of the same gene responsible for *rolling Nagoya*, as ataxia is seen only in *Cacna1a*$^{tg\text{-}la}$ homozygotes [Alonso et al., 2008], as well as a SCA14 transgenic model [Zhang et al, 2009]. Thus, there is a double dissociation regarding ataxia and paw-clasping, some mutants with both signs, some with ataxia without clasping, some clasping without ataxia. We propose that limb-clasping results from a functional interaction between the cerebellum and the basal ganglia that may be understood by analyzing neuro-chemical changes in mutant mice.

Conversely, neurochemical changes in cerebellum may be responsible for behavioral signs in mice with basal ganglia pathology. In particular, altered motor behavior was associated with abnormal expression of glycosyltransferase genes in the cerebellum of the R6/1 transgenic model of Huntington's disease [Denny et al, 2010]. Moreover, cerebellar wet weight and total ganglioside concentration was lower in these transgenic mice than wild-type controls. Likewise, neuropathologic changes in the cerebellum and striatum were discerned by MRI in the R6/2 transgenic [Sawiak et al, 2009], with polyglutamine aggregates found in both structures for both R6/2 transgenics and a *Hdh*$_{Q150}$ knock-in [Woodman et al, 2007]. Moreover, the endogenous excitotoxin, quinolinate, and the free radical generator, 3-hydroxykynurenine, were elevated in both striatum and cerebellum of R6/2 mice [Guidetti et al, 2006]. *HD*/Q89 *and HD*/Q48 transgenics also showing limb-clasping have transgene expression in both cerebellum and striatum [Reddy et al, 1999]. There is also evidence in mice of a role for the cerebellum in conjunction with the basal ganglia with respect to dystonic movements [Neychev et al, 2008]. Thus, cerebellar effects in basal ganglia pathology may be due to anterograde or retrograde transsynaptic changes or else to the direct action of the mutated gene in the cerebellum.

Motor Activity

In view of the akinesia and bradykinesia seen in patients with Parkinson's disease [Marsden, 1982] and striatal dopamine depletion with hypoactivity seen after MPTP injections in mice [Schwarting et al, 1999], one expects to find hypoactivity in other mouse models of this disease. This result was obtained in the deletion $SNCA_{A53T}$ transgenic with truncated human α-synuclein and reduced SNc dopamine neuronal numbers [Wakamatsu et al, 2008], the $SNCA_{120}$ transgenic with truncated human α-synuclein and reduced striatal dopamine concentrations [Tofaris et al, 2006], and a $SNCA_{\mathrm{A53T}}$ transgenic driven by the murine *Prp* promoter [George et al, 2008], whereas the $SNCA_{\mathrm{A30P}}$ transgenic driven by the murine *Prp* promoter had lower vertical but not horizontal activity [Freichel et al, 2007]. Moreover, two different exon 3 *Park2* null mutants were hypoactive in the open-field [Itier et al, 2003; Zhu et al, 2007], as well as $UCHL1_{\mathrm{I93M}}$ transgenic mice in their home-cage [Setsuie et al, 2007].

Because of their reduced striatal dopamine concentrations [Roffler-Tarlov and Graybiel, 1986; Roffler-Tarlov et al., 1996; Triarhou et al., 1988], one also expects ataxic $Girk2^{Wv}$ mutants to be hypoactive, a result found when compared with littermate controls in a T-maze [Lalonde et al, 1988a] and an open-field [Strazielle et al, 2006]. However, $Rora^{sg}$ mutants with normal dopamine concentrations in dorsal striatum [Roffler-Tarlov and Graybiel, 1986] were also hypoactive [Lalonde et al, 1988b], presumably due to their ataxia. On the contrary, ataxic $Grid2^{Lc}$ mutants, also with normal dopamine concentrations in dorsal striatum [Reader et al, 1998], had normal activity levels relative to controls in the same apparatus [Lalonde et al, 1986]. These results indicate that ataxia alone is not sufficient to cause hypoactivity, activity measures reflecting the degree of ataxia, more severe in $Rora^{sg}$ than $Grid2^{Lc}$. In $Rora^{sg}$, COX activity increased in red nucleus and VTA, two midbrain cerebellar efferent regions [Deiss et al, 2000]. Like $Rora^{sg}$, COX activity augmented in red nucleus of $Grid2^{Lc}$ mutants [Strazielle et al, 1998], presumably as a consequence of Purkinje cell atrophy shared by both, but not in VTA, crucially involved in motor activity. On the other hand, both $Rora^{sg}$ and $Girk2^{Wv}$ mutants are hypoactive and have higher COX activity in VTA. Another possibility to explain behavioral differences is that, unlike $Grid2^{Lc}$, COX activity decreased in several thalamic nuclei of $Rora^{sg}$ mutants, including the midline, crucial for behavioral activation [Deiss et al, 2000].

In view of the biphasic response (more activity at a young age, less activity at an older age) seen in Huntington's disease [Bates et al, 2002; Harper, 1996], one expects to find the same outcome in murine Huntington models, a result reported in R6/1 [Bolivar et al, 2004] and R6/2 [Lüesse et al, 2001] transgenic mice in the open-field. The same biphasic response was reported with respect to rearing responses in Hdh_{Q94} knock-in mice [Menalled et al, 2003].

Motor Coordination

Patients with Parkinson's disease are subject to falls [Cole et al, 2010]. Relative to controls, these patients had higher stride timing variability, reduced arm swing, and walked with a more stooped posture, with fallers being particularly vulnerable to impaired control of the head and trunk. Therefore, motor coordination deficits on tests requiring balance and equilibrium are expected from experimental models of this disease. As expected, *SNCA* transgenic mice with A30P [Yavich et al, 2004; Gomez-Isla et al, 2003; Freichel et al, 2007], A53T [Gispert et al, 2003; van der Putten et al, 2000], and Y39C [Zhou et al, 2008] mutations were deficient relative to wild-type on the rotorod test, requiring walking in synchrony with a moving beam, as well as *Pitx3/ak* mice relative both to wild-type and mutant mice with retinal degeneration [Ardayfio et al, 2008]. The role of dopamine in this skill is indicated by the finding of a deficit in mice chronically injected with a MPTP dose causing lower striatal dopamine levels without hypoactivity [Luchtman et al, 2009].

In a similar fashion to Parkinsonians, patients with Huntington's disease were subject to lower stepping times and poorer dynamic balance than controls [Goldberg et al, 2010]. As expected, R6/1 [Hansson et al, 2001; Hodges et al 2008; van Dellen et al, 2000], R6/2 [Carter et al, 1999; Hickey et al, 2005; Lüesse et al, 2001], HDH_{Q48} [Guidetti et al, 2001], and HDH_{Q89} [Guidetti et al, 2001] transgenic mice were deficient relative to wild-type on the rotorod, as well as the Hdh_{Q150} knock-in [Heng et al, 2007; Lin et al, 2001]. On the contrary, Hdh_{Q92} knock-in mice were not deficient on the rotorod [Trueman et al, 2007; Wheeler et al, 2000], probably due to fewer polyglutamine repeats than the previous model. Other tests sensitive to deficits in Parkinson [Fleming et al, 2004; Goldberg et al, 2003] and Huntington [Carter et al, 1999; Heng et al, 2007; Lin et al, 2001; van Dellen et al, 2000] murine models include the stationary beam.

In a similar fashion to patients with basal ganglia disorders, SCA patients are more subject to postural instability than controls [Küng et al, 2009]. The number of falls in SCA patients were associated with ataxia severity but also some non-ataxic symptoms [Fonteyn et al, 2010]. In parallel to basal ganglia models, deficits in balance and coordination on the rotorod and other tests are a feature of SCA models such as $Grid2^{Lc}$, $Rora^{sg}$, and $Girk2^{Wv}$ [Lalonde and Strazielle, 2007a,b]. Likewise, *SCA1*/Q82 transgenic mice, containing 82 CAG repeats of mutated human *SCA1* driven by the Purkinje-cell specific *Pcp2/L7* promoter [Burright et al, 1995], were impaired on the rotorod as early as 5 weeks of age, prior to ataxia, when the main histopathological markers are cytoplasmic vacuoles in Purkinje cells [Clark et al, 1997]. Thus, rotorod deficits are found in SCA models without forebrain dopamine losses and prior to ataxia.

Spatial Orientation

The Morris water maze is conducted to specify the contribution of brain regions in spatial learning and visuomotor coordination [Morris et al, 1982], the first evaluated by a hidden platform task solved on the basis of spatial cues and the second a visible platform one with local cues. The spatial subtest is hippocampus-mediated [Morris et al, 1982], while the dorsal striatum [Martel et al, 2007] and cerebellum [Lalonde and Strazielle, 2007b] mediate visuomotor control, though depending on lesion site a dissociation is sometimes found between deficient hidden and intact visible platform performance in cerebellar-lesioned mice and rats. The impact of dopamine is illustrated by findings of impaired visuomotor guidance in rats with 6-hydroxydopamine-induced lesions in SNc [Ferro et al, 2005].

In accord with spatial deficits reported in patients with Parkinson's disease [Bowen et al, 1972; Hietanen et al, 1988], acquisition of the hiddden platform subtest was slowed down in a *Park2* knockout model [Zhu et al, 2007]. Moreover, relative to wild-type controls and mutant mice with retinal degeneration, *Pitx3/ak* mice were deficient in left-right discrimination learning in a water-filled T-maze [Ardayfio et al, 2008]. In accord with spatial deficits reported in patients with Huntington's disease [Boll et al, 1974; Mohr et al, 1991], R6/2 mice had impaired acquisition of place learning in the Morris maze [Lione et al, 1999; Lüesse et al, 2001; Murphy et al, 2000], though their visuomotor guidance was normal [Lione et al, 1999; Lüesse et al, 2001].

Water maze deficits are also a feature of SCA models, of a spatial nature in $Rora^{sg}$ and a visuomotor one in $Grid2^{Lc}$ and $Girk2^{Wv}$ [Lalonde and Strazielle, 2007]. The deficits may be accrued in $Girk2^{Wv}$ because of the added SNc damage and in $Grid2^{Lc}$ because of the more severe cerebellar cortical damage relative to $Rora^{sg}$. In addition to $Rora^{sg}$, spatial orientation was dissociated from visuomotor control in $Agtpbp1^{pcd}$ mutants, mainly characterized by Purkinje cell degeneration [Goodlett et al, 1992].

Conclusion

Genetically modified mice with lesions of the basal ganglia have an abnormal limb-clasping reflex, together with changes in motor activity and deficits in motor coordination and spatial orientation or visuomotor control. Although not necessarily due to the same reason, these anomalies are reproduced in mutant mice with cerebellar atrophy, indicating interrelations between these two brain regions. This hypothesis is supported by findings of neurochemical changes in basal ganglia in cerebellar mutant mice. Conversely, neurochemical changes in cerebellum may be responsible for behavioral signs in mice with basal ganglia pathology.

Acknowledgments

This research was funded by a grant from the Natural Sciences and Engineering Research Council of Canada to R.L.

References

Alonso, I; Marques, JM; Sousa, N; Sequeiros, J; Olsson, IA; Silveira, I. Motor and cognitive deficits in the heterozygous leaner mouse, a Cav2.1 voltage-gated Ca2+ channel mutant. *Neurobiol Aging* 2008, 29, 1733-43.

Ardayfio, P; Moon, J; Leung, KK; Youn-Hwang, D; Kim, KS. Impaired learning and memory in Pitx3 deficient aphakia mice, a genetic model for striatum-dependent cognitive symptoms in Parkinson's disease. *Neurobiol Dis* 2008, 31, 406-12.

Aronin, N; Chase, K; Young, C; Sapp, E; Schwarz, C; Matta, N; Kornreich, R; Landwehrmeyer, B; Bird, E; Beal, MF; Vonsattel, J-P; Smith, T; Carraway, R; Boyce, FM; Young, AB; Penney, JB; DiFiglia, M. CAG expansion affects the expression of mutant Huntingtin in the Huntington's disease brain. *Neuron* 1995, 15, 1193-201.

Bates, G; Harper, PS; Jones, L. eds. *Huntington's disease.* 3rd ed. Oxford: England, Oxford University Press, 2002.

Blatt, GJ; Eisenman, LM. A qualitative and quantitative light microscopic study of the inferior olivary complex of normal, *reeler*, and *weaver* mutant mice, *J Comp Neurol* 1985, 232, 117-28.

Bolivar, VJ; Manley, K; Messer, A. Early exploratory behavior abnormalities in R6/1 Huntington's disease transgenic mice. *Brain Res* 2004, 1005, 29-35.

Boll, TJ; Heaton, R; Reitan, RM. Neuropsychological and emotional correlates of Huntington's chorea. *J Nerv Ment Dis* 1974, 158, 61-9.

Bostan, AC ; Dum, RP ; Strick, PL. The basal ganglia communicate with the cerebellum. *Proc Natl Acad Sci USA* 2010, 107, 8452-6.

Botez-Marquard, T; Botez MI. Cognitive behavior in heredodegenerative ataxias. *Eur Neurol* 1993, 33, 351-7.

Bowen, FP; Hoehn, MM; Yahr, MD. Parkinsonism, alterations in spatial orientation as determined by a route-walking test. *Neuropsychologia* 1972, 10, 355-61.

Browne, SE. Mitochondrial dysfunction and oxidative damage in Huntington's disease. In, MF Beal; N Howell; I Bodis-Wollner. Eds. *Mitochondria and free radicals in neurodegenerative diseases.* New York: Wiley-Liss, 1997, 361-80.

Burright, EN; Clark, HB; Servadio, A; Matilla, T; Feddersen, RM; Yunis, WS; Duvick, LA; Zoghbi, HY; Orr, HT. *SCA1* transgenic mice: a model for neurodegeneration caused by an expanded CAG trinucleotide repeat. *Cell* 1995, 82, 937-48.

Butcher, LL; Wolf, NJ. Cholinergic neurons and networks revisited. In: Paxinos G, editor. *The rat nervous system.* Amsterdam: Elsevier; 2004; 1257-68.

Butters, N; Wolfe, J; Martone, M; Granholm, E; Cermak, LS. Memory disorders associated with Huntington's disease; verbal recall; verbal recognition and procedural memory. *Neuropsychologia* 1985, 23, 729-43.

Butters, N; Sax, D; Montgomery, K; Tarlow, S. Comparison of the neuropsychological deficits associated with early and advanced Huntington's disease. *Arch Neurol* 1978, 35, 585-9.

Caddy, KWT; Biscoe, TJ. Structural and quantitative studies on the normal C3H and *Lurcher* mutant mouse. *Philos Trans Roy Soc Lond (Biol)* 1979, 287, 167-201.

Carter, RJ; Lione, LA; Humby, T; Mangiarini, L; Mahal, A; Bates, GP; Dunnett, SB; Morton, AJ. Characterization of progressive motor deficits in mice transgenic for the human Huntington's disease mutation. *J Neurosci* 1999, 19, 3248-57.

Cemal, CK; Carroll, CJ; Lawrence, L; Lowrie MB; Ruddle P; Al-Mahdawi S; King RH; Pook MA; Huxley C; Chamberlain S. YAC transgenic mice carrying pathological alleles of the MJD1 locus exhibit a mild and slowly progressive cerebellar deficit. *Hum Mol Genet* 2002, 11, 1075-94.

Chesselet, M-F. In vivo alpha-synuclein overexpression in rodents; a useful model of Parkinson's disease. *Exp Neurol* 2008, 209, 22-7.

Chevalier, G; Deniau, JM. Inhibitory nigral influence on cerebellar evoked responses in the rat ventromedial thalamic nucleus. *Exp Brain Res* 1982, 48, 369-76.

Chou, A-H; Yeh, T-H; Ouyang, P; Chen, YL; Chen, SY; Wang, HL. Polyglutamine-expanded ataxin-3 causes cerebellar dysfunction of SCA3 transgenic mice by inducing transriptional dysregulation. *Neurobiol Dis* 2008, 31, 89-101.

Chou, A-H; Chen, C-Y; Chen, S-Y; Chen, W-J ; Chen, Y-L ; Weng, Y-S ; Wang, H-L. Polyglutamine-expanded ataxin-7 causes cerebellar dysfunction by inducing transcriptional dysregulation. *Neurochem Int* 2010, 56, 329-39.

Clark, HB; Orr, HT. Spinocerebellar ataxia type 1-modeling the pathogenesis of a polyglutamine neurodegenerative disorder in transgenic mice. *J Neuropathol Exp Neurol* 2000, 59, 265-70.

Clark, HB; Burright, EN; Yunis, WS; Larson, S; Wilcox, CC; Hartman, B; Matilla, A; Zoghbi, HY; Orr, HT. Purkinje cell expression of a mutant allele of SCA1 in transgenic mice leads to disparate effects on motor behaviors, followed by a progressive cerebellar dysfunction and histological alterations. *J Neurosci* 1997, 17, 7385-95.

Cole, MH; Silburn, PA; Wood, JM; Worringham, CJ; Kerr, GK. Falls in Parkinson's disease: kinematic evidence for impaired head and trunk control. *Mov Disord* 2010, 25, 2369-78.

Deiss, V; Dubois, M; Lalonde, R; Strazielle, C. Cytochrome oxidase activity in the olfactory system of *staggerer* mutant mice. *Brain Res* 2000, 910, 126-33.

Denny, CA ; Desplats, PA ; Thomas, EA ; Seyfried, TN. Cerebellar lipid differences between R6/1 transgenic mice and humans with Huntington's disease. *J Neurochem* 2010, 115, 748-58.

Dubois, B; Pillon, B. Cognitive deficits in Parkinson's disease. *J Neurol* 1997, 244, 2-8.

Fernagut, PO; Diguet, E; Bioulac, B; Tison, F. MPTP potentiates 3-nitropropionic acid-induced striatal damage in mice; reference to striatonigral degeneration. *Exp Neurol* 2004, 185, 47-62.

Ferro, MM; Bellissimo, MI; Anselmo-Franci, JA; Angellucci, ME; Canteras, NS; Da Cunha, C. Comparison of bilaterally 6-OHDA- and MPTP-lesioned rats as models of the early phase of Parkinson's disease: histological, neurochemical, motor and memory alterations. *J Neurosci Methods* 2005, 148, 78-87.

Fleming, SM; Fernagut, PO; Chesselet, MF. Genetic mouse models of parkinsonism; strengths and limitations. *NeuroRx* 2005, 2, 495-503.

Fleming, SM; Salcedo, J; Fernagut, PO; Rockenstein, E; Masliah, E; Levine, MS; Chesselet, MF. Early and progressive sensorimotor anomalies in mice overexpressing wild-type human alpha-synuclein. *J Neurosci* 2004, 24, 9434-40.

Fonteyn, EM; Schmitz-Hübsch, T; Verstappen, CC; Baliko, L; Bloem, BR; Boesch, S; Bunn, L; Charles, P; Dürr, A; Filla, A; Giunti, P; Globas, C; Klockgether, T; Melegh, B; Pandolfo, M; De Rosa, A; Schöls L; Timmann, D; Munneke, M; Kremer, BP; van de Warrenburg, BP. Falls in spinocerebellar ataxias: Results of the EuroSCA Fall Study. *Cerebellum* 2010, 9, 232-9.

Freichel, C; Neumann, M; Ballard, T; Müller, V; Woolley, M; Ozmen, L; Borroni, E; Kretzschmar, HA; Haass, C; Spooren, W; Kahle, PJ. Age-dependent cognitive decline and amygdala pathology in alpha-synuclein transgenic mice. *Neurobiol Aging* 2007, 28, 1421-35.

Garden, GA; Libby, RT; Fu, YH; Kinoshita, Y; Huang, J; Possin, DE; Smith, AC; Martinez, RA; Fine, GC; Grote, SK; Ware, CB; Einum, DD; Morrison, RS; Ptacek, LJ; Sopher, BL; La Spada, AR. Polyglutamine-expanded ataxin-7 promotes non-cell-autonomous Purkinje cell degeneration and displays proteolytic cleavage in ataxic transgenic mice. *J Neurosci* 2002, 22, 4897-905.

Garrard, P; Martin, NH; Giunti, P; Cipolotti, L. Cognitive and social cognitive functioning in spinocerebellar ataxia: a preliminary characterization. *J Neurol* 2008, 255, 398-405.

George, S; van den Buuse, M; San Mok, S; Masters, CL; Li, QX; Culvenor, JG. Alpha-synuclein transgenic mice exhibit reduced anxiety-like behaviour. *Exp Neurol* 2008, 210, 788-92.

Giolli, RA; Gregory, KM; Suzuki, DA; Blanks, RH; Lui, F; Betelak, KF. Cortical and subcortical afferents to the nucleus reticularis tegmenti pontis and basal pontine nuclei in the macaque monkey. *Vis Neurosci* 2001, 18, 725-40.

Gispert, S; Del Turco, D; Garrett, L; Chen, A; Bernard, DJ; Hamm-Clement, J; Korf, HW; Deller, T; Braak, H; Auburger, G; Nussbaum, RL. Transgenic mice expressing mutant A53T human alpha-synuclein show neuronal dysfunction in the absence of aggregate formation. *Mol Cell Neurosci* 2003, 24, 419-29.

Goldberg, A; Schepens, SL; Feely, SM; Garbern, JY; Miller, LJ; Siskind, CE; Conti, GE. Deficits in stepping response time are associated with impairments in balance and mobility in people with Huntington disease. *J Neurol Sci* 2010, 298, 91-5.

Goldberg, MS; Fleming, SM; Palacino, JJ; Cepeda, C; Lam, HA; Bhatnagar, A; Meloni, EG; Wu, N; Ackerson, LC; Klapstein, GJ; Gajendiran, M; Roth, BL; Chesselet, MF; Maidment, NT; Levine, MS; Shen, J. Parkin-deficient mice exhibit nigrostriatal deficits but not loss of dopaminergic neurons. *J Biol Chem* 2003, 278, 436, 28-35.

Gomez-Isla, T; Irizarry, MC; Mariash, A; Cheung, B; Soto, O; Schrump, S; Sondel, J; Kotilinek, L; Day, J; Schwarzschild, MA; Cha, JH; Newell, K; Miller, DW; Uéda, K; Young, AB; Hyman, BT; Ashe, KH. Motor dysfunction and gliosis with preserved dopaminergic markers in human alpha-synuclein A30P transgenic mice. *Neurobiol Aging* 2003, 24, 245-58.

Goodlett, CR; Hamre, KM; West, JR. Dissociation of spatial navigation and visual guidance performance in *Purkinje cell degeneration* (*pcd*) mutant mice. *Behav Brain Res* 1992, 47, 129-41.

Graybiel, AM. The basal ganglia. *Trends Neurosci* 1995, 18, 60-2.

Guidetti, P; Charles, V; Chen, EY; Reddy, PH; Kordower, JH; Whetsell, WO Jr; Schwarcz, R; Tagle, DA. Early degenerative changes in transgenic mice expressing mutant huntingtin involve dendritic abnormalities but no impairment of mitochondrial energy production. *Exp Neurol* 2001, 169, 340-50.

Guidetti, P; Bates, GP; Graham, RK; Hayden, MR; Leavitt, BR; MacDonald, ME; Slow, EJ; Wheeler, VC; Woodman, B; Schwarcz, R. Elevated brain 3-hydroxykynurenine and quinolinate levels in Huntington disease mice. *Neurobiol Dis* 2006, 23, 190-7.

Hammond, C; Rouzaire-Dubois, B; Féger, J; Jackson, A; Crossman, AR. Anatomical and electrophysiological studies on the reciprocal projections between the subthalamic nucleus and nucleus tegmenti pedunculopontinus in the rat. *Neuroscience* 1983, 9, 41-52.

Hansson, O; Guatteo, E; Mercuri, NB; Bernardi, G; Li, XJ; Castilho, RF; Brundin, P. Resistance to NMDA toxicity correlates with appearance of nuclear inclusions;

behavioural deficits and changes in calcium homeostasis in mice transgenic for exon 1 of the Huntington gene. *Eur J Neurosci* 2001, 14, 1492-504.

Harper, PS. *Huntington's disease.* London: WB Saunders, 1996.

Heckroth, JA. Quantitative morphological analysis of the cerebellar nuclei in normal and *Lurcher* mutant mice. I. Morphology and cell number; *J Comp Neurol* 1994, 343, 173-82.

Helmich, RC; Janssen, MJ; Oyen, WJ; Bloem, BR; Toni, I. Pallidal dysfunction drives a cerebellothalamic circuit into Parkinson tremor. *Ann Neurol* 2011, 69, 269-81.

Heng, MY; Detloff, PJ; Albin, RL. Rodent genetic models of Huntington disease. *Neurobiol Dis* 2008, 32, 1-9.

Heng, MY; Tallaksen-Greene, SJ; Detloff, PJ; Albin RL. Longitudinal evaluation of the Hdh(CAG)150 knock-in murine model of Huntington's disease. *J Neurosci* 2007, 27, 8989-98.

Herrup, K. Role of *staggerer* gene in determining cell number in cerebellar cortex. I. Granule cell death is an indirect consequence of *staggerer* gene action. *Dev Brain Res* 1983, 11, 267-74.

Herrup, K; Mullen, RJ. Regional variation and absence of large neurons in the cerebellum of the *staggerer* mouse. *Brain Res* 1979, 172, 1-12.

Herrup, K; Trenkner, E. Regional differences in cytoarchitecture of the *weaver* cerebellum suggest a new model for *weaver* gene action. *Neuroscience* 1987, 23, 871-85.

Hickey, MA; Gallant, K; Gross, GG; Levine, MS; Chesselet, MF. Early behavioral deficits in R6/2 mice suitable for use in preclinical drug testing. *Neurobiol Dis* 2005, 20, 1-11.

Hietanen, M; Teräväinen, H. The effect of age of disease onset on neuropsychological performance in Parkinson's disease. *J Neurol Neurosurg Psychiatry* 1988, 51, 244-9.

Hirano, A; Dembitzer, HM. Cerebellar alterations in the *weaver* mouse. *J Cell Biol* 1973, 56, 478-86.

Hodges, A; Hughes, G; Brooks, S; Elliston, L; Holmans, P; Dunnett, SB; Jones, L. Brain gene expression correlates with changes in behavior in the R6/1 mouse model of Huntington's disease. *Genes Brain Behav* 2008, 7, 288-99.

Hoshi, E; Tremblay, L; Féger, J; Carras, PL; Strick, PL. The cerebellum communicates with the basal ganglia. *Nat Neurosci* 2005, 8, 1491-3.

Hwang, DY; Ardayfio, P; Kang, UJ; Semina, EV; Kim, KS. Selective loss of dopaminergic neurons in the substantia nigra of *Pitx3*-deficient aphakia mice. *Mol Brain Res* 2003, 114, 123-31.

Itier, JM; Ibanez, P; Mena, MA; Abbas, N; Cohen-Salmon, C; Bohme, GA; Laville, M; Pratt, J; Corti, O; Pradier, L; Ret, G; Joubert, C; Periquet, M; Araujo, F; Negroni, J; Casarejos, MJ; Canals, S; Solano, R; Serrano, A; Gallego, E; Sanchez, M; Denefle, P; Benavides, J; Tremp, G; Rooney, TA; Brice, A; Garcia de Yebenes, J. Parkin gene inactivation alters behaviour and dopamine neurotransmission in the mouse. *Hum Mol Genet* 2003, 12, 2277-91.

Kageyama, Y; Yamamoto, S; Ueno, M; Ichikawa, K. [A case of adult-onset Huntington disease presenting with spasticity and cerebellar ataxia, mimicking spinocerebellar degeneration, Japanese]. *Rinsho Shinkeigaku* 2003, 43, 16-9.

Kahle, PJ. alpha-Synucleinopathy models and human neuropathology; similarities and differences. *Acta Neuropathol* 2008, 115, 87-95.

Kita, H; Kitai, ST. Efferent projections of the subthalamic nucleus in the rat: light and electron microscopic analysis with the PHA-L method. *J Comp Neurol* 1987, 260, 435-52.

Küng, UM; Horlings, CG; Honegger, F; Kremer, HP; Bloem, BR; van De Warrenburg, BP; Allum, JH. Postural instability in cerebellar ataxia: correlations of knee, arm and trunk movements to center of mass velocity. *Neuroscience* 2009, 159, 390-404.

Lalonde, R. Motor abnormalities in *weaver* mutant mice. *Exp Brain Res* 1987a, 65, 479-81.

Lalonde, R. Motor abnormalities in *staggerer* mutant mice. *Exp Brain Res* 1987b, 68, 417-20.

Lalonde, R; Strazielle, C. Brain regions and genes affecting postural control. *Prog Neurobiol* 2007a, 81, 45-60.

Lalonde, R; Strazielle, C. Spontaneous and induced mouse mutations with cerebellar dysfunctions: behavior and neurochemistry. *Brain Res* 2007b, 1140, 51-74.

Lalonde, R; Strazielle, C. Brain regions and genes affecting limb-clasping responses. *Brain Res Rev* 2011, 67, 252-9.

Lalonde, R; Manseau, M; Botez, MI. Spontaneous alternation and exploration in *Weaver* mutant mice. *Behav Brain Res* 1988a, 31, 111-4.

Lalonde, R; Manseau, M; Botez, MI. Spontaneous alternation and exploration in *staggerer* mutant mice. *Behav Brain Res* 1988b, 27, 273-6.

Lalonde, R; Lamarre, Y; Smith, AM; Botez, MI. Spontaneous alternation and habituation in *Lurcher* mutant mice. *Brain Res* 1986, 362, 161-4.

Landsend, AS; Amiry-Moghaddam, M; Matsubara, A; Bergersen, L; Usami, S; Wenthold, RJ; Ottersen, OP. Differential localization of delta glutamate receptors in the rat cerebellum: coexpression with AMPA receptors in parallel fiber-spine synapses and absence from climbing fiber-spine synapses. *J Neurosci* 1997, 17, 834-42.

Lee, FJS; Liu, F. Genetic factors involved in the pathogenesis of Parkinson's disease. *Brain Res Rev* 2008, 58, 354-64.

Lin, CH; Tallaksen-Greene, S; Chien, WM; Cearley, JA; Jackson, WS; Crouse, AB; Ren, S; Li, XJ; Albin, RL; Detloff, PJ. Neurological abnormalities in a knock-in mouse model of Huntington's disease. *Hum Mol Genet* 2001, 10, 137-44.

Lione, LA; Carter, RJ; Hunt, MJ; Bates, GP; Morton, AJ; Dunnett, SB. Selective discrimination learning impairments in mice expressing the human Huntington's disease mutation. *J Neurosci* 1999, 19, 10428-37.

Lozano, AM; Dostrovsky, J; Chen, R; Ashby, P. Deep brain stimulation for Parkinson's disease: disrupting the disruption. *Lancet Neurol* 2002, 1, 225-31.

Luchtman, DW; Shao, D; Song, C. Behavior, neurotransmitters and inflammation in three regimens of the MPTP mouse model of Parkinson's disease. *Physiol Behav* 2009, 98, 130-8.

Lüesse, HG; Schiefer, J; Spruenken, A; Puls, C; Block, F; Kosinski, CM. Evaluation of R6/2 HD transgenic mice for therapeutic studies in Huntington's disease; behavioral testing and impact of diabetes mellitus. *Behav Brain Res* 2001, 126, 185-95.

Mangiarini, L; Sathasivam, K; Seller, M; Cozens, B; Harper, A; Hetherington, C; Lawton, M; Trottier, Y; Lehrach, H; Davies, SW; Bates, GP. Exon 1 of the HD gene with an expanded CAG repeat is sufficient to cause a progressive neurological phenotype in transgenic mice. *Cell* 1996, 87, 493-506.

Marsden, CD. Basal ganglia disease. *Lancet* 1982, 2, 1141-7.

Martel, G; Blanchard, J; Mons, N; Gastambide, F; Micheau, J; Guillou, JL. Dynamic interplays between memory systems depend on practice: the hippocampus is not always the first to provide solution. *Neuroscience* 2007, 150, 743-53.

Masliah, E; Rockenstein, E; Veinbergs, I; Mallory, M; Hashimoto, M; Takeda, A; Sagara, Y; Sisk, A; Mucke, L. Dopaminergic loss and inclusion body formation in alpha-synuclein mice; implications for neurodegenerative disorders. *Science* 2000, 287, 1265-9.

Meco, G; Gasparini, M; Doricchi, F. Attentional functions in multiple system atrophy and Parkinson's disease. *J Neurol Neurosurg Psychiatry* 1996, 60, 393-8.

Menalled, L; Zanjani, H; MacKenzie, L; Koppel, A; Carpenter, E; Zeitlin, S; Chesselet, MF. Decrease in striatal enkephalin mRNA in mouse models of Huntington's disease. *Exp Neurol* 2000, 162, 328-42.

Menalled, LB; Sison, JD; Wu, Y; Olivieri, M; Li, XJ; Li, H; Zeitlin, S; Chesselet, MF. Early motor dysfunction and striosomal distribution of huntingtin microaggregates in Huntington's disease knock-in mice. *J Neurosci* 2002, 22, 8266-76.

Menalled, LB; Sison, JD; Dragatsis, I; Zeitlin, S; Chesselet, MF. Time course of early motor and neuropathological anomalies in a knock-in mouse model of Huntington's disease with 140 CAG repeats. *J Comp Neurol* 2003, 465, 11-26.

Moers-Hornikx, VM; Vles, JS; Tan, SK; Cox, K; Hoogland, G; Steinbusch, WM; Temel, Y. Cerebellar nuclei are activated by high-frequency stimulation of the subthalamic nucleus. *Neurosci Lett* 2011, 496, 111-5.

Mohr, E; Brouwers, P; Claus, JJ; Mann, UM; Fedio, P; Chase, TN. Visuospatial cognition in Huntington's disease. *Mov Disord* 1991, 6, 127-32.

Morris, RG; Garrud, P; Rawlins, JN; O'Keefe, J. Place navigation impaired in rats with hippocampal lesions. *Nature* 1982, 297, 681-3.

Mure, H; Hirano, S; Tang, CC; Isaias, IU; Antonini, A; Ma, Y; Dhawan, V; Eidelberg, D. Parkinson's disease tremor-related metabolic network: characterization, progression, and treatment effects. *Neuroimage* 2011, 54, 1244-53.

Murphy, KP; Carter, RJ; Lione, LA; Mangiarini, L; Mahal, A; Bates, GP; Dunnett, SB; Morton, AJ. Abnormal synaptic plasticity and impaired spatial cognition in mice transgenic for exon 1 of the human Huntington's disease mutation. *J Neurosci* 2000, 20, 5115-23.

Neychev, VK; Fan, X; Mitev, VI; Hess, EJ; Jinnah, HA. The basal ganglia and cerebellum interact in the expression of dystonic movement. *Brain* 2008, 131, 2499-509.

Ni, Z; Pinto, AD; Lang, AE; Chen, R. Involvement of the cerebellothalamocortical pathway in Parkinson disease. *Ann Neurol* 2010, 68, 816-24.

Nunes, I; Tovmasian, LT; Silva, RM; Burke, RE; Goff, SP. Pitx3 is required for development of substantia nigra dopaminergic neurons. *Proc Natl Acad Sci USA* 2003, 100, 4245-50.

Parent, A; Hazrati, LN. Functional anatomy of the basal ganglia. I. The cortico-basal ganglia-thalamo-cortical loop. *Brain Res Rev* 1995, 20, 91-127.

Parent, A; Hazrati, LN. Functional anatomy of the basal ganglia. II. The place of subthalamic nucleus and external pallidum in basal ganglia circuitry. *Brain Res Rev* 1995, 20, 128-54.

Patil, N; Cox, DR; Bhat, D; Faham, M; Myers, RM; Peterson A. A potassium channel mutation in *weaver* mice implicates membrane excitability in granule cell differentiation. *Nature Genet* 1995, 11, 126-9.

Perciavalle, V; Berretta, S; Raffaele, R. Projections from the intracerebellar nuclei to the ventral midbrain tegmentum in the rat. *Neuroscience.* 1989, 29, 109-19.

Reader, TA; Strazielle, C; Botez, MI; Lalonde, R. Brain dopamine and amino acid concentrations in *Lurcher* mutant mice. *Brain Res Bull* 1998, 45, 489-93.

Reddy, PH; Charles, V; Williams, M; Miller, G; Whetsell, WO Jr; Tagle, DA. Transgenic mice expressing mutated full-length HD cDNA: a paradigm for locomotor changes and selective neuronal loss in Huntington's disease. *Philos Trans R Soc Lond B Biol Sci* 1999, 354, 1035-45.

Reddy, PH; Williams, M; Charles, V; Garrett, L; Pike-Buchanan, L; Whetsell, WO Jr; Miller, G; Tagle, DA. Behavioural abnormalities and selective neuronal loss in HD transgenic mice expressing mutated full-length HD cDNA. *Nat Genet* 1998, 20, 198-202.

Richfield, EK; Thiruchelvam, MJ; Cory-Slechta, DA; Wuertzer, C; Gainetdinov, RR; Caron, MG; Di Monte, DA; Federoff, HJ. Behavioral and neurochemical effects of wild-type and mutated human alpha-synuclein in transgenic mice. *Exp Neurol* 2002, 175, 35-48.

Roffler-Tarlov, S; Graybiel, AM. Expression of the *weaver* gene in dopamine-containing neural systems is dose-dependent and affects both striatal and nonstriatal regions, *J Neurosci* 1986, 6, 3319-30.

Roffler-Tarlov, S; Martin, B; Graybiel, AM; Kauer, JS. Cell death in the midbrain of the murine mutation *weaver*. *J Neurosci* 1996, 16, 1819-26.

Roos, RAC. Huntington's disease. In: Vinken PJ, Bruyn GW, Klawans HL editors. *Handbook of Clinical Neurology;* vol 49; Extrapyramidal disorders. Amsterdam: Elsevier; 1986; 315-326.

Rosas, HD; Koroshetz, WJ; Chen, YI; Skeuse, C; Vangel, M; Cudkowicz, ME; Caplan, K; Marek, K; Seidman, LJ; Makris, N; Jenkins, BG; Goldstein, JM. Evidence for more widespread cerebral pathology in early HD: an MRI-based morphometric analysis. *Neurology* 2003, 60, 1615-20.

Ruigbrok, TJH. Precerebellar nuclei and red nucleus. In: Paxinos G, editor. *The rat nervous system*. Amsterdam: Elsevier; 2004; 167-204.

Saint-Cyr, JA; Taylor, AE; Lang, AE. Procedural learning and neostriatal dysfunction in man. *Brain* 1988, 111, 941-59.

Sawiak, SJ ; Wood, NI ; Williams, GB ; Morton, AJ ; Carpenter, TA. Voxel-based morphometry in the R6/2 transgenic mouse reveals differences between genotypes not seen with manual 2D morphometry. *Neurobiol Dis* 2009, 33, 20-7.

Schwarting, RK; Sedelis, M; Hofele, K; Auburger, GW; Huston, JP. Strain-dependent recovery of open-field behavior and striatal dopamine deficiency in the mouse MPTP model of Parkinson's disease. *Neurotox Res* 1999, 1, 41-56.

Sen, S; Kawaguchi, A; Truong, Y; Lewis, MM; Huang, X. Dynamic changes in cerebello-thalamo-cortical motor circuitry during progression of Parkinson's disease. *Neuroscience* 2010, 166, 712-9.

Setsuie, R; Wang, YL; Mochizuki, H; Osaka, H; Hayakawa, H; Ichihara, N; Li, H; Furuta, A; Sano, Y; Sun, YJ; Kwon, J; Kabuta, T; Yoshimi, K; Aoki, S; Mizuno, Y; Noda, M; Wada, K. Dopaminergic neuronal loss in transgenic mice expressing the Parkinson's disease-associated UCH-L1 I93M mutant. *Neurochem Int* 2007, 50, 119-29.

Shults, CW; Rockenstein, E; Crews, L; Adame, A ; Mante, M; Larrea, G; Hashimoto, M; Song, D; Iwatsubo, T; Tsuboi, K; Masliah, E. Neurological and neurodegenerative alterations in a transgenic mouse model expressing human alpha-synuclein under oligodendrocyte promoter; implications for multiple system atrophy. *J Neurosci* 2005, 25, 10689-99.

Skinner, PJ; Koshy, BT; Cummings, CJ; Klement, IA; Helin, K; Servadio, A; Zoghbi, HY; Orr, HT. Ataxin-1 with an expanded glutamine tract alters nuclear matrix-associated structures. *Nature* 1997, 389, 971-74.

Smeyne, RJ; Goldowitz, D. Development and death of external granular layer cells in the *weaver* mouse cerebellum: a quantitative study. *J Neurosci* 1989, 9, 1608-20.

Smidt, MP; Smits, SM; Burbach, JP. Homeobox gene *Pitx3* and its role in the development of dopamine neurons of the substantia nigra. *Cell Tissue Res* 2004, 318, 35-43.

Snider, RS; Maiti, A; Snider, SR. Cerebellar pathways to ventral midbrain and nigra. *Exp Neurol* 1976, 53, 714-28.

Strazielle, C; Krémarik, P; Ghersi-Egea, J-F; Lalonde, R. Regional brain variations of cytochrome oxidase activity and motor coordination in *Lurcher* mutant mice. *Exp Brain Res* 1998, 121, 35-45.

Strazielle, C; Lalonde, R; Amdiss, F; Botez, MI; Hébert, C; Reader, TA. Distribution of dopamine transporters in basal ganglia of cerebellar ataxic mice [^{125}I]RTI-121 quantitative autoradiography. *Neurochem Int* 1998, 32, 61-8.

Strazielle, C; Deiss, V; Naudon, L; Raisman-Vozari, R; Lalonde, R. Regional brain variation of cytochrome oxidase activity and motor coordination in Girk2^{WV} (*Weaver*) mutant mice. *Neuroscience* 2006, 142, 437-49.

Takahashi, E; Niimi, K; Itakura, C. Neonatal motor functions in *Cacna1α* mutant *rolling* Nagoya mice. *Behav Brain Res* 2010, 207, 273-9.

Takahashi, E; Niimi, K; Itakura, C. Motor coordination impairment in aged heterozygous rolling Nagoya, Cav2.1 mutant mice. *Brain Res* 2009, 1279, 50-7.

Tofaris, GK; Garcia Reitböck, P; Humby, T; Lambourne, SL; O'Connell, M; Ghetti, B; Gossage, H; Emson, PC; Wilkinson, LS; Goedert, M; Spillantini, MG. Pathological changes in dopaminergic nerve cells of the substantia nigra and olfactory bulb in mice transgenic for truncated human alpha-synuclein(1-120): implications for Lewy body disorders. *J Neurosci* 2006, 26, 3942-50.

Triarhou, LC; Norton, J; Ghetti, B. Mesencephalic dopamine cell deficit involves areas A8; A9 and A10 in *weaver* mutant mice. *Exp Brain Res* 1988, 70, 256-65.

Trueman, RC; Brooks, SP; Jones, L; Dunnett, SB. The operant serial implicit learning task reveals early onset motor learning deficits in the Hdh knock-in mouse model of Huntington's disease. *Eur J Neurosci* 2007, 25, 551-8.

Unger, EL; Eve, DJ; Perez, XA; Reichenbach, DK; Xu, Y; Lee, MK; Andrews, AM. Locomotor hyperactivity and alterations in dopamine neurotransmission are associated with overexpression of A53T mutant human alpha-synuclein in mice. *Neurobiol Dis* 2006, 21, 431-43.

van Dellen, A; Blakemore, C; Deacon, R; York, D; Hannan, AJ. Delaying the onset of Huntington's in mice. *Nature* 2000, 404, 721-2.

van den Munckhof, P; Luk, KC; Ste-Marie, L; Montgomery, J; Blanchet, PJ; Sadikot, AF; Drouin, J. Pitx3 is required for motor activity and for survival of a subset of midbrain dopaminergic neurons. *Development* 2003, 130, 2535-42.

van der Putten, H; Wiederhold, KH; Probst, A; Barbieri, S; Mistl, C; Danner, S; Kauffmann, S; Hofele, K; Spooren, WP; Ruegg, MA; Lin, S; Caroni, P; Sommer, B; Tolnay, M; Bilbe, G. Neuropathology in mice expressing human alpha-synuclein. *J Neurosci* 2000, 20, 6021-9.

Wakamatsu, M; Ishii, A; Iwata, S; Sakagami, J; Ukai, Y; Ono, M; Kanbe, D; Muramatsu, S; Kobayashi, K; Iwatsubo, T; Yoshimoto, M. Selective loss of nigral dopamine neurons induced by overexpression of truncated human alpha-synuclein in mice. *Neurobiol Aging* 2008, 29, 574-85.

Wetts, R; Herrup, K. Interaction of granule, Purkinje and inferior olivary neurons in *Lurcher* chimeric mice. II. Granule cell death. *Brain Res* 1982, 250, 358-62.

Wheeler, VC; Gutekunst, CA; Vrbanac, V; Lebel, LA; Schilling, G; Hersch, S; Friedlander, RM; Gusella, JF; Vonsattel, JP; Borchelt, DR; MacDonald ME. Early phenotypes that presage late-onset neurodegenerative disease allow testing of modifiers in Hdh CAG knock-in mice. *Hum Mol Genet* 2002, 11, 633-40.

Wheeler, VC; Auerbach, W; White, JK; Srinidhi, J; Auerbach, A; Ryan, A; Duyao, MP; Vrbanac, V; Weaver, M; Gusella, JF; Joyner, AL; MacDonald, ME. Length-dependent gametic CAG repeat instability in the Huntington's disease knock-in mouse. *Hum Mol Genet* 1999, 8, 115-22.

Wheeler, VC; White, JK; Gutekunst, CA; Vrbanac, V; Weaver, M; Li, XJ; Li, SH; Yi, H; Vonsattel, JP; Gusella, JF; Hersch, S; Auerbach, W; Joyner, AL; MacDonald, ME. Long glutamine tracts cause nuclear localization of a novel form of huntingtin in medium spiny striatal neurons in HdhQ92 and HdhQ111 knock-in mice. *Hum Mol Genet* 2000, 9, 503-13.

Woodman, B; Butler, R; Landles, C; Lupton, MK; Tse, J; Hockly, E; Moffitt, H; Sathasivam, K; Bates, GP. The Hdh(Q150/Q150) knock-in mouse model of HD and the R6/2 exon 1 model develop comparable and widespread molecular phenotypes. *Brain Res Bull* 2007, 72, 83-97.

Yamamoto, T; Hassler R; Huber, C; Wagner, A; Sasaki, K. Electrophysiologic studies on the pallido- and cerebellothalamic projections in squirrel monkeys *(saimiri sciureus). Exp Brain Res* 1983, 51, 77-87.

Yavich, L; Tanila, H; Vepsäläinen, S; Jäkälä, P. Role of alpha-synuclein in presynaptic dopamine recruitment. *J Neurosci* 2004, 24, 11165-70.

Zhang, Y; Snider, A; Willard, L; Takemoto, DJ; Lin, D. Loss of Purkinje cells in the PKCγ H101Y transgenic mouse. *Biochem Biophys Res Commun* 2009, 378, 524-8.

Zhou, W; Milder, JB; Freed, CR. Transgenic mice overexpressing tyrosine-to-cysteine mutant human alpha-synuclein; a progressive neurodegenerative model of diffuse Lewy body disease. *J Biol Chem* 2008, 283, 9863-70.

Zhu, XR; Maskri, L; Herold, C; Bader, V; Stichel, CC; Güntürkün, O; Lübbert, H. Non-motor behavioural impairments in parkin-deficient mice. *Eur J Neurosci* 2007, 26, 1902-11.

Zuo, J; De Jager, PI; Takahashi, KA; Jiang, W; Linden, DJ; Heintz, N. Neurodegeneration in *Lurcher* mutant mice caused by mutation in the delta 2 glutamate receptor gene; *Nature* 1997, 388, 769-73.

In: Striatum: Anatomy, Functions and Role in Disease ISBN 978-1-61942-384-8
Editors: Hugo T. Maldonado and Ignacio M. Ortega

Chapter V

Striatal Dysfunction and Social Cognition

Clare M. Eddy
Department of Neuropsychiatry, The Barberry National Centre for Mental Health, Birmingham, UK

Abstract

The last few decades of clinical research have revolutionised our view of the striatum, such that current understanding of the functions of this structure extend far beyond an exclusive influence on processes involved in motor control. By virtue of connections between the striatum and the prefrontal cortex, which form cortico-striato-thalamo-cortical circuits or frontostriatal pathways, changes in the functioning of the striatum can exert a critical influence on a range of aspects of human cognition. The study of cognitive functioning in patients with Movement Disorders has demonstrated how striatal dysfunction can impair memory, attention and executive functions. More recently, attention has turned towards the abilities of these patients to reason about aspects of social cognition. Research to date has revealed that individuals with disorders such as Parkinson's disease, Huntington's disease and Tourette syndrome can demonstrate difficulties in reasoning about human emotion and social interaction, including poor recognition of emotional facial expressions, misinterpretation of story character's intentions and difficulties in judging socially appropriate behaviours. These alterations in Theory of Mind implicate a role for the striatum in supporting cognitive processes which allow us to understand people's mental states, and emphasise the need to develop more precise and inclusive models of frontostriatal circuitry.

Frontostriatal Circuitry and the Neural Substrates of Social Cognition

In their original model of frontostriatal circuitry, Alexander et al (1986) describe the involvement of the striatum in five parallel cortico-striato-thalamo-cortical circuits. These circuits are formed by neurons originating in different regions of the frontal cortex, which project to the striatum, the globus pallidus and substantia nigra, before returning to the frontal cortex via the thalamus. Dysfunction of the subcortical components within a circuit are expected to result in deficits that resemble those that would be observed if the cortical area involved in the circuit was damaged directly (Middleton and Strick, 2000).Two of the frontal regions involved in Alexander et al.'s circuits are the supplementary motor and oculomotor cortex, which play an important role in motor functions. However, other frontostriatal circuits involve non-motor regions of the frontal cortex, such as dorsolateral prefrontal cortex (DLPFC), lateral orbitofrontal cortex (OFC) and anterior cingulate cortex (ACC). The model of frontostriatal circuitry proposed by Alexander et al. therefore allows us to consider how changes in the functioning of frontostriatal circuitry may affect not only motor processes, but also cognitive, social and emotional processes which are reliant on the latter prefrontal brain regions.

Social cognition has been described as "the sum of those processes that allow individuals of the same species (conspecifics) to interact with one another" (Frith and Frith, 2007, pp. R724), and involves a collection of abilities including Theory of Mind (ToM): the ability to understand mental states, such as beliefs and emotions. Studies indicate that healthy participants activate medial prefrontal cortex when engaged in a ToM task (e.g. Fletcher et al, 2005) and lesion studies have further established a specific role for orbitofrontal cortex (in addition to the amygdala) in social cognition (Stone et al, 1998; Stone et al, 2003). Dysfunction within frontostriatal circuitry involving these neural regions could therefore result in deficits in social cognition.

Clinical and developmental studies have highlighted a critical role for executive functions such as working memory and response inhibition during social cognitive tasks involving ToM (Carlson et al, 2002; Henry et al, 2006). While the importance of inhibition may rest in successful suppression of one's own mental state in order to take another's perspective (Samson et al, 2005), working memory is likely to contribute to performance by providing a basis for the holding in mind of multiple perspectives (Gordon and Olson, 1998). Standard executive tasks involving inhibition and working memory activate anterior cingulate cortex and dorsolateral prefrontal cortex (Aleman and van't Wout, 2008; Nathaniel-James et al, 1997) respectively. Dysfunction within frontostriatal circuitry involving anterior cingulate or dorsolateral prefrontal cortex could therefore to disrupt processes involved in social cognition indirectly, through problems with executive functions.

In Movement Disorders such as Parkinson's disease (PD), Huntington's disease (HD) and Tourette syndrome (TS), the principle site of neural dysfunction is thought to be the striatum. Changes in the functioning of striatal regions lead to characteristic motor symptoms through alterations in functioning within frontostriatal motor circuits. In the hypokinetic condition PD, degeneration of dopaminergic neurons in the substantia nigra characteristic motor symptoms include tremor, rigidity and bradykinesia. Both the inherited neurodegenerative condition HD and the chronic neurodevelopmental condition TS may be considered hyperkinetic disorders. However, HD involves chorea, whereas patients with TS experience motor and phonic tics. Experimental studies have shown that in addition to these motor symptoms, cognitive changes further characterise these conditions. PD and HD are both associated with a range of deficits in executive functioning and subcortical dementia which becomes apparent with disease progression, while TS is generally linked to much more subtle difficulties with attention and inhibitory processes (Eddy et al, 2009). Since it has been established that the impact of striatal dysfunction is not restricted to movement, more recent attention has turned to the performance of patients with Movement Disorders on tasks involving emotion and social reasoning. We now turn to the findings yielded by exploration of social cognition in Movement Disorders over the last couple of decades, before considering their implications for our understanding of the role of the striatum in this area of cognition which is so critical to human functioning and individual experience.

Investigating Social Cognition in Movement Disorders

Parkinson's Disease

In PD, dysfunction within frontostriatal pathways could affect ToM performance through executive deficits. For example, difficulties with working memory as a result of dysfunction involving dorsolateral prefrontal cortex are common in PD (e.g. Gilbert et al, 2005) and Monetta et al (2008) showed that patients with PD can exhibit more general deficits in inference generation as a result of working memory dysfunction. ToM deficits could therefore arise through more general problems with inferential reasoning. However, if striatal dysfunction was to extend to affect circuitry involving medial orbitofrontal cortex, it could be that patients with PD would exhibit specific deficits in ToM *per se*.

A few studies have reported evidence of ToM deficits in PD, including deficits in understanding false belief (Mengelberg and Siegert, 2003). Saltzman et al (2000) reported that patients' ToM deficits were related to executive deficits. Oher studies have reported no such link. These include a study conducted by Bodden et al (2010), which found patients with PD exhibited most difficulties with second order ToM. As second order ToM involves inferring one character's belief about another character's mental state, it is likely to make greater memory and executive demands than first order ToM, which involves reasoning about one character's mental state. However, Bodden et al. found no evidence that these difficulties with second order ToM were linked to executive dysfunction.

Peron et al (2009) reported evidence of difficulties in recognizing socially inappropriate behaviors in PD. Patients with advanced PD who did not exhibit signs of dementia performed poorly on a faux pas task. These difficulties indicated that some patients found it difficult to correctly judge the social appropriateness of story characters' remarks. However, patients at an earlier stage of the disease performed similarly to controls on the faux pas task. Findings from our laboratory support the likelihood that the understanding of faux pas is likely to be intact in early-stage PD (Eddy, 2009).

Other reports have investigated recognition of emotional facial expressions in PD (Clark et al 2008; Suzuki et al, 2006; Yoshimura et al, 2005). In one study (Peron et al, 2009) patients with PD did not differ from controls on the 'Reading the Mind in the Eyes Test' (developed by Baron-Cohen et al, 2001), which involves recognition of complex mental states (e.g. anxiety, interest, desire) from photographs of the eye region of the face. However, other studies have documented conflicting findings providing evidence of a deficit on this task (Bodden et al, 2010; Mimura et al, 2006).

It has been suggested (Peron et al, 2009) that the understanding of cognitive mental states (cognitive ToM) such as intentions or beliefs could be more vulnerable to PD than the understanding of emotions (affective ToM). One explanation for deficits in cognitive ToM being more common in PD may lie in the role of executive functions. One study of patients with frontal lesions (Shamay-Tsoory and Aharon Peretz, 2007) provided evidence for largely separate neuroanatomical substrates for affective and cognitive ToM, and impairments in cognitive ToM were more often associated with lesions to dorsolateral prefrontal cortex, a region important for executive functions. Specific difficulties with cognitive ToM could occur because PD is associated with executive deficits, and cognitive ToM relies more on executive functioning than affective ToM. However, some authors (e.g. Bodden et al, 2010) report that patients' difficulties can encompass problems with both cognitive ToM and affective ToM.

Problems with social cognition in PD appear to extend to pragmatic communication (McNamara and Durso, 2003), including poor comprehension of metaphor (Monetta and Pell, 2007) and sarcasm (Monetta et al, 2009). ToM deficits could underlie patients' impaired comprehension of pragmatic language such as metaphors and sarcasm, because the accurate interpretation of non-literal language involves appreciation of the speaker's mental state. However, the ability to hold in mind different interpretations of pragmatic remarks again highlight an important role for executive functions such as working memory in task performance. Monetta et al (2009) found that patients with PD performed poorly on first and second-order belief questions during a pragmatic comprehension task. These difficulties were related to poor performance on measures of working memory and verbal fluency, so executive deficits are likely to have resulted in the ToM difficulties and poor understanding of non-literal language.

A series of experiments involving patients with PD conducted at our clinic documented no deficit on a faux pas task (Eddy, 2009), but did reveal impairment understanding character's false belief on a simple forced choice vignette task. Manipulation of tasks aimed at reducing working memory demands improved patients' performance, demonstrating that failure to meet incidental task demands can lead to deficits on ToM tasks in PD. These findings imply that patients' deficits are not always found to be related to performance on executive tasks.

In summary, although studies demonstrate that patients with PD can exhibit impairments in a range of aspects of social cognition, there is currently not enough evidence to firmly establish whether these difficulties reflect deficits in ToM *per se*. Furthermore, studies also need to address the potential effect of dopaminergic medications on patients' performance.

Huntington's Disease

HD involves a selective pattern of degeneration that begins in the caudate, and progresses from dorsal to ventral regions of the striatum. Patients' executive deficits (Montoya et al, 2006) implicate dysfunction within frontostriatal pathways, with working memory, inhibitory and set-shifting deficits likely to reflect dysfunction of dorsolateral prefrontal cortex and anterior cingulate cortex (Aleman and van't Wout, 2008; Peterson et al, 1999; Vanderhasselt et al, 2006[a,b]). According the Alexander et al's (1986) model of frontostriatal circuitry, dysfunction of the caudate could affect circuitry involving lateral orbitofrontal cortex, but more medial regions of the frontal cortex may only be implicated when striatal degeneration encompasses more ventral regions of the striatum, later in the disease course.

Patients with HD show changes in mood including emotional lability (Duff et al, 2010) and reduced empathy for others (Snowden et al, 2003). These changes could contribute to the breakdown of interpersonal relationships which some families affected by HD appear to experience (Snowden et al, 2003).

Many studies have revealed deficits in the recognition of emotional facial expressions in HD. Some authors have provided evidence for greater deficits in the recognition of disgust. Sprengelmeyer et al (1997) found mild impairments in the recognition of a number of emotional expressions in HD, but patients exhibited a more severe deficit for disgusted faces. Gray et al (1997) found that this deficit extended to huntingtin gene carriers. Further support for the vulnerability of disgust was provided by Wang et al (2003), who reported a similar 'differentially severe impairment' for disgust expressions in both patients with HD and patients with Wilson's disease (another disorder associated with basal ganglia dysfunction). However, other reports have indicated that patients sometimes exhibit most impairment in the recognition of facial expressions of fear (Milders et al, 2003) or anger (Henley et al, 2008; Snowden et al, 2008). The expression recognition deficits exhibited by gene carriers can also extend to anger, fear and sadness (Johnson et al, 2007).

One explanation for these mixed findings is that patients with HD could exhibit a general impairment in facial emotion recognition and that greater impairments are found for certain emotions because they are more difficult to recognize. This possibility was supported by evidence of mild deficits on more general face perception measures in HD (e.g. Wang et al, 2003). However, another study that employed a wide range of tasks reported no effect of item difficulty (Snowden et al, 2008).

Another possible reason for the inconsistency of facial emotion recognition impairments reported across studies is variation in the pattern of neurodegeneration across different samples. That is, particular study samples could exhibit greater degeneration in neural substrates involved in recognising particular negative emotions. For example, the ventral striatum may play an important role in the recognition of angry faces (Calder et al, 2004), while the amygdala is linked to the recognition of fearful expressions (Adolphs et al, 2002). Specific deficits with disgust in HD patients and presymptomatic gene carriers have been linked to a reduced response in left dorsal anterior insula (Hennenlotter et al, 2004). However, Henley et al (2008) report that poor recognition of faces depicting a range of expressions (angry, disgusted, surprised and fearful) was associated with striatal volume loss, and it was a deficit in recognizing fear, rather than disgust, which was related to insula degeneration.

Reports indicate that brain regions associated with recognizing a particular emotion in another are likely to be involved in the direct experience of that emotion (Adolphs, 2002). A few studies have therefore investigated patients' emotional responses to emotion-provoking stimuli. Disgust has been most studied, and disgust deficits in HD have been observed in response to pictures, olfactory and gustatory stimuli (Hayes et al., 2007; Mitchell et al, 2005). In one study (Snowden et al, 2008), poor recognition of disgust from other peoples' faces and voices was observed alongside reduced disgust response to written scenarios that elicited this emotion in controls. In another study, disgust responses to pictures and stories were not significantly different for patients and controls (Eddy et al, 2011[a]). However, patients with HD gave significantly lower fear ratings in response to both pictures and stories that reliably elicited this emotion in matched controls. One limitation of this study was that recognition of other's emotions was not also tested in this sample.

Only a few studies have investigated perspective taking and more complex aspects of ToM in HD. In one study, patients exhibited abnormal interpretations of real-life social situations (Naarding et al, 2001) and in another (Snowden et al, 2003) made faulty inferences in response to tasks involving social interactions. A later study found that patients with HD exhibited difficulty on a story task which involved reasoning about characters' intentions (Brüne et al, 2011). Findings from our laboratory indicate that HD can also be associated with deficits in reading mental states from pictures of the eyes, and in making judgments about socially inappropriate behavior on the faux pas task (Eddy, Sira Mahalingappa & Rickards, 2011). While executive deficits could contribute to these results, we found that patients with HD were still significantly poorer than healthy matched controls at recognizing socially inappropriate remarks when ToM errors linked to errors on associated memory and comprehension questions were excluded from analysis. Dysfunction of the amygdala may contribute to problems understanding faux pas (Stone et al, 2003), so if patients' errors were linked to deficits in ToM *per* se, they could implicate dysfunction within frontostriatal circuitry involving this region in HD.

Tourette Syndrome

In addition to tics, patients with TS can exhibit urges to mirror other peoples' speech or gestures (echolalia/echopraxia) or make offensive remarks or gestures (coprolalia/ copropraxia). Co-morbid psychiatric disorders including obsessive-compulsive disorder and attention-deficit hyperactivity disorder are very common (Cavanna et al, 2009; Leckman, 2002; Robertson, 2000). Kurlan et al (1996) describe non-obscene socially inappropriate symptoms (NOSIS), which are characterised by urges to act in a socially inappropriate way or make socially inappropriate remarks including insults. Both the social relevance of some of the symptoms seen in TS, and reported striatal abnormalities which could implicate frontostriatal dysfunction (e.g. Singer et al, 1993; Peterson et al, 2003), prompt investigation of social cognition in this patient group.

Two early studies investigating ToM included a group of patients with TS. The first included these patients as a control group (Baron-Cohen et al, 1997) and reported no deficits. The second (Channon et al, 2004) assessed patients with TS on two tasks involving ToM which contained examples of non-literal language (ToM is considered to be important for the understanding of non-literal language, as interpretation relies on consideration of the speaker's mental state in addition to the words that are used). No deficits were reported on these tasks. However, this finding may have reflected lack of sensitivity in the measures used.

Later studies documented evidence of impaired performance on ToM tasks in TS. Eddy et al (2010)[a] showed that patients with TS can understand simple false belief, but exhibit significant difficulty when asked to make judgments about the social appropriateness of behavior during the faux pas task (from Stone et al, 1998; Gregory et al, 2002). Patients made errors both in failing to recognize faux pas, and in stating faux pas was present in control stories. A later study replicated the deficit in understanding faux pas in a new sample of patients with TS (Eddy et al, 2010[b]) and further demonstrated impairments in understanding examples of non-literal language, such as sarcasm and metaphor. A third study (Eddy et al,

2011[b]) tested the performance of eighteen patients with TS on four tasks involving ToM. One task was the Reading the Mind in the Eyes task, and another was a task which involved selecting facial expressions based on matching and contrasting emotions (gloating and envy). Patients also completed a multiple choice task which involved understanding the joke in humorous cartoons (i.e. thinking about cartoonist's intentions), and a version of the Ultimatum game, an economic decision making task linked to ToM. Patients with TS exhibited significant deficits on all four tasks in comparison to a matched control group. Furthermore, ToM deficits were present in uncomplicated TS (patients without co-morbid conditions).

Most of TS patients' difficulties on social cognitive tasks appear to reflect unconventional interpretations of social interactions rather than a failure to infer mental states. For example, where patients signalled faux pas had occurred when it had not, or inferred that the protagonist's offensive remark was deliberate (Eddy et al, 2010[a]). Such errors indicate that differences are apparent in the way that patients reason about social interaction and make attributions about the motives and intentions behind social behaviour. It could be that patients with TS exhibit increased emotional reactivity when tasks highlight conflict within social interaction, such as situations where one person may be negatively affected by another person's actions. This could help explain why patients with TS were more likely to reject offers of money during the Ultimatum Game (Eddy et al, 2011[b]), where an unfair proposer offered them an ultimatum choice of an unfair share of money or nothing. Increased emotional reactivity in response to stimuli associated with negative emotion could lead to reduced 'logical' control over decision making within social or emotional contexts in TS.

One possible explanation for TS patients' difficulties on social cognitive tasks is inhibitory dysfunction. Patients with uncomplicated TS (without co-morbid behavioural problems) exhibit inhibitory deficits on the Hayling task (Burgess and Shallice, 1996), as shown by a number of studies (Channon et al, 2003; Channon et al, 2004; Channon et al, 2006). It has been suggested that appreciating another's mental state often requires inhibition of one's own perspective (Samson et al, 2005), and developmental studies have found links between performance on ToM tasks and inhibitory tasks (e.g. Carlson et al, 2002). Indeed, the same inhibitory processes recruited during executive tasks may contribute to performance on ToM tasks (Saxe et al., 2006). In the previous studies reporting ToM changes in TS, patients with TS exhibited mild inhibitory impairments on the Hayling task (Eddy et al, 2010[a]), and a Stroop task (Eddy et al, 2010[b]) and on a verbal fluency measure (Eddy et al, 2011[b]). However, the deficits revealed on ToM tasks seemed largely independent of executive dysfunction.

If patients' deficits on ToM tasks do reflect changes in ToM *per* se, this may suggest activation changes within frontostriatal pathways involving ventromedial prefrontal cortex (including orbitofrontal cortex), as dysfunction of this region can impair performance on the faux pas task (Stone et al, 1998), reasoning about socially competitive emotions (Shamay-Tsoory et al, 2007) and decision making during the Ultimatum game (Koenigs & Tranel, 2007).

Role of the Striatum in Social Cognition

Many studies have documented that patients with striatal dysfunction linked to the Movement Disorders PD, HD or TS can exhibit evidence of difficulties on tasks involving social cognition. This implies that the striatum must make a contribution to processes involved in recognising emotional facial expressions, understanding intentions in social interaction, judging the appropriateness of social behaviour and reasoning about complex mental states.

The precise nature of striatal dysfunction within patients with different Movement Disorders is thought to vary, so patients with PD, HD and TS may exhibit different patterns of dysfunction within frontostriatal circuits involving regions activated during social cognitive tasks, such as dorsolateral prefrontal cortex, orbitofrontal cortex and amygdala. Different patterns of frontostriatal dysfunction could be linked to different patterns of impairment across social cognitive tasks, or different reasons for impairment on a task (e.g. executive problems or ToM deficits *per se*).

Although only tentative conclusions can be drawn from the available literature, patients with different Movement Disorders do appear to demonstrate some differences in task performance. Patients with PD and HD can both exhibit difficulties in recognising emotional facial expressions. However, while patients with TS appear to exhibit difficulty on more complex tasks of this nature (e.g. The Reading the Mind in the Eyes test), studies have yet to document evidence of difficulties in recognising basic emotions from faces. Appreciation of basic false belief can be impaired in PD, and needs further investigation in HD, but appears intact in TS. The understanding of socially inappropriate behaviour has also been assessed in patients with all three disorders. There is mixed evidence in terms of the performance of patients with PD, which suggests understanding is intact in early-stage patients and impaired later on. Preliminary indications indicate impairment in HD, and deficits are fairly well established in TS. In terms of cognitive versus affective ToM, it may be questioned whether both are affected in PD, HD seems likely to affect both forms of ToM, and patients with TS seem to exhibit more evidence of difficulty on tasks involving processes related to emotion.

One important contribution to the observed performance differences across these patient groups is likely to be the level of executive dysfunction. Patients with PD and HD exhibit more extensive executive problems than those with TS. If executive function was more important for cognitive ToM, this could help explain why patients with PD and HD may perform more poorly on simple false belief tasks than patients with TS. Although further investigations are needed, the impact of executive deficits would be in accordance with likely greater dysfunction within frontostriatal pathways involving dorsolateral prefrontal cortex in PD and HD.

If neuroimaging studies can document alterations in brain regions thought to be important for ToM but perhaps less activated during executive performance, this could offer insight into whether patients' deficits could be classified as deficits in ToM *per se*. Such brain regions could include orbitofrontal cortex and the amygdala. Patients with TS tend to demonstrate most difficulty on ToM tasks involving affective information, which may be in line with evidence from neuroimaging studies which report alterations affecting medial prefrontal regions, such as the anterior cingulate (Muller-Vahl et al, 2009) and orbitofrontal cortex (Braun et al, 1995), and the amygdala (Peterson et al, 2007). In HD, one study showed that changes in circuitry involving the caudate and lateral orbitofrontal cortex may contribute to difficulties with facial emotion recognition (Henley et al, 2008), and changes in fear experience could indicate amygdala dysfunction (Eddy et al, 2011[a]). In PD, evidence of impairments on the faux pas task in patients with later stage PD (Peron et al, 2009) may indicate involvement of medial orbitofrontal cortex is more likely at a more advanced stage of the disease. However, one study reported that orbitofrontal and amygdalar presynaptic dopaminergic functions may be altered in early PD (Ouchi et al, 1999).

In summary, although the striatum is not thought of as a core neural substrate for social cognition, it appears to make a critical contribution to performance on social cognitive tasks. This may be through alterations in the functioning of frontostriatal circuitry needed for executive functioning, or circuitry involving regions thought to subserve processes specific to ToM *per se*. Whether the striatum is considered to make a direct or indirect impact on social cognitive performance will depend on whether one's conceptualisation of the neuroanatomical substrates underlying social cognition consists of individual nodes or networks.

Study Limitations and Remaining Questions

There are limitations associated with comparing the performance of patients with different Movement Disorders as studies vary in terms of methodology. Indeed, although striatal dysfunction is thought to be similar in different patients with a particular Movement Disorder, these patient groups are far from homogenous. For example, in PD, executive performance may vary considerably across individuals. In HD, age of onset and speed of disease progression also vary according to CAG repeat length. In TS, patients exhibit different clinical profiles in terms of the nature of tic symptoms and severity, and accompanying co-morbid disorders. These variations make it difficult to compare studies involving individuals with the same disorder, and inconsistencies in study findings are likely to reflect the influence of such variables.

A specific difficulty associated with investigating social cognition already highlighted in this chapter is the association between this collection of abilities and higher cognitive or executive function. Executive deficits are so far proving difficult to disentangle from abilities such as ToM. In fact, aspects of executive function may largely prove to be inseparable from ToM and form an integral part of the social reasoning process. However, more efforts could be made to reduce incidental executive demands and compare performance across verbal and non-verbal tasks. Future research should address these challenges in order to determine whether it could be established that patients' deficits reflect deficits in ToM *per se*.

An additional problem with assessment is that the reasons behind patients' difficulties on social cognitive tasks may vary. The noted deficits in faux pas for instance, may lead one to expect that patients with TS and HD are similar in relation to their difficulties in understanding socially inappropriate behaviour. However, there may be subtle differences which lead to the same errors. For example, patients with TS seem to be particularly sensitive to social exchanges and sometime over analyse the motivations and meanings behind social interaction. In contrast, patients with HD seem more insensitive to emotional information and find it more difficult to take anothers' perspective. The differences in the way these patient groups respond to social and emotional information can both result in misinterpretations of social interaction but the underlying basis for patients' misunderstandings are not equivalent.

Complexities associated with interpreting patients' performance highlight the importance of task selection. Greater attention should be given to what the social cognitive tasks used in a study are measuring. For example, some tasks (e.g. faux pas tasks) may be completed using stored knowledge as opposed to online reasoning, and tasks which assess more spontaneous aspects of social cognition may reveal different performance to those which cue individuals or ask them to pick between multiple answers. Future research should aim to test well described sample of individuals on batteries of social cognitive tasks which assess different aspects or stages involved in social cognition, including tasks with matched control trials which offer greater insight into the impact of more general cognitive limitations.

Our ability to draw conclusions about the likely neural basis of patients' deficits is also limited. Although models of frontostriatal circuitry such as that provided by Alexander et al (1986) provide a useful basis for understanding deficits in social cognition in Movement Disorders, more precise and inclusive models are needed to help understand the role of different parts of the orbitofrontal cortex (i.e. medial and lateral) and subcortical structures such as the amygdala, neural regions which play a key role in social cognition. For example, dysfunction of the striatum could affect the amygdala indirectly via the action of frontostriatal pathways that terminate in orbitofrontal cortex, which in turn sends projections to the amygdala. However, the striatum also has the potential to affect the functioning of the amygdala more directly, via the intralaminar nucleus of the thalamus. Future research should aim to combine functional MRI and structural neuroimaging techniques which consider the integrity of connections between brain regions. Such studies will make a valuable contribution to our understanding of the precise neural basis of patients' deficits and further elucidate the role of the striatum in social cognition.

References

Adolphs, R. (2002). Neural systems for recognizing emotion. *Current Opinion in Neurobiology*, 12, 169-177.

Aleman, A. and van't Wout, M. (2008). Repetitive transcranial stimulation over the right dorsolateral prefrontal cortex disrupts digit span task performance. *Neuropsychobiology*, 57, 1-2, 44-48.

Alexander, G.E., Delong, M.R. and Strick, P.L. (1986) Parallel organization of functionally segregated circuits linking basal ganglia and cortex [Review]. *Annual_Review of Neuroscience*, 9, 357-381.

Baron-Cohen, S. Wheelwright, S. and Joliffe, T. (1997). Is there a "language of the eyes"? Evidence from normal adults, and adults with autism or asperger's syndrome. *Visual Cognition*, 4, 3, 311-331.

Baron-Cohen, S., Wheelwright, S., Hill, J., Raste, Y. and Plumb, I. (2001). The "Reading the Mind in the Eyes" Test Revised Version: A study with normal adults, adults with Asperger's syndrome or high-functioning autism. *Journal of Child Psychology and Psychiatry and Allied Disciplines*, 42, 2, 241-251.

Braun, A.R., Randolph, C., Stoetter, B., Mohr, E., Cox, C., Vladar, K., Sexton, R., Carson, R.E., Herscovitch, P. and Chase, T.N. (1995). The functional neuroanatomy of Tourette's Syndrome: An FDG-PET study. II: Relationships between regional cerebral metabolism and associated behavioral and cognitive features of the illness. *Neuropsychopharmacology*, 13, 2, 151-168.

Brüne, M., Blank, K., Witthaus, H., Saft, C. (2011). "Theory of mind" is impaired in Huntington's disease. *Movement Disorders,* 26(4), 671-8.

Burgess P.W. and Shallice, T. (1996). Response suppression, initiation and strategy use following frontal lobe lesions. *Neuropsychologia*, 34, 263-273.

Calder, A.J., Keane, J., Lawrence, A.D. and Manes, F. (2004). Impaired recognition of anger following damage to the ventral striatum. *Brain*, 127, 1958-1969.

Carlson, S.M., Moses, L.J. and Breton, C. (2002). How specific is the relation between executive function and theory of mind? Contributions of inhibitory control and working memory. *Infant and Child Development*, 11, 2, 73-92.

Cavanna, A.E., Servo, S., Monaco, F. and Robertson, M.M. (2009). More than tics: the behavioral spectrum of Gilles de la Tourette syndrome. *Journal of Neuropsychiatry and Clinical Neurosciences*, 21, 13-23.

Channon, S., Gunning, A., Frankl, J., and Robertson, M.M. (2006). Tourette's Syndrome (TS): Cognitive performance in adults with uncomplicated TS. *Neuropsychology*, 20, 1, 58-65.

Channon, S., Pratt, P. and Robertson, M. (2003). Executive function, memory and learning in Tourette's syndrome. *Neuropsychology*, 17, 247-254.

Channon, S., Sinclair, E., Waller, D., Healey, L., and Robertson, M.M. (2004). Social cognition in Tourette's Syndrome: Intact Theory of Mind and impaired inhibitory functioning. *Journal of Autism and Developmental Disorders*, 34, 6, 669-677.

Clark, U.S., Neargarder, S. and Cronin-Golomb, A. (2008). Specific Impairments in the Recognition of emotional facial expressions in Parkinson's Disease. *Neuropsychologia*, 46, 2300-2309.

Duff, K., Paulsen, J.S., Beglinger, L.J., Langbehn, D.R., Wang, C., Stout, J.C., Ross, C.A.,

Aylward, E., Carlozzi, N.E., Queller, S; Predict-HD Investigators of the Huntington.

Study Group. (2010). "Frontal" behaviors before the diagnosis of Huntington's disease andtheir relationship to markers of disease progression: evidence of early lack of awareness. Journal of Neuropsychiatry and Clinical Neurosciences, 22(2), 196-207.

Eddy, C.M., Rizzo, R. and Cavanna, A.E. (2009). Neuropsychological Aspects of Tourette Syndrome: A Review. *Journal of Psychosomatic Research*, 603, 503-513.

Eddy, C.M., Mitchell, I.J., Beck, S.R., Cavanna, A.E. and Rickards, H. (2010)[a]. Altered Attribution of Intention in Tourette Syndrome. *Journal of Neuropsychiatry and Clinical Neurosciences*, 22, 3, 348-351.

Eddy, C.M., Mitchell, I.J., Beck, S.R., Cavanna, A.E. and Rickards, H.E (2010)[b]. Impaired comprehension of nonliteral language in Tourette Syndrome. *Cognitive and Behavioral Neurology*, 23, 178–184.

Eddy, C.M, Mitchell, I.J, Beck, S.R, Cavanna, A.E, and Rickards, H. (2011)[a]. Altered subjective fear responses in Huntington's Disease. *Parkinsonism and Related Disorders*, 17, 386-389.

Eddy, C.M., Mitchell, I.J., Beck, S.R., Cavanna, A.E, and Rickards, H.E. (2011)[b]. Social Reasoning in Tourette syndrome. *Cognitive Neuropsychiatry*, 18, 1-22.

Eddy, C.M. (2009). 'Social Cognition in Disorders of the Basal Ganglia'. Ph.D. Thesis. University of Birmingham, UK.

Eddy, C.M., Siramahalingappa, S. and Rickards, H.E. Theory of Mind in Huntington's Disease [Abstract]. *Clinical Genetics,* 80, S1, 41.

Fletcher, P.C., Happé, F., Frith, U., Baker, S.C., Dolan, and R.J., Frackowiak, R.S. and Frith, C.D. (1995). Other minds in the brain: a functional imaging study of ''Theory of Mind'' in story comprehension. *Cognition*, 57, 109-128.

Frith, U. and Frith, C.D. (2003). Social Cognition in Humans. Current Biology 17, R724–R732.

Gilbert, B., Belleville, S., Bherer, L. and Chouinard, S. (2005). Study of verbal working memory in patients with Parkinson's disease. *Neuropsychology*, 19, 1, 106-114.

Gordon, A.C.L. and Olson, D.R. (1998). The relation between theory of mind and the capacity to hold in mind. *Journal of Experimental Child Psychiatry*, 68, 70-83.

Gray, J.M., Young, A.W., Barker, W. A., Curtis, A., and Gibson, D. (1997). Impaired recognition of disgust in Huntington's disease gene carriers. *Brain*, 120, 2029–2038.

Gregory, C. , Lough, S., Stone, V.E., Erzinclioglu, S., Martin, L., Baron-Cohen, S. and Hodges, J. (2002). Theory of mind in frontotemporal dementia and Alzheimer's disease: Theoretical and practical implications. *Brain*, 125, 752-64.

Hayes, C.J., Stevenson, R.J. and Coltheart, M. (2007). Disgust and Huntington's disease. *Neuropsychologia*, 45, 1135-1151.

Henley, S.M.D., Wild, E.J., Hobbs, N.Z., Warren, J.D., Frost, C., Scahill, R.I., Ridgway, G.R., MacManus, D.G., Barker, R.A., Fox, N.C. and Tabrizi, S.J. (2008). Defective emotion recognition in early HD is neuropsychologically and anatomically generic. *Neuropsychologia*, 46, 2152-2160.

Hennenlotter, A., Schroeder, U., Erhard, P., Haslinger, B., Stahl, R., Weindl, A., von Einsiedel, H.G., Lange, K.W. and Ceballos-Baumann, A.O. (2004). Neural correlates associated with impaired disgust processing in presymptomatic Huntington's disease. *Brain*, 127, 1446-1453.

Henry, J.D., Phillips, L.H., Crawford, J.R., Ietswaart, M. and Summers, F. (2006). Theory of Mind following traumatic brain injury: The role of emotion recognition and executive dysfunction. *Neuropsychologia*, 44, 1623-1628.

Johnson, S.A., Strafella, A.P. and Zatorre, R.J. (2007). The role of the dorsolateral prefrontal cortex in bimodal divided attention: Two transcranial magnetic stimulation studies. *Journal of Cognitive Neuroscience*, 19, 6, 907-920.

Koenigs, M. and Tranel, D. (2007). Irrational economic decision making after ventromedial prefrontal damage - evidence from the Ultimatum Game. *The Journal of Neuroscience*, 27, 4, 951-956.

Kurlan, R., Daragfari, C., Como, P.G., McDermott, M.P., Trinidad, K.S., Roddy, S., Brower, C.A. and Robertson, M.M. (1996). Non-obscene socially inappropriate behavior in Tourette's Syndrome. *Journal of Neuropsychiatry and Clinical Neurosciences*, 8, 311-317.

Leckman, J.F. (2002). Tourette's Syndrome. *The Lancet*, 360, 9345, 1577-1586.

McNamara, P. and Durso, R. (2003). Pragmatic communication skills in patients with Parkinson's disease. *Brain and Language*, 84, 414-423.

Mengelberg, A. and Siegert, R.J. (2003). Is theory-of-mind impaired in Parkinson's disease? *Cognitive Neuropsychiatry*, 8, 191-209.

Middleton, F.A. and Strick, P.L. (2000). Basal ganglia and cerebellar loops: motor and cognitive circuits. *Brain Research Reviews*, 31, 236-250.

Milders, M. Crawford, J.R., Lamb, A. and Simpson, S.A. (2003). Differential deficits in expression recognition in gene-carriers and patients with Huntington's disease. *Neuropsychologia*, 41, 1484-1492.

Mimura, M., Oeda, R. and Kawamura, M. (2006). Impaired decision making in Parkinson's disease. *Parkinsonism and Related Disorders*, 12, 169-175.

Mitchell, I. J., Boyce, S., Sambrook, M. A. and Crossman, A. R. (1992). A 2-deoxyglucose study of the effects of dopamine agonists on the parkinsonian primate brain: implications for the neural mechanisms that mediate dopamine agonist-induced dyskinesia. *Brain*, 115, 809-824.

Monetta, L. and Pell, M.D. (2007). Effects of verbal working memory deficits on metaphor comprehension in patients with Parkinson's disease. *Brain and Language*, 101, 80-89.

Monetta, L., Grindrod, C.M. and Pell, M.D. (2008). Effects of working memory capacity on inference generation during story comprehension in adults with Parkinson's disease. *Journal of Neurolinguistics*, 21, 400-417.

Monetta, L., Grindrod, C.M. and Pell, M.D. (2009). Irony comprehension and theory of mind deficits in patients with parkinson's disease. *Cortex*, 45972-981.

Montoya A, Price BH, Menear M, Lepage M. Brain imaging and cognitive dysfunctions in Huntington's disease. J Psychiatry Neurosci. 2006 Jan;31(1):21-9.

Muller-Vahl, K.R., Kaufmann, J., GrossKruetz, J., Dengler, R., Emrich, H.M. and Peschel, T. (2009). Prefrontal and anterior cingulate abnormalities in Tourette Syndrome: Evidence from voxel-based morphometry and magnetization transfer imaging. *BMC Neurosciences*, 10, 47.

Naarding, P., Kremer, H.P.H. and Titman, F.G. (2001). Huntington's disease: a review of the literature on prevalence and treatment of neuropsychiatric phenomena. *European Psychiatry*, 16, 439-445.

Nathaniel-James, D.A., Fletcher, P. and Frith, C.D. (1997). The functional anatomy of verbal initiation and suppression using the Hayling Test. *Neuropsychologia*, 35, 559-566.

Ouchi, Y., Yoshikawa, E., Okada, H., Futatsubashi, M., Sekine, Y., Iyo, M. and Sakamoto, M. (1999). Alterations in binding site density of dopamine transporter in the striatum, orbitofrontal cortex, and amygdala in early Parkinson's disease: compartment analysis for beta-CFT binding with positron emission tomography. *Annals of Neurology*, 45(5), 601-10.

Peron, J., Vicente, S., Leray, E., Drapier, S., Drapier, D., Cohen, R., Bisuel, I., Rouaud, T., Le Jeune, F., Sauleau, P. and Verin, M. (2009). Are dopaminergic pathways involved in theory of mind? A study in Parkinson's disease. *Neuropsychologia*, 47, 406-414.

Peterson, B. S., Thomas, P., Kane, M. J., Scahill, L. Zhang, H., and Bronen, R. (2003). Basal ganglia volumes in patients with Tourette's syndrome. *Archives of General Psychiatry*, 60, 415–424.

Peterson, B.S., Choi, H.A., Hao, X., Amat, J.A., Zhu, H., Whiteman, R., Lui, J., Xu, D. and Bansal, R. (2007). Morphological features of the amygdala and hippocampus in children and adults with Tourette Syndrome. *Archives of General Psychiatry*, 64, 11, 1281-1291.

Peterson, B.S., Skudlarski, P., Gatersby, J.C., Zhang, H.P., Anderson, A.W. and Gore, J.C. (1999). An fMRI study of stroop word-color interference: Evidence for cingulate subregions subserving multiple distributed attentional systems. *Biological Psychiatry*, 45, 10, 1237-1258.

Robertson, M.M. (2000). Tourette Syndrome, associated conditions and the complexities of treatment. *Brain*, 123, 425-462.

Saltzman, J., Strauss, E., Hunter, M. and Archibald, S. (2000). Theory of mind and executive functions in normal aging and Parkinson's disease. *Journal of the International Neurological Society*, 6, 7, 781-788.

Samson, D., Apperly, I.A., Kathirgamanathan, U. and Humphreys, G. W. (2005). Seeing it my way: a case of a selective deficit in inhibiting self perspective. *Brain*, 128, 1102-1111.

Saxe, R., Schulz, L.E. and Jiang, Y.V. (2006). Reading minds versus following rules: Dissociating theory of mind and executive control in the brain. *Social Neuroscience*, 1, 3-4, 284-298.

Shamay-Tsoory, S. G., Tibi-Elhanany, Y., and Aharon-Peretz, J. (2007). The green-eyed monster and malicious joy: The neuroanatomical bases of envy and gloating (schadenfreude). *Brain*, 130, 1663-1678.

Shamay-Tsoory, S.G. and Aharon Peretz, J. (2007). Dissociable prefrontal networks for cognitive and affective theory of mind: A lesion study. *Neuropsychologia*, 45, 3054-3067.

Singer, H.S., Reiss, A.L., Brown, J.E., Aylward, E.H., Shin, B., Chee, E., Harris, E.L., Reader, M.J., Chase, G.A., Bryan, R.N. and Denckla, M.B. (1993). Volumetric MRI changes in basal ganglia of children with Tourette's syndrome. *Neurology*, 43, 950-956.

Snowden, J.S., Austin, N.A., Sembi, S., Thompson, J.C., Crauford, D. and Neary, D. (2008). Emotion recognition in Huntington's disease and frontotemporal dementia. *Neuropsychologia*, 46, 2638-2649.

Snowden, J.S., Gibbons, Z.C., Blackshaw, A., Doubleday, E., Thompson, J., Crauford, D., Foster, J., Happé, F. and Neary, D. (2003). Social cognition in frontotemporal dementia and Huntington's disease. *Neuropsychologia*, 41, 688-670.

Sprengelmeyer, R., Young, A.W., Sprengelmeyer, A., Calder, A.J., Rowland, D. and Perrett, D. (1997). Recognition of facial expressions: Selective impairment of specific emotions in Huntington's disease. *Cognitive Neuropsychology*, 14, 6, 839-879.

Stone, V.E., Baron-Cohen, S., and Knight, R.T. (1998). Frontal lobe contributions to Theory of Mind. *Journal of Cognitive Neuroscience*, 10, 640-656.

Stone, V.E., Baron-Cohen, S., Calder, A., Keane, J. and Young, A. (2003). Acquired theory of mind impairments in individuals with bilateral amygdala lesions. *Neuropsychologia*, 41, 209-220.

Suzuki, A., Hoshino, T., Shigemasu, K. and Kawamura, M. (2006). Disgust specific impairment of facial expression recognition in Parkinson's disease. *Brain*, 129, 707-717.

Vanderhasselt, M.A., De Raedt, R., Baeken, C., Leymen, L. and D'haenen, H. (2006)a. The influence of rTMS over the left dorsolateral prefrontal cortex on stroop task performance. *Experimental Brain Research*, 169, 2, 279-283.

Vanderhasselt, M.A., De Raedt, R., Baeken, C., Leyman, L. and D'haenen, H. (2006)b. The influence of rTMS over the right dorsolateral prefrontal cortex on intentional set switching. *Experimental Brain Research*, 172, 4, 561-565.

Wang, K., Hoosain, R., Yang, R.M., Meng, Y. and Wang, C-Q. (2003). Impairment of recognition of disgust in Chinese with Huntington's or Wilson's disease. *Neuropsychologia*, 41, 527-537.

Yoshimura, N., Kawamura, M., Masaoka, Y. and Homma, I. (2005). The amygdala of patients with Parkinson's disease is silent in response to fearful facial expressions. *Neuroscience*, 131, 523e34.

In: Striatum: Anatomy, Functions and Role in Disease
Editors: Hugo T. Maldonado and Ignacio M. Ortega
ISBN 978-1-61942-384-8

Chapter VI

Striatum: Structure, Function and Role in Diseases

Dian-shuai Gao and Jin Gao*
Department of Neurobiology and Anatomy,
Xuzhou Medical College, Jiangsu, China

Abstract

The corpus striatum consists of the caudate nucleus, putamen and globus pallidus. the putamen and globus pallidus were once considered as an entity, termed the lentiform nucleus. However, it is now known that the caudate nucleus and the putamen both develop from the telencephalon, share a common chemocytoarchitecture connections, and sometimes are referred to as the neostriatum; while the globus pallidus develop from the diencephalon and is called as paleostriatum. However, the striatum can also be differentiated into dorsal and ventral striatum based on the limbic inputs and also on cyto- and chemoarchitectonic characteristics. The dorsal striatum forms a continuous and large mass including the caudate and the putamen; the ventral stritum contains the nucleus accumbens and the olfactory tubercle.

Neurons of striatum are mainly medium-sized multipolar cells, mixed with a smaller number of large multipolar cells, the dendrites of both medium and large cells may be either spiny or non-spiny. The most common neurons (usually 75% of the total) are medium-sized cells with spiny dendrites, containing γ-aminobutyric acid (GABA), enkephalin, or substance P/dynorphin as their transmitters. The remaining medium-sized striatal neurons are aspiny, these cells contain acetylcholinesterase (AChE), choline acetyltransferase (CAT), somatostatin and neuropeptide Y, and appear to synapse with striatal projection neurons. Large neurons with spiny dendrites contain AChE and CAT, and most of them are intrinsic neurons.

The major input and output pathways of the striatum have been well established. The most important afferent, in terms of quantities of axons, is the corticostriatal connections.

* Correspondence to: Dian-shuai Gao, Department of Neurobiology and Anatomy, Xuzhou Medical College, 84 Huaihai West Road, Xuzhou, Jiangsu, 221002, China. Phn: 86-516-8277-1525. Fax: 86-516-8583-1817 E-mail: dshgao@vip.sina.com; gaojin82@126.com.

Another well known afferent is the nigrostriatal connections. The striatum also receives afferents from the thalamus, subthalamic nucleus and the external globus pallidus. The output pathway is made up of the striato-pallidonigral bundle and this projection comprises successively the external and internal globus pallidus, the pars compacta of the substantia nigra, and the pars reticulate of substantia nigra. Among these targets upon, the external globus pallidus does not send axons outside the system, while the others send axons to the superior colliculus, passing through different parts of thalamus then, and reaching different parts of cortex finally.

Disorders of the striatum, such as Parkinson's disease and dyskinesias, are principally characterized by abnormalities of movement, muscle tone and posture. However, it is also thought that non motor functions (eg. learning, memory, drug addiction and Obsessive compulsive disorder and et al) are associated with the striatum.

Introduction

The basal ganglia (or basal nuclei) are a group of nuclei of varied origin in the brains of vertebrates that act as a cohesive functional unit. They are situated at the base of the forebrain and strongly connected with the cerebral cortex, thalamus and other brain areas.The basal ganglia include the striatum, claustrum, and amygdaloid complex. These three parts collectively form a functional complex involved in the control of movement and motivational aspects of behaviour. The striatum is the important part of the basal ganglia. The striatum, also known as the corpus striatum, neostriatum, or striate nucleus, is a subcortical part of the forebrain. It’s the principal input structure of the basal ganglia system. In primates (including humans), the striatum is divided by a white matter tract called the internal capsule into two sectors called the caudate nucleus and putamen.

The caudate nuclei are located near the center of the brain, sitting astride the thalamus. There is a caudate nucleus within each hemisphere of the brain. Individually, they resemble a C-shape structure with a wider "head" at the front, tapering to a "body" and a "tail". Sometimes a part of the caudate nucleus is referred to as the "knee". The head and body of the caudate nucleus form part of the floor of the anterior horn of the lateral ventricle. After the body travels briefly towards the back of the head, the tail curves back toward the anterior, forming the roof of the inferior horn of the lateral ventricle. This means that a coronal section that cuts through the tail will also cross the body and head of the caudate nucleus. The putamen along with the caudate nucleus forms the dorsal striatum.

The striatum have complex connections with other parts of the brain through the ‘input’ and ‘output’ structures. The ‘input’ of the striatum is said that it can receive the majority of afferents of the neuraxis from cortex and substantia nigra pars compacta of the brain. Its principal efferent connections of the striatum are to the globus pallidus and pars reticulata of the substantia nigra, then to other parts of the brain. Thus, the globus pallidus and, more particularly, its medial segment, together with the pars reticulata of the substantia nigra are regarded as the main ‘output’ structure.

Disorders of the striatum are principally characterized by the abnormalities of movement system, though it can affect not only one system of the body. In clinic, there is a wide spectrum of the abnormalities of the movement system ranging from poverty of movement and hypertonia (Parkinson’s disease) to abnormal involuntary movements (dyskinesias). The underlying pathophysiological mechanisms that mediate these disorders have been much studied in recent years. This has led to the introduction of new rational therapeutic strategies for both medical and neurosurgical treatment of movement disorders.

The Anatomy Structure of Striatum

The structural composition of striatum is different according to different criteria. At the beginning, people think that the striatum consists of the caudate nucleus, putamen and globus pallidus, which are all highly cellular and well vascularized. Because of their close proximity, the putamen and globus pallidus were once considered as an entity, termed the lentiform nucleus. However, it is now known that the caudate nucleus and putamen are traversed by numerous small bundles of axons, and the caudate nucleus and putamen both develop from the telencephalon and share a common chemocytoarchitecture and connections, they are referred to jointly as the neostriatum or simply the striatum. The globus pallidus is itself divided into two segments, the external segment and the internal segment, separated by the internal medullary lamina. While the globus pallidus develop from the diencephalon and is called as paleostriatum (Figure 1 and Figure 2).

It is especially important to note that the striatum can also be divided into dorsal and ventral striatum on the basis of specific cortical, thalamic （Voorn *et al*; 2004） . To date, few structural or functional markers uniquely characteristic for either of the two regions have been identified. In the literature, the striatum can also be differentiated into dorsal and ventral striatum based on the limbic inputs and also on cyto- and chemoarchitectonic characteristics. The dorsal striatum forms a continuous and large mass including the caudate and the putamen; the ventral striatum contains the nucleus accumbens and the olfactory tubercle, although, some sources also include the ventromedial parts of the caudate nucleus and putamen (Voorn *et al*, 2004; Ubeda-Bañon *et al*, 2007; Martin, 2003).

The medium-sized multipolar cells are the principal neurons of the striatum, which occupy 90% of the total cells of striatum. There are a small number of large multipolar cells among these medium-sized multipolar cells. Both medium and large neurons have sepherical dendritic trees (spiny or non-spiny), which receive the synaptic terminal of many striatal afferents(Wilson, 2004; Stocco *et al*, 2010).

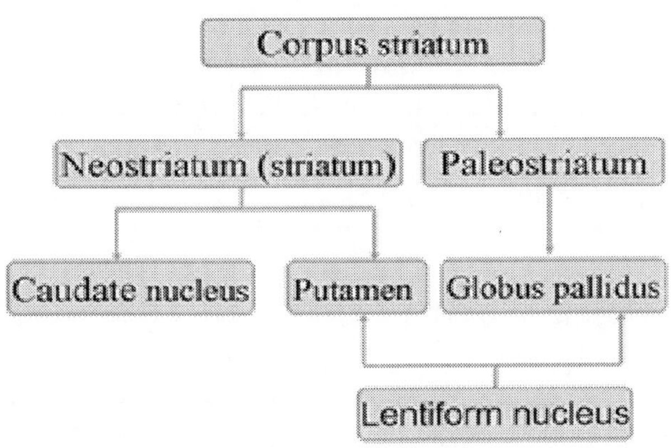

Figure 1. Terminology and relationship of the structures forming the corpus striatum.

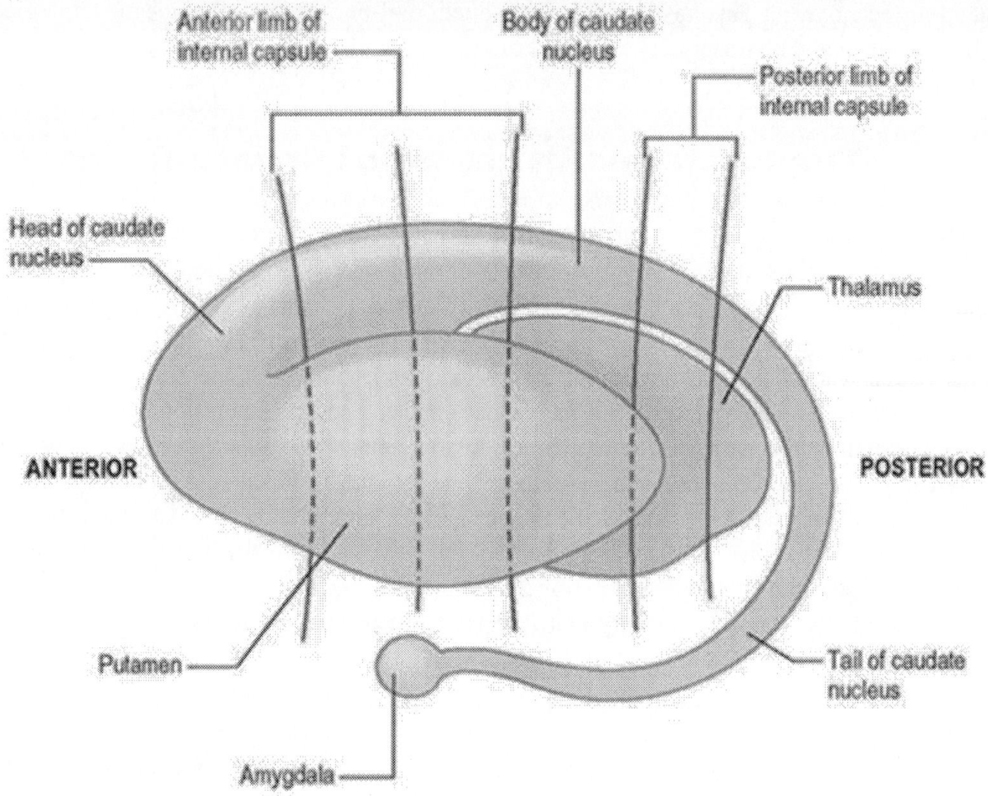

Figure 2. The striatum within the left cerebral hemisphere. (This photograph comes from Crossman AR, Neary D 2000 Neuroanatomy, 3rd edn. Edinburgh: Churchill Livingstone).

Different neurons utilize different substance as their transmitter. For example, the major medium-sized cells (usually 75% of the total medium-sized cells) use γ-aminobutyric acid (GABA) or enkephalin or substance P/dynorphin as their transmitter, these neurons are the major striatal efferent neurons.

The remaining medium-sized neurons are aspiny cells that contain acetylcholinesterase (AChE), choline acetyltransferase (CAT) and somatostatin. Large neurones contain AChE and CAT. Neuroactive chemicals are not distributed uniformly in the striatum. For example, the caudal part of the striatum contains the highest concentrations of glutamic acid decarboxylase (GAD), while rostral part contains the highest concentrations of substance P, acetylcholine (ACh) and dopamine (Gerfen, 1988; Haber, 1986; Semba *et al*, 1987; McGinty, 2007; McGeer *et al*, 1984; Yelnik *et al*, 1997).

The Major Connections of the Striatum

The major input and output pathways of the mammalian striatum have been well established. The general connections of the striatum can be made that the dorsal striatum is predominantly connected with motor and associative areas of the cerebral cortex, whilst the ventral striatum is connected with the limbic system and orbitofrontal and temporal cortices.

For both dorsal and ventral striatum, the pallidum and substantia nigra pars reticulata are key efferent structures. The fundamental arrangement is the same for both divisions. The cerebral cortex projects to the striatum, which in turn projects to the pallidum and substantia nigra pars reticulata, and efferents from the pallidum and substantia nigra pars reticulata influence the cerebral cortex and the superior colliculus (Figure 3).

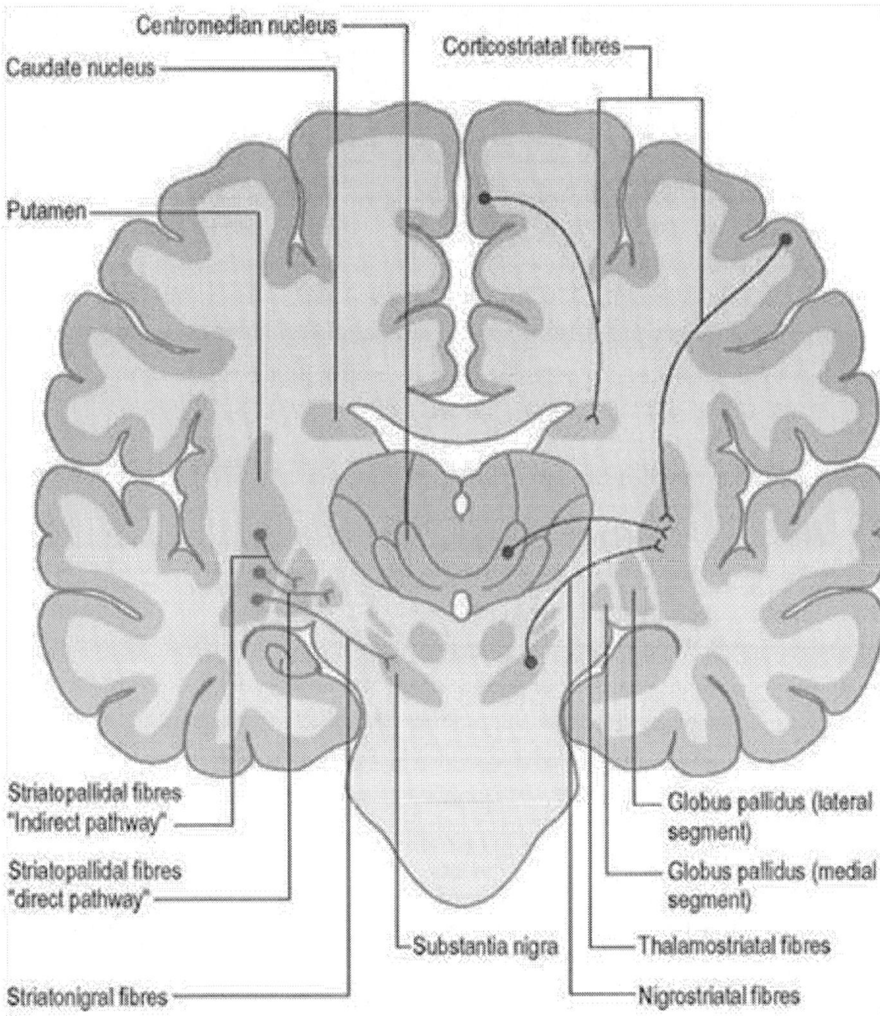

Figure 3. Connections of the striatum. The major afferent projections to the striatum are shown on the right and major efferent projections from the striatum on the left. (This photograph comes from Gray's Anatomy, 40th Edition, Susan Standring).

Afferent Connections of Dorsal Striatum

The most important afferent in terms of quantity of axons is the corticostriatal connection. Many parts of the neocortex innervate the dorsal striatum. The cortical pyramidalneurons projecting to the striatum are located in layer II-IV, but the most dense projections come from layer V (Rosell and Giménez-Amaya , 1999). They end mainly on the spines of the spiny neurons. They are glutamatergic, exciting striatal neurons. The greater part of these inputs to the dorsal striatum is derived from the frontal and parietal lobes, that from the occipitotemporal cortex being relatively small. Thus, the orbitofrontal association cortex projects to the inferior part of the head of the caudate nucleus, which lies next to the ventral striatum. The dorsolateral frontal association cortex and frontal eye fields project to the rest of the head of the caudate nucleus, and much of the parietal lobe projects to the body of the nucleus. The somatosensory and motor cortices project predominantly to the putamen (Carmichael *et al*, 1996; Flaherty *et al*, 1994; Goldman-Rakic *et al*, 1986; Haber *et al*, 1995; Kunzle, 1975).

The dorsal striatum also receives afferents from other areas of the brain except the cerebral cortex. The glutamatergic inputs to the dorsal striatum come from the polysensory intralaminar thalamus. The dopaminergic inputs to the dorsal striatum are derived from the substantia nigra pars compacta. The serotoninergic afferents to the striatum are derived from the dorsal raphe nucleus, and the noradrenergic inputs to the striatum are derived from the locus coeruleus (Flores-Barrera, 2010; Dahlström, 1964; Joel, 2000; Abigail *et al*,1986; Tao and Auerbach,1995; Nygren and Olson,1977). These aminergic inputs appear to modulate the responses of the striatum to cortical and thalamic afferent influences.

Afferent Connections of Ventral Striatum

The ventral striatum is the primary target of cortical afferents from limbic cortices, including allocortex, and from limbic associated regions. Thus, the hippocampus and orbitofrontal cortex project to the nucleus accumbens and the olfactory, entorhinal, anterior cingulate and temporal visual cortices project to both the nucleus accumbens and olfactory tubercle in varying degrees. The tubercle also receives afferents from the amygdale (Carmichael ST, 1996; Flaherty AW, 1994; Haber SN, 1995; Ferreira TL, 2008; Marín et al, 1997; Newman and Winans, 1980).

Efferent Connections of Dorsal Striatum

The efferent connections are made up of the striatum along with the regions to which it projects directly, via the striato-pallidonigral bundle. The striato-pallidonigral bundle is a very dense bundle of sparsely myelinated axons, giving a whitish appearance. This projection comprises successively the globus pallidus, and the substantia nigra. Efferents from the striatum pass to both segments of the globus pallidus and to the substantia nigra, where they end in a topically ordered fashion.

One outflow from the dorsal striatum is to the globus pallidus（Flaherty AW, 1994; Kunzle H, 1978）. Different striatal cells project their fibres to different segment of the pallidal (lateral or external). Neurons which co-localize GABA and enkephalin project their fibres to the lateral pallidum, these neurons influence the activity of striatum output neurons in the medial pallidum via the subthalamic nucleus, they are described as 'indirect pathway'. Other neurons, which contain GABA and substance P/dynorphin, project directly to the medial pallidum and are therefore described as the 'direct pathway' (McGinty JF, 2007; Flaherty AW, 1994; Nambu A, 2004; Kemp and Powell,1971; Durieux *et al*,1986) .

Another outflow from the dorsal striatum project to the pars reticulata of the substantia nigra (Mailly *et al*, 2003; Durieux *et al*, 1986) . This also has both direct and indirect pathways, via the lateral pallidum and subthalamic nucleus.

Efferent Connections of Ventral Striatum

Fibres come from the ventral striatum project to the ventral pallidum and the substantia nigra pars reticulata. In the latter case, the connection is both direct and indirect via the subthalamic nucleus. The projections from the pars reticulata are as described for the dorsal system, but axons from the ventral pallidum reach the thalamic mediodorsal nucleus (which projects to cingulate and prefrontal association cortex) and midline nuclei (which project to the hippocampus). Ventral pallidal axons also reach the habenular complex of the limbic system (Gray's Anatomy, 40th Edition, Susan Standring).

Circuit Connections

In conclusion, all of the input and output fribres constitute the circuit connections. The circuit can be divided into direct pathway and indirect pathway (Figure 4).

In the direct pathway, cortical cells project excitatory inputs to the striatum, which in turn projects inhibitory neurons onto the cells of the SNr-GPi complex. The SNr-GPi complex projects directly onto the thalamus through the inhibitory ansa lenticularis pathway. The striatal inhibition of the SNr-GPi complex coupled with SNr-GPi inhibition of the thalamus therefore results in a net reduction of inhibition of the thalamus via the striatum. The thalamus projects excitatory glutamatergic neurons to the cortex itself. The direct pathway, therefore, results in the excitation of the motor cortex by the thalamus.

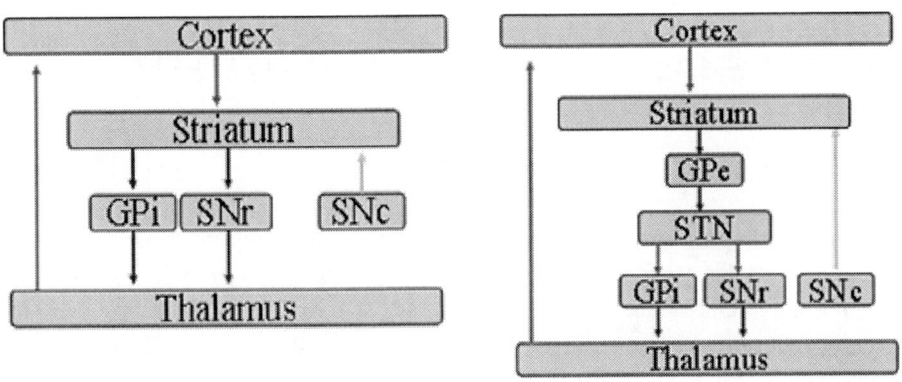

Figure 4. Connections of the striatum. The major direct pathway of the striatum are shown on the left and the major indirect pathway are shown on the right. Connectivity diagram showing excitatory glutamatergic pathways as red, inhibitory GABAergic pathways as blue, and modulatory dopaminergic pathways as orange. (Abbreviations: GPi: internal globus pallidus; GPe: external globus pallidus; STN: subthalamic nucleus; SNr: substantia nigra reticulata; SNc: substantia nigra compacta).

Once stimulated, the cortex projects its own excitatory outputs to the brain stem and ultimately muscle fibers via the lateral corticospinal tract (Hauber, 1998; Bolam *et al*, 2000).

The indirect pathway also starts from neurons in the striatum. Once stimulated by the cortex, striatal neurons in the indirect pathway project inhibitory axons onto the cells of the globus pallidus externa (GPe), which tonically inhibits the subthalamic nucleus (STN). This inhibition (by the striatum) of the inhibitory projections of the GPe, results in the net reduction of inhibition of the STN. The STN, in turn, projects excitatory inputs to the SNr-GPi complex (which inhibits the thalamus). The end-result is inhibition of the thalamus and, therefore, decreased stimulation of the motor cortex by the thalamus and reduced muscle activity. The direct and indirect pathways are therefore antagonist in their functions (Wilson, 2004; Hauber, 1998; Bolam *et al*, 2000).

The antagonistic functions of the direct and indirect pathways are modulated by the substantia nigra pars compacta (SNc), which produces dopamine. Special D1-receptors in the basal ganglia are excited by dopamine, favoring the direct pathway, whereas specialized D2-receptors in the basal ganglia are inhibited in presence of dopamine and favor the indirect pathway. Through these mechanisms the body is able to maintain balance between excitation and inhibition of motion (Wilson, 2004).

Pathophysiology of Striatum Disorders

The striatum occupy the core of the basal ganglia and consist of evolutionarily conserved motor nuclei that form recurrent circuits critical for motivation and motor planning. As far as their role in movement control is concerned, a reasonable definition is that they function to promote and support patterns of behaviour and movement that are appropriate in the prevailing circumstances and to inhibit unwanted or inappropriate behaviour and movements. Some diseases can exemplify this notion, when people suffer from Parkinson's disease, they will lose their ability to initiate and execute wanted movements, people can not prevent unwanted movements when they have Huntington's disease. Disorders of the striatum are principally characterized by abnormalities of movement, muscle tone and posture, however, Current studies have shown that non motor functions are also associated with the striatum, such as learning, memory, drug addiction, and post-traumatic stress disorder.

Parkinson's Disease

Though disorders of striatum can lead to abnormal functions of motor and non-motor system, Parkinson's disease is the most common pathological condition. It is characterized by akinesia, muscular rigidity and tremor. The primary symptoms of Parkinson's disease result from greatly reduced activity of dopamine-secreting cells caused by cell death in the pars compacta region of the substantia nigra (Obeso *et al*, 2008) . Because of these dopaminergic neurons project their fibres to the striatum by nigrostriatal pathway, when these neurons degenerate, the associated axon terminals are lost in the striatum and dopamine levels are severely reduced, dopamine receptors which are located upon medium spiny neurons are also spared, so, the dopamine pathway is depleted.

Dopamine appears to have a dual action on medium spiny striatal neurones. It inhibits those of the indirect pathway and excites those of the direct pathway. Consequently, when dopamine is lost from the striatum, the indirect pathway becomes overactive and the direct pathway becomes underactive. Overactivity of the striatal projection to the lateral pallidum results in inhibition of pallidosubthalamic neurones and, consequently, overactivity of the subthalamic nucleus. Subthalamic efferents mediate excessive excitatory drive to the medial globus pallidus and substantia nigra pars reticulata. This is exacerbated by underactivity of the GABAergic, inhibitory direct pathway. Overactivity of basal ganglia output then inhibits the motor thalamus and its excitatory thalamocortical connections. While this description is little more than a first approximation of the underlying pathophysiology, this model of the basis of parkinsonian symptoms has led to the introduction of new neurosurgical approaches to the treatment of Parkinson's disease, based upon lesioning and deep brain stimulation of the medial globus pallidus and subthalamic nucleus (Gray's Anatomy, 40th Edition, Susan Standring).

Now, there are several methods to treat this disease. The most common method is medical treatment. The discovery in 1960 that the death of DAnergic neurons in substantia nigra parc compacta opened the way for the development of pharmaceutical therapies regulating DA synaptic transmittion. These have induced the levodopa (L-DOPA; L-dihydroxyphenylalanine) treatment, or upon dopamine agonists (Birkmayer and HornykiewirL, 1961; Birkmayer and HornykiewirL, 1962; Lieberman and Goldslein, 1985; Goelz, 1990; Lees, 1994). Before the advent of levodopa therapy, neurosurgery for this disease was commonplace (Gross *et al*, 1999). The globus pallidus and thalamus are favoured targets for chemical or thermal lesions, current studies showed that the pedunculopontine nucleus was also a good target for this disease (Lozano, 2000). Implantation of deep-brain electrodes is also a kind of methods which can therapy Parkinson's disease, through this method high-frequency pulses generated by a pacemaker could inhibit cells in the vicinity. Taking this way can avoid making permanent brain lesions, and make bilateral surgery safer (Bronstein et al, 2011)

Dystonia

Another manifestation of striatum dysfunction is dystonia. Dystonia is a neurological sign characterized by involuntary, prolonged twisting and turning movements that are frequently stereotyped and repetitive, and produce characteristic abnormal postures.

Dystonia may occur as a consequence of levodopa treatment in Parkinson's disease or inherited disease (e.g. early-onset torsion, or Oppenheim's dystonia, an autosomal dominant disorder most commonly associated with a mutation in the DYT1 gene that encodes torsinA) or caused by other factors such as lead poisoning or reaction to pharmaceutical drugs. Though the precise pathophysiological basis of dystonia is unclear, the abnormality of GABA and dopamine may play an important role for the development of dystonia. In 2007, Levy and Hallett found the deficient level of GABA in the cortex and striatum of patients with adult-onset primary dystonia, which leaded to the reduced activity of GABAergic neurons in primary dystonia (Levy and Hallett, 2002). The dopamine receptor (especially the D2) also reduced in patients with dystonia (Carbon et al,2009; Beukers et al,2009).The deficient GABA levels could be consistent with reduced dopaminergic neurotransmission in the putamen, since dopamine receptors mostly inhibit the GABAergic striatal medium spiny neurons (Levy and Hallett, 2002; Carbon et al, 2009). The discovery of genetic mutations underlying inherited forms of dystonia (such as TOR1A and SGCE genes) is a relatively recent development that holds great promise for contributing to our understanding of the pathogenesis of primary dystonia. These discoveries have already provided some exciting insights into the molecular basis of primary dystonia, the identification of these dystonia-related genes has provided some interesting clues into potential relationships between different forms of dystonia, and the cell biological mechanisms that could underlie the abnormal CNS function or development that is believed to cause primary dystonia (Lauren *et al*, 2009).

Medical treatment has been limited to minimizing the symptoms of the disorder as there is yet no successful treatment for its cause(Sherman and Chaudhuri, 2010; Lubarr and Bressman, 2011). Though the neurosurgery for this disease can relieve some symptoms (such as the denervation of selected muscles), the destruction of nerves in the limbs or brain is not reversible. Recently, Implantation of deep-brain electrodes has proven successful in a number of cases of severe generalised dystonia(Bronte-Stewart, 2003; Aziz and Green, 2009).

Learning, Memory and Language Processing

Before 21th century, scientists think that novel behaviors are mediated primarily in cortex and that the development of automaticity is a process of transferring control to subcortical structures. However, more recently, much evidence suggests that subcortical structures, such as the striatum, make significant contributions to learning and memory. Many studies have found that it plays different roles of dorsal and ventral striatum in learning and memory. The dorsal striatum are associated with skill learning, response-based learning, and instrumental conditioning involving both goal-directed and habitual responding (Yin and Knowlton, 2006; Wickens *et al*, 2007; Grahn *et al*, 2008; Yin *et al*, 2008, 2009; F. Gregory Ashby, 2011). The ventral striatum play its roles in spatial learning, pavlovian conditioning, and pavlovian-instrumental transfer, among other types of learning (Parkinson *et al*, 2000; Corbit *et al*, 2001; Roitman *et al*, 2005; Ito *et al*, 2008).

The striatal subregions participate in these types of learning as part of at least 3 distinct circuits: an “associative” circuit involving associative cortical regions (e.g. medial prefrontal cortex) connectons to the dorsomedial striatum/caudate; a “sensorimotor” circuit involving sensory and motor cortex connections to the dorsolateral striatum/putamen; and a “limbic” circuit involving limbic cortex, basolateral amygdala and hippocampal connections to the ventral striatum/nucleus accumbens (Yin and Knowlton, 2006; Yin *et al*, 2008). Indeed, it can be argued that the striatum as a whole participates in most types of learning through participation in the actions of these circuits.

While the role of cortical areas in linguistic processing is relatively well established, the role of sub-cortical structures such as the striatum, and the way they impact language processing, is still controversial.

Indeed, studies using both patient sustaining striatal damage and functional brain imaging with healthy subjects have suggested that the striatum is involved in various aspects of language comprising phonology (Tettamanti *et al*, 2005; Teichmann *et al*,2009), word morphology (Ullman *et al*, 1997; Teichmann *et al*, 2005; Vannest *et al*, 2005; Teichmann *et al*, 2006) and syntax (Moro *et al*, 2001; Friederici and Kotz, 2003; Teichmann *et al*, 2005), rule and lexical as well as arithmetic (Marc Teichmann, 2008).

Drug Addiction

Drug addiction is also associated with the dysfunction of the striatum. Drug addiction is defined primarily on the basis of behavioral abnormalities, that is, loss of control over drug use and compulsive seeking and taking despite the knowledge of its adverse consequences (Nestler, 2004a). Chronic drug exposure causes long-lasting neuroadaptive changes in the brain at the molecular and cellular levels, which may contribute to compulsive drug use and relapse (Chao and Nestler, 2004; Nestler, 2004b). Some drugs, such as cocaine or methamphetamine, can cause the nerve cells to release abnormally large amounts of natural neurotransmitters (mainly dopamine) or to prevent the normal recycling of these brain chemicals, which is needed to shut off the signaling between neurons.

Dopamine release in the ventral striatum is a common characteristic of acute responses to addictive substances. It is generally assumed that addictive drugs take control of dopaminergic signals in the nucleus accumbens (and other dopamine-innervated limbic areas) (Pontieri *et al*, 1996; Zhang *et al*, 2009). As a person continues to overstimulate the dopamine pathway, the brain adapts to the overwhelming surges in dopamine by producing less of the hormones or by reducing the number of receptors in the pathway. As a result, the chemical's impact on the pathway is lessened, reducing the drug-abuser's ability to enjoy the things that previously brought pleasure. This decrease compels those addicted to the dopaminergic-effect of the drug, to increase the drug consumption in order to re-create the earlier or initial experiences and to bring their "feel-good" hormone level back to normal —an effect known as tolerance. Development of dopamine tolerance can eventually lead to profound changes in neurons and brain circuits, with the potential to severely compromise the long-term health and functioning of a person's brain (http://www.drugabuse.gov/infofacts/understand.html). In addition, although clinical work has used DA receptor agonists and antagonists to treat drug-seeking behavior, their side effects preclude widespread use.

Recent work has focused more on the role of other receptors such as glutamate and-aminobutyricacid (GABA). Studies have shown that advanced stages of addiction, seem to depend mostly on adaptations in cortical glutamatergic projections to the nucleus accumbens (Wolf, 2002; Kelley, 2004; Kalivas and Volkow, 2005). In more recently, the findings of other receptor systems, especially the NMDA receptors are involved in drug addiction, opens new therapeutic avenues (Lu *et al*, 1999; Simoes *et al*, 2007; Kerdsan *et al*, 2009; MA *et al*, 2009).

Obsessive Compulsive Disorder

Obsessive–compulsive disorder (OCD) is a chronic anxiety disorder characterised by recurrent obsessions and compulsions aimed at reducing the distress caused by obsessional thinking. Lesions, functional neuro-imaging, and neuropsychological studies have indicated that the cortex- striatum-thalamus-cortex circuitry (A circuit linking the orbitofrontal cortex, caudate nucleus, globus pallidus, and the thalamus, known as the CSTC loop) may have a key role in the pathogenesis of OCD (Aouizerate *et al*,2004). The overall output of this pathway is inhibitory and is thought to serve as a counterweight to the excitatory positive feedback loop as described in this article. This inhibitory pathway also receives serotonergic projections from the midbrain into the striatum. These connections are hypothesized to contribute to the affective anxiety component of OCD symptoms. One would then expect OCD symptoms to appear when the CSTC loop is abnormally decreased (too little inhibition) (Shah *et al*, 2008). The clinical studies also shown the striatum are associated with the development of the OCD. For example, PET scanning studies in man have shown that sufferers from OCD exhibit abnormal activity in the prefrontal cortex and caudate nuclei. Recent SDM meta-analyses of voxel-based morphometry studies also have found people with OCD have increased grey matter volumes in bilateral lenticular nuclei, extending to the caudate nuclei(Joaquim and David, 2009; Joaquim *et al*, 2010).

The molecular mechanism of OCD is not known nowadays. However, neurotransmitters, such as dopamine and serotonin, may contribute to OCD. Dopamine receptors in the striatum have been also suggested to have a modulatory role (Saxena *et al*, 1998). For example, the dopamine D_2 receptors in OCD patients are down regulated compared with controls (Denys *et al*, 2004; Moresco *et al*, 2006). The serotonin is now a kind of prevailing transmitter associated with the OCD. This is largely based on the efficacy of serotonin reuptake inhibitors (SRIs) in the disorder. Independent studies have consistently found unusual dopamine and serotonin activity in various regions of the brain in individuals with OCD. These can be defined as dopaminergic hyperfunction in the prefrontal cortex and serotonergic hypofunction in the basal ganglia (Wee *et al*, 2004; Kim *et al*, 2007; Harsányi *et al*, 2007).

Behavioral therapy, cognitive behavioral therapy, and medications should be regarded as first-line treatments for OCD (Doctor's Guide, 2007). Psychodynamic psychotherapy may help in managing some aspects of the disorder. Electroconvulsive therapy has been found effective in severe and refractory cases (Cybulska *et al*, 2006). For some, medication, support groups and psychological treatments fail to alleviate obsessive–compulsive symptoms. These patients may choose to undergo psychosurgery as a last resort. In this procedure, a surgical lesion is made in an area of the brain. In one study, 30% of participants benefited significantly from this procedure (Barlow and Durand, 2006).Deep-brain stimulation is possible surgical options that do not require destruction of brain tissue (Shah *et al*, 2008).

References

Abigail M. Snyder1, Michael J. Zigmond2, Raymond D. Lund1.Sprouting of serotoninergic afferents into striatum after dopamine-depleting lesions in infant rats: A retrograde transport and immunocytochemical study.*The Journal of Comparative Neurology* 1986; 245(2):274–281.

Aouizerate, B. et al. Pathophysiology of obsessive-compulsive disorder: a necessary link between phenomenology, neuropsychology, imagery and physiology. *Prog. Neurobiol* 2004.;72: 195–221.

Ab Radua, Joaquim; van den Heuvel, Odile A.; Surguladze, Simon; Mataix-Cols, David. Meta-analytical comparison of voxel-based morphometry studies in obsessive-compulsive disorder vs other anxiety disorders. *Archives of General Psychiatry* 2010;67(7):701–711.

Aziz TZ, Green AL.Dystonia: a surgeon's perspective.Parkinsonism Relat Disord.2009;15 Suppl 3:S75-80.

Aoulzerate B, Cuny E, Martln-Guehl C, Guehl D, Amleva H,Benazzouz A, et al. Deep brain stimulation of the ventral cau-date nucleus in the treatment of obsessive-compulsive disorder and maior depression. *J. Neurosure* 2004:101:682-6.

Bronstein JM, Tagliati M, Alterman RL, et al. Deep brain stimulation for Parkinson disease: an expert consensus and review of key issues. *Arch. Neurol* 2011 ;68 (2): 165.

Barlow, D. H. and V. M. Durand. *Essentials of Abnormal Psychology*. California: Thomson Wadsworth, 2006.

Birkmayer, W. and HornykiewirL, O. The L-3,4-dioxyphenylalanine (DOPA)-effect in Parkinson-akinesia. Wien Klin Wochenschr.1961; (10)73:787-8.

Birkmayer, W. and HornykiewirL, O. Der L-Dopa Effekt beim Parkinson-Syndrom des Menschen. Zur Palhogenese and Behandlung der Parkinson-Akinese. *Arch. Psyichiat. Nervenkr* 1962; 203:560-574.

Bolam J, Hanley J, Booth P, et al. Synaptic organization of the basal ganglia. *Anat* 2000;196:527-542.

Carmichael ST, Price JL. Limbic connections of the orbital and medial prefrontal cortex in macaque monkeys. *Comp. Neurol.* 1996;363: 615-641.

Carpenter MB, Peter P. Nigrostriatal and nigrothalamic fibers in the rhesus monjey. *Comp. Neurol.* 1971 ;144: 93-116.

C.H. Kima, K.A. Cheond, M.-S. Kood, e, Y.H. Ryub, J.D. Leeb, J.W. Changc, H.S. Leea. Dopamine Transporter Density in the Basal Ganglia in Obsessive-Compulsive Disorder, Measured with[123I]IPT SPECT before and after Treatment with Serotonin Reuptake Inhibitors. *Neuropsychobiology* 2007;55:156-162.

Chikama M, McFarland N, Amaral DG, Haber SN. Insular cortical projections to functional regions of the striatum correlate with cortical cytoarchitectonic organization in the primate. *Neurosci* 17: 9686-9705.

Dahlström A, Fuxe K . Localization of monoamines in the lower brain stem. *Experientia* 1964;20: 398–399.

Durieux PF, Schiffmann SN, de Kerchove d'Exaerde A.Front Neuroanat. *Targeting neuronal populations of the striatum* 2011;5:40.

Doctor's Guide. New guidelines to set standards for best treatment of OCD. Doctor's Guide Publishing, Ltd.2007.

Dr A. M. Lozano. The pedunculopontine nucleus and Parkinson's disease.*Brain* 2000; 123 (9):1767-1783.

Dr R. M. Zweig MD1, W. R. Jankel PhD2, J. C. Hedreen MD1, R. Mayeux MD3, D. L. Price MD1,2,4.The pedunculopontine nucleus in Parkinson's disease.*Annals of Neurology* 1989; 26(1): 41–46.

Eva M Cybulska. Obsessive Compulsive disorder, the brain and electroconvulsive therapy. *British Journal of Hospital Medicine* 2006;67(2):77-82.

Friederici and Kotz, 2003 A.D. Friederici and S.A. Kotz. The brain basis of syntactic processes, functional imaging and lesion studies. *Neuroimage* 20 (1) 2003 :8–17.

Flaherty AW, Graybiel AM . Input-output organization of the sensorimotor striatum in the squirrel monkey. *Neurosci* 1994;14: 599-610.

Flores-Barrera E, Vizcarra-Chacón BJ, Tapia D, Bargas J, Galarraga E. Different corticostriatal integration in spiny projection neurons from direct and indirect pathways. *Front Syst Neurosci.*2010;10(4):15.

Ferreira TL ; Shammah-Lagnado SJ;Bueno OF. The indirect amygdala-dorsal striatum pathway mediates conditioned freezing: insights on emotional memory networks. *Neuroscience* 2008.153(1):84-94.

Goldman-Rakic PS, Selemon LD. Topography of corticostriatal projections in nonhuman primates and implicatinos for functional parcellation of the neostriatum. *Cerebral cortex* 1986; (5) 4447-466.

Gerfen CR. Synaptic organization of the striatum. *Electron Microsc. Tech.* 1988;10(3):265-81.

Graybiel, A. M. and Rauch, S. L. Toward a neurobiology of obsessive-compulsive disorder. *Neuron* 2000;28:343–347 .

Goelz, C. G. Dopaminergic agonises in Lhe Lreaunenl of Parkinson's disease. *Neurology* 1990;46: 50-57.

Gross CE, Boraud T, Guehl D, Bioulac B, Bezard E.From experimentation to the surgical treatment of Parkinson's disease: prelude or suite in basal ganglia research? *Prog. Neurobiol.* 1999 ; 59(5):509-32.

Haber SN, Kunishio K, Mizobuchi M, Lynd-Balta E. The orbital and medial prefrontal circuit through the primate basal ganglia. *Neurosci.* 1995;15: 4851-4867.

Hauber W. Involvement of basal ganglia transmitter systems in movement initiation. *Prog. Neurobiol* 1998;45:507-540.

Haber SN. Neurotransmitters in the human and nonhuman primate basal ganglia. *Hum. Neurobiol.* 1986; 5(3):159-68.

Harsányi A, Csigó K, Demeter G, Németh A.New approach to obsessive-compulsive disorder: dopaminergic theories. *Psychiatr. Hung.* 2007;22(4):248-58.

Helen Bronte-Stewart. Surgical therapy for dystonia. Current Neurology and *Neuroscience Reports* 2003; 3(4): 296-305.

Janet M. Kemp and T. P. S. Powell.The Connexions of the Striatum and Globus Pallidus: Synthesis and Speculation. *Phil. Trans. R. Soc. Lond. B* 1971; 262 (845): 441-457.

Kunishio K,Haber SN. Primate cingulostriatal projection:limbic striatal versus sensorimotor striatal input.*Comp. Neurol.* 1994;350:337-356.

Kunzle H. Bilateral projections from precentral motor cortex to the putamen and other parts of the basal ganglia. An autoradiographic study in Macaca fascicularis. *Brain Res.* 1975;88:195-209.

Kunzle H. An autoradiographic analysis of the efferent connections from premotor and adjacent prefrontal regions (areas 6 and 9)in Macaca fascicularis. *Brain Behav. Evol.* 1978;185-234.

Lauren M. Tanabe, Connie E. Kim, Noga Alagem and William T. Dauer. Primary dystonia: molecules and mechanisms. *Nat. Rev. Neurol.* 2009;5:598–609.

Levy, L. M. and Hallett, M. Impaired brain GABA in focal dystonia. *Ann. Neurol.* 2002;51:93–101.

Lees,A. J. Levodopa substitution: the gold standard. *Clin.Neuropharmac* 1994;17: S1-S6.

Lieberman, A. N. and Goldslein,M. Bromocripline in Parkinson's disease. *Pharmac.Rev.* 1985;37,217-227.

Joel D ; Weiner I. The connections of the dopaminergic system with the striatum in rats and primates: an analysis with respect to the functional and compartmental organization of the striatum. *Neuroscience* 2000;96(3):451-74.

Lars-Göran Nygren and Lars Olson.A new major projection from locus coeruleus: The main source of noradrenergic nerve terminals in the ventral and dorsal columns of the spinal cord. *Brain Research* 1977;132(1): 85-93.

McGinty JF. Co-localization of GABA with other neuroactive substances in the basal ganglia. *Prog. Brain Res*.2007;160:273-84.

McGeer EG, Staines WA, McGeer PLCan. Neurotransmitters in the basal ganglia. *Neurol. S*ci.1984;11(1):89-99.

Martin, John Joseph. *Neuroanatomy: text and atlas*. New York: McGraw-Hill 2003:393.

M. Carbon, M. Niethammer, S. Peng, D. Raymond, V. Dhawan, T. Chaly, Y. Ma, S. Bressman and D. Eidelberg.Abnormal striatal and thalamic dopamine neurotransmission: Genotype- related features of dystonia. *Neurology* 2009;72:2097-2103.

Moro A, Tettamanti M, Perani D, Donati C, Cappa SF, and Fazio F.Syntax and the brain: disentangling grammar by selective anomalies. *NeuroImage* 2001;13: 110-118.

Ma YY, Cepeda C, Cui CL. The role of striatal NMDA receptors in drug addiction. *Int. Rev. Neurobiol*.2009;89:131-46.

Marc Teichmann, Emmanuel Dupoux, Sid Kouider, and Anne-Catherine Bachoud-Lévi.The Role of the Striatum in Processing Language Rules: *Evidence from Word Perception in Huntington's Disease* 2006;18(9): 1555-1569.

Marc Teichmann,Emmanuel Dupoux, Sid Kouider, Pierre Brugières, Marie-Françoise Boissé,Sophie Baudic, Pierre Cesaro, Marc Peschanski1 and Anne-Catherine Bachoud-Lévi. The role of the striatum in rule application: the model of Huntington's disease at early stage. *Brain* 2005;128 (5): 1155-1167.

Marc Teichmann, Isabelle Darcyd, Anne-Catherine Bachoud-Levi and Emmanuel Dupoux. The role of the striatum in phonological processing. Evidence from early stages of Huntington's disease. *Cortex*. 2009;45(7):839-49.

Naomi Lubarr and Susan Bressman. *Treatment of Generalized Dystonia*.2011; 13(3): 274-289.

NIDA InfoFacts. *Understanding Drug Abuse and Addiction*. National Institutes of Health 2008.

National Collaborating Centre for Chronic Conditions, ed. Symptomatic pharmacological therapy in Parkinson's disease. *Parkinson's Disease*. London: Royal College of Physicians 2006.

Nic J. van der Wee, M.D., Henk Stevens, M.D., Ph.D., Johannes A. Hardeman, M.D., Rene C. Mandl, M.S., Damiaan A. Denys, M.D., Harold J. van Megen, M.D., Ph.D., René S. Kahn, M.D., Ph.D., and Herman M. Westenberg, Ph.D.Enhanced Dopamine Transporter Density in Psychotropic-Naive Patients With Obsessive-Compulsive Disorder Shown by [123I] ß-CIT SPECT. *Am. J. Psychiatry* 2004; 161:2201-2206.

Nambu, A. A new dynamic model of the cortico-basal ganglia loop. *Prog. Brain Res.* 2004; 143: 461-466.

Oscar Marín1, Agustín González1 .Wilhelmus J.A.J. Smeets2.Basal ganglia organization in amphibians: Afferent connections to the striatum and the nucleus accumbens.*Comparative Neurology* 1997; 378(1):16-49.

Obeso JA, Rodríguez-Oroz MC, Benitez-Temino B, et al. Functional organization of the basal ganglia: therapeutic implications for Parkinson's disease. *Mov. Disord* 2008; 23 (Suppl 3): S548–59.

Pontieri, F. E., Tanda, G., Orzi, F.,andDi Chiara, G.. Effects of nicotine on the nucleus accumbens and similarity to those of addictive drugs. *Nature* 1996; 382: 255-257.

Pieter Voorn, Louk J. M. J. Vanderschuren, Henk J. Groenewegen, Trevor W. Robbins and Cyriel M. A. Pennartz.Putting a spin on the dorsal-ventral divide of the striatum. *Trends in Neurosciences* 2004; 27 (8) 1: 468-474.

Philippe Mailly,Stéphane Charpier,Annie Menetrey, and Jean-Michel Deniau.Three-Dimensional Organization of the Recurrent Axon Collateral Network of the Substantia Nigra Pars Reticulata Neurons in the Rat. *The Journal of Neuroscience* 2003; 23(12):5247-5257.

Pieter Voorn, Louk J. M. J. Vanderschuren, Henk J. Groenewegen, Trevor W. Robbins and Cyriel M. A. Pennartz. Putting a spin on the dorsal-ventral divide of the striatum. *Trends in Neurosciences* 2004;27(8):468-474.

Richard Newman, Sarah Schilling Winans.An experimental study of the ventral striatum of the golden hamster. I. Neuronal connections of the nucleus accumbens. *The Journal of Comparative Neurology* 1980;191(2):167–192.

R. Tao and S.B. Auerbach.Involvement of the dorsal raphe but not median raphe nucleus in morphine-induced increases in serotonin release in the rat forebrain. *Neuroscience* 1995;68(2): 553-561.

R.M. Beckstead, a and C.J. Cruza.Striatal axons to the globus pallidus, entopeduncular nucleus and substantia nigra come mainly from separate cell populations in cat .*Neuroscience* 1986;19(1):147-158.

Rosell A, Giménez-Amaya JM . Anatomical re-evaluation of the corticostriatal projections to the caudate nucleus: a retrograde labeling study in the cat. *Neurosci. Res.* 1999;34(4):257–69.

Stocco, Andrea; Lebiere, Christian; Anderson, John R. Conditional routing of information to the cortex: A model of the basal ganglia's role in cognitive coordination. *Psychological Review* 2010; 117 (2): 541–74.

Semba K, Fibiger HC, Vincent SR. Neurotransmitters in the mammalian striatum: neuronal circuits and heterogeneity. *Can J Neurol Sci.* 1987;14(3):386-94.

Radua, Joaquim; Mataix-Cols, David. Voxel-wise meta-analysis of grey matter changes in obsessive–compulsive disorder. *British Journal of Psychiatry* 2009;195 (5): 393–402.

R. J. Beukers and J. Booij and N. Weisscher and F. Zijlstra and T. A. M. J. van Amelsvoortand M. A. J. Tijssen. Reduced striatal D receptor binding in myoclonus–dystonia. *Eur. J. Nucl. Med. Mol. Imaging* 2009; 36:269–274.

Rosalie Sherman and K Ray Chaudhuri.Current Treatment Options in Neurology Dystonia. *Movement Disorders in Clinical Practice* 2010;49-66.

Rosell A, Giménez-Amaya JM. Anatomical re-evaluation of the corticostriatal projections to the caudate nucleus: a retro grade labeling study in the cat. *Neurosci. Res.* 1999;34 (4): 257–69.

Shah DB, Pesiridou A, Baltuch GH, Malone DA, O'Reardon JP. Functional neurosurgery in the treatment of severe obsessive compulsive disorder and major depression: overview of disease circuits and therapeutic targeting for the clinician. *Psychiatry* (Edgmont) 2008; 5(9):24-33.

Tettamanti M, Moro A, Messa C, Moresco RM, Rizzo G, Carpinelli A, Matarrese M, Fazio F, Perani D.Basal ganglia and language: phonology modulates dopaminergic release. *Neuroreport.* 2005 15;16(4):397-401.

Ubeda-Bañon I, Novejarque A, Mohedano-Moriano A, et al. Projections from the posterolateral olfactory amygdala to the ventral striatum: neural basis for reinforcing properties of chemical stimuli. *BMC Neuroscience* 2007, 8:103.

Ullman MT, Corkin S, Coppola M, Hickok G, Growdon JH,Koroshetz WJ, et al. A neural dissociation within language:evidence that the mental dictionary is part of declarative memory, and that grammatical rules are processed by the procedural system. *Journal of Cognitive Neuroscience* 1997; 9: 266-276.

Vannest J, Polk TA, and Lewis RL. Dual-route processing of complex words: new fMRI evidence from derivational suffixation. *Cognitive, Affectiue and Behavioral Neuroscience* 2005; 5: 67-76.

Wilson, C.J. Basal Ganglia In: G. M. Shepherd (ed.) *The Synaptic Organization of the Brain.* Oxford University Press, Oxford 2004: 361-414.

Yelnik J, Francois C, Percheron G. Spatial relationships between striatal axonal endings and pallidal neurons in macaque monkeys. *Adv. Neurol.* 1997;74:45-56.

Zhang T, Zhang L, Liang Y, Siapas AG, Zhou FM, Dani JA.Dopamine signaling differences in the nucleus accumbens and dorsal striatum exploited by nicotine. *Neurosci.* 2009; 29(13):4035-43.

In: Striatum: Anatomy, Functions and Role in Disease
Editors: Hugo T. Maldonado and Ignacio M. Ortega
ISBN 978-1-61942-384-8

Chapter VII

Effects of Experience on Striatal Morphology

Paola De Bartolo[1,2], Francesca Gelfo[2], Lorena Burello[1,2] and Laura Petrosini[1,2]
[1]Department of Psychology, "Sapienza" University of Rome, Rome, Italy
[2]I.R.C.C.S. S. Lucia Foundation, Rome, Italy

Abstract

The neostriatum is considered a key-structure in the induction of goal-directed movements or in the suppression of movements. A complex neuronal network regulates these functions by involving different cell populations, such as spiny projection neurons and several types of aspiny interneurons. This chapter will focus on anatomical features of striatal cells and their circuitries to better understand how morphology sustains striatal activities.

Lifespan experience has been demonstrated to affect brain function inducing plastic remodelling of brain structure. Such a form of plasticity consists in cerebral adaptation to always changing information by means of generation of new synapses or reorganization of existing neuronal circuits in response to environmental experience. Moreover, brain plastic properties are heavily recruited to restore impaired abilities when damage occurs. This fundamental topic will be faced up in relation to experience-dependent morphological changes in striatal neurons, considering the involvement of the neostriatum in a number of motor-related diseases.

Introduction

The basal ganglia are a group of subcortical nuclei involved in a variety of processes including motor, associative, cognitive and mnemonic functions. The dorsal division of basal ganglia consists of the neostriatum (or caudate-putamen), the globus pallidus, the subthalamic nucleus and the substantia nigra. In addition to these structures - which are associated with motor and associative functions - there is a ventral division of the basal ganglia (ventral striatum or nucleus accumbens; ventral pallidum and ventral tegmental area) that is associated with limbic functions.

This chapter will focus the attention on the neostriatum that is the major division of the basal ganglia. It receives the majority of afferent inputs and is arguably the principal site within the basal ganglia where information processing occurs. This issue will be faced up by reviewing evidence arising from animal studies.

Morphological Features of Neostriatal Neurons

The neostriatum receives input from the whole of the cortical mantle. The cortico-striatal axons mainly innervate the GABAergic (γ-aminobutyric acid) medium-sized densely spiny neurons (MSNs), which account for the large majority of neostriatal neurons. In turn, these MSNs project preferentially to the output nuclei (the internal segment of globus pallidus and the pars reticulate of substantia nigra) of the basal ganglia (*direct pathway*) or to the external segment of globus pallidus and thence to the output nuclei (*indirect pathway*).

The remaining neurons of the neostriatum are interneurons. They have been classified, based on morphology, neurochemistry and physiology, into one population of cholinergic cells and at least three distinct types of GABAergic interneurons. The GABAergic interneurons colocalize the calcium binding proteins parvalbumin or calretinin, or neuropeptide Y, somatostatin and NADPH diaphorase (Kawaguchi, 1993). There are two major potential sources of inhibition acting on MSNs in the neostriatum: *feedforward inhibition* from the GABAergic interneurons and *feedback inhibition* from the axon collaterals of the MSNs themselves.

MSNs. Striatal projection cells are MSNs. Soma diameter of these neurons is about 15 μm and their collaterals branch from their axons before the axons exit the neostriatum. They account for the 90-95% of the total population of the striatal neurons, utilize GABA as their major neurotransmitter and are subdivided into two major populations on the basis of their projection region, pattern of axonal collateralization and their neurochemical content. One population projects preferentially to the output nuclei of the basal ganglia (*direct pathway*) and expresses - in addition to GABA - the neuropeptides substance P and dynorphin and the D1 subtype of dopamine receptors. The second subpopulation projects almost exclusively to the globus pallidus (*indirect pathway*) and expresses enkephalin and the D2 subtype of dopamine receptors. Evidence from morphological studies - such as Golgi impregnation and intracellular filling of neurons - demonstrated that MSNs also give rise to extensive local axon collaterals, one of the major synaptic targets of which are other MSNs. This is supported by the findings that terminals display immunoreactivity for the neuropeptides expressed by MSNs - such as substance P or enkephalin - possess the morphological features of MSNs terminals and make symmetric synaptic contact with the dendrites, spines and soma of MSNs. The early anterograde degeneration studies demonstrated that corticostriatal terminals form asymmetric synapses primarily with dendritic spines. The fact that MSNs are the major spine-bearing neurons in the neostriatum indicates that these cells are likely to be the major target of cortico-striatal projections. It has been proposed that an individual cortical neuron makes very few synaptic contacts with an individual neostriatal neuron, that there is a high degree of convergence of cortical neurons onto individual striatal neurons but close neighbors do not share common cortical inputs. The activation of cortico-striatal neurons leads to the release of glutamate, activation of both AMPA and NMDA receptors that are localized almost exclusively within the synapse which leads to a depolarization of the neuron; a train of action potentials follows if there is sufficient convergent excitatory input to an individual MSN.

The excitatory cortical input to MSNs is modulated by the many other inputs to spiny neurons, including those from extrinsic sources and from local interneurons. Details of local interneurons are described below.

For further information see: Bolam, Hanle, Boot, and Bevan, 2000; Kawaguchi, 1993; Kawaguchi, 1997.

GABAergic interneurons. As mentioned above, there are three subtypes of neostriatal GABAergic interneurons and together comprise about 2% of the total neostriatal cell population.

The best characterized are those that express the calcium binding protein parvalbumin (PV). On the basis of their electrophysiological properties they are referred to as fast-spiking interneurons (FSIs). Their soma (round or oval) average 16-18 μm in diameter and issue aspiny dendrites that branch modestly. There is some morphological heterogeneity, with one subtype exhibiting a smaller soma and a relatively restricted and varicose dendritic arborization in the region of 200-300 μm in diameter, and the other displaying a larger cell body and a more extended non-varicose dendritic field of 500-600 μm in diameter. The neurons are characterized by an extremely dense local axonal plexus surrounding and extending beyond the dendritic field of the cell of origin that is heavily invested with presynaptic buttons. Unbiased stereological estimates of FS interneurons put their numbers at about 0.7% of the total in rat neostriatum. The strong medio-lateral gradient in PV-positive axons and terminals suggests that these cells might be more integral to functioning in the lateral neostriatum than those in the medial neostriatum. The neurons are similar in many ways to PV-expressing GABAergic interneurons in cortex and hippocampus. They exert powerful monosynaptic inhibition of MSNs through multiple perisomatic synapses and are themselves electronically coupled by way of gap junctions. FSIs receive a powerful excitatory input from the cortex that is different in character from the input received by MSNs, GABAergic input from MSNs and other interneurons. They also receive a cholinergic input. The predominant synaptic target of the FSI is the MSN. Single spikes in FSIs produce large unitary inhibitory postsynaptic potentials (IPSPs) in MSNs of about 1mV, and short bursts of action potentials in FSIs lead to IPSPs that can summate up to about 7mV in MSNs. The IPSP representing the *feedforward inhibition* from FSIs is strong enough to delay or completely suppress firing in MSNs, and is much larger and more powerful at the soma than the IPSP produced by the axon collaterals of the MSNs (*feedback inhibition*).

A second kind of neostriatal GABAergic interneurons colocalizes the calcium binding protein calretinin. These neurons represent 0.8% of neostriatal neurons in rat. They are of medium size, possess few, aspiny, infrequently branching dendrites and are relatively sparse in the caudal components of neostriatum. There are no electrophysiological data from intracellularly labeled neurons identified as calretinin-positive, so their electrophysiological profile remains unknown.

The third kind of GABAergic interneurons is distinguished by the absence of calcium binding proteins and by the presence of NPY, somatostatine, nitric oxide synthase and NADPH diaphorase. These neurons are of medium size and comprise about 0.8% of neostriatal cells in rats. They have the least dense axonal arborizations of any of the striatal interneurons. The neurons receive both cholinergic and dopaminergic input and are characterized electrophysiologically by low threshold calcium spikes and prolonged calcium dependent plateau potentials. They have therefore been termed persistent and low-threshold spike neurons. Single action potentials in the cell produce large inhibitory postsynaptic current.

For further information see: Kawaguchi, 1993; Kawaguchi, Wilson, Augood, and Emson, 1995; Koòs and Tepper, 1999; Plotkin, Wu, Chesselet, and Levine, 2005; Tepper and Bolam, 2004; Tepper, Tecuapetla, Koòs, and Ibàñez-Sandoval, 2010; Tepper, Wilson, and Koòs, 2008.

Cholinergic interneurons. The largest neurons in the neostriatum, with a somatic diameter that can be in excess of 40 μm are the giant cholinergic aspiny neurons. In the rat they comprise only about 0.3% of the striatal neurons. These cells have large polygonal or fusiform cell bodies and emit three-six thick, smooth primary dendrites that branch moderately to form a dendritic arborization up to 1 mm in diameter. Excitatory inputs arise from cortex and thalamus. The neurons also receive GABAergic inputs from MSNs as well as dopaminergic inputs from the substantia nigra. The dense and widespread local axons collateral plexus of a cholinergic interneuron is largely restricted to the neostriatal matrix where it primarily targets the MSNs, although GABAergic interneurons also receive cholinergic synaptic inputs. *In vivo* they fire tonically but irregularly in response to excitatory synaptic inputs because they are relatively depolarized and their resting potential is close to the spike threshold. It has been proposed that cholinergic interneurons participate in the modulation of MSNs activity and hence the functioning of the neostriatal circuits that underlie reward-based learning and/or motivated behavior.

For further information see: Kawaguchi, 1993; Kawaguchi, Wilson, Augood, and Emson, 1995; Tepper and Bolam, 2004.

Experience-Dependent Structural Plasticity in the Brain

The nervous system is a continuously changing structure with powerful plastic properties. Across the entire lifespan, experience-dependent neuroplasticity underlies learning of new competencies in response to ever-changing environmental experiences. In fact, sensory, cognitive and motor stimulations arising from environment have a key-role in refining neuronal circuitries required for brain function.

Most of our understanding of the environmental effects on brain is a result of research on laboratory rodents, in which housing environment complexity is manipulated. Typically, laboratory rats live in small cages with one or two cage mates and with food and water provided *ad libitum*. These conditions are compatible with growth and health that are "normal" by present animal care standards. However, in wildlife, rats live in and deal with much more complex environments. In this regard, for the first time during the 1940's Hebb described a form of environmental complexity in a neuroscientific context. He compared rats allowed to roam freely in his home with rats left in laboratory cages, showing that "free" rats displayed improved problem-solving capacities (Hebb, 1947).

It wasn't until the late 1950's that the American psychologist Rosenzweig and his colleagues rendered the environmental enrichment (EE) a scientific and testable concept, developing an experimental protocol for rats (Rosenzweig, Krech, Bennet and Diamond, 1962; Rosenzweig, 1966; Rosenzweig and Bennett, 1978). An enriched environment is defined as "a combination of complex inanimate and social stimulation". Four basilar components are needed and handled: social interaction, environmental exploration, exposition to novelty and physical activity. Thus, usually "enriched" animals are housed in large cages containing a large number of conspecifics (10-14), giving them opportunities to establish complex social relationships. Furthermore, the animals are constantly stimulated since they may interact with a great variety of objects (tunnels, materials for nest construction, wheels for travel and running, tubes, ladders, toys) that are frequently renewed to ensure an increasingly diverse environment. The provision of food and water is changed over time to encourage environmental exploration and exposure to new things. It must be stressed, however, that an enriched environment is enriched only in comparison to standard laboratory conditions, that is only in relation to the state of relative deprivation associated with rearing in small cages with perhaps only one other conspecific (Sale, Berardi, and Maffei, 2009).

Changes in cerebral structure as a result of EE have been observed in cortical weight and thickness, dimension of cerebral hemispheres, extension of dendritic branching, density of dendritic spines and size of synaptic contact areas (Greenough, Black, and Wallace, 1987; Kolb, Forgie, Gibb, Gorny, and Rowntree, 1998). These parameters are considered valid indicators of neuronal plasticity. In fact, the dendritic surface receives more than 95% of the synapses of a neuron, so the change in the number of synapses can be inferred by measuring the extent of dendritic trees. Furthermore, synaptic density reflects the distribution of dendritic spines on the dendrites because of more than 90% of the synapses involving dendritic spines; by using the count of dendritic spines, it is possible to have a reasonable estimate of synapse counts. The exposure to a protracted enrichment of animals from weaning onward induces a sharp increase in the spine density and dendritic arborizations both in parietal and in frontal cortices (Leggio et al., 2005; Gelfo, De Bartolo, Giovine, Petrosini, and Leggio, 2009). Furthermore, EE increases hippocampal neurogenesis and the integration of these newly born cells into functional circuits (Kempermann, Kuhn, and Gage, 1997; Bruel-Junrgeman, Laroche, and Rampon, 2005). A wide range of research on the molecular mechanisms of EE effects have been aimed at finding promising molecules that reproduce the beneficial effects of enriched experience. Following the early studies by Rosenzweig who showed an increase of the cholinergic system in response to EE, other neurotransmitter systems, such as the serotoninergic and noradrenergic systems, have been reported to be affected by EE. A group of molecules particularly sensitive to environmental stimuli are the neurotrophins, factors strongly implicated in the structural and functional plasticity during development and adulthood (Gelfo et al., 2010; Sale, Berardi, and Maffei, 2009). EE also increases the expression of synaptic proteins, such as the presynaptic vesicle protein synaptophysin and postsynaptic density-95 protein (PSD-95) (Lambert, Fernandez, and Frick, 2005), consistently with EE-induced enhancement of experience-dependent synaptogenesis. Furthermore, EE induces alterations of the expression of NMDA and AMPA receptor subunits, which are integral for glutamatergic signalling (Naka, Narita, Okado, and Narita, 2005), consistently with evidence that EE evokes increased synaptic plasticity (Nithianantharajah and Hannan, 2006). Such structural and molecular EE-induced modifications have been demonstrated to impact on behavior. Enriched subjects show greater abilities to adapt or to cope with highly conflicting and demanding environmental situations (De Bartolo et al., 2008; Foti et al., 2010; Leggio et al., 2005; Mandolesi et al., 2008). In addition, exposure to enriched environment is able to counteract the cognitive decline associated with aging (Van Praag, Kempermann, and Gage, 2000) and to decrease anxiety and increase exploratory activity (De Bartolo et al., 2008; Foti et al., 2010; Leggio et al., 2005; Mandolesi et al., 2008).

EE elicits beneficial effects not only in intact subjects – as described above – but also in brain lesioned subjects. Namely, exposure to enriched living conditions subsequent to lesion results in improved behavioral outcomes on several sensori-motor tasks following focal ischemic injury, status epilepticus, or subicular lesion (see Petrosini et al., 2009 for a review). EE used as rehabilitative technique is reported to stabilize or improve functional outcomes after cholinergic damage or in transgenic mouse models of Alzheimer's, Huntington's and Parkinson's Diseases (see Nithianantharajah and Hannan, 2006 for a review). A number of studies determined if a cerebral reserve could be "built up" to face up pathology or aging by exposing subjects to complex experiences before brain lesion or aging. Indeed, previously enriched animals can show no or reduced cognitive impairment following pathological events, and EE animals show restored synaptic connectivity or neurogenesis (Mandolesi et al., 2008; Nithianantharajah and Hannan, 2011; Petrosini et al., 2009; Van Dellen, Cordery, Spires, Blakemore and Hannan, 2008).

Structural Effects of Complex Experiences in the Neostriatum

Studies on Healthy Subjects

Exposure to an EE has been shown to induce marked plastic changes in the brain. The positive effects of enriched environmental stimulation are not limited to primary sensory pathways, association area and hippocampal formation – as already described – but may also entail neostriatal structures.

Despite no large-scale studies concerning the neostriatum has been described, Thiriet et al. (2008) provided a detailed demonstration that rearing mice in an enriched environment from weaning to adulthood induced a complex pattern of transcriptional changes in the neostriatum. Gene transcripts that were influenced by EE in a cDNA array analysis belonged to classes of genes playing a role in cell proliferation and differentiation, intracellular signalling, structural changes and cell metabolism. Among genes involved in cellular signalling, it is worth of note that the protein kinase C (PKC) lambda was up-regulated by EE. Indeed, PKC lambda is known to participate in synaptic plasticity and then can play a role in the structural changes induced by EE. Another gene found to be up-regulated by EE is the dynamin 1-like (DMN-1L) that has been shown to be involved in synaptic vesicle recycling. Thus, its up-regulation in enriched animals may indicate increased synaptic vesicle recycling associated with increased synaptic plasticity. EE also regulated other genes involved in cell structure changes (synaptotagmin-like 4, Actinin alpha 3, Decorin, Actin alpha 2) and remodeling of axonal connections (GPI-anchored membrane protein 1, Tissue inhibitor 4, Vasodilator-stimulated phosphoprotein). Altogether, these results indicate that gene transcript alterations of enriched animals are related to long-lasting adaptations in neostriatal morphology.

As a further matter, responsiveness of the neostriatum to the environmental complexity has been demonstrated even when the EE period started in adulthood. Studies indicated that adult animals acutely exposed to EE showed a striking neostriatal up-regulation of mRNA products of the activity-regulated cytoskeletal protein (arc) (Pinaud, Penner, Robertson, and Currie, 2001) and the nerve growth factor induced gene-A (NGFI-A) (Pinaud et al., 2002). These are both immediate early genes postulated to be involved in the early genetic steps of neural plasticity leading to more stable structural modifications. Namely, arc translation takes place in polyribosomal complexes located in the post-synaptic density and then the protein encoded by this gene is thought to be involved in plastic changes of dendritic configuration. NGFI-A (also known as zif-268, Krox-24, Egr-1 or ZENK), instead, is able to regulate the expression of two key proteins for synaptic function as synapsin I and II. Therefore, the EE-induced up-regulation of arc and NGFI-A in adulthood supports a life-long neostriatal sensitivity to experience as well as a reorganization of neostriatal neurons in response to enhanced environmental complexity.

Interestingly, morphological studies not only confirm the profound remodeling suggested by gene and mRNA alterations but also indicate that different classes of neostriatal neurons exhibit different modalities of structural plasticity following a similar exposure to a complex environment.

The MSNs have been the most frequently analyzed neostriatal neurons. It has been showed that morphological plasticity of these neurons after a rearing in enriched environment was not affected when two measures of neuronal growth were considered: total cell volume and total dendritic length (Faherty, Kerley, and Smeyne, 2003). Instead, a similar EE protocol greatly affected morphology of MSNs when a different parameter of plasticity, i.e. dendritic spine density was analyzed. Animals reared in complex environments displayed indeed spine density increased of about 30% in comparison to animals individually reared (Comery, Shah, and Greenough, 1995). This plastic change has been related to an enhancement of motor activity during complex environment exposure. Subsequently, the same research group has further detailed this observation by considering EE-induced alterations in the density of multiple-headed dendritic spines (Comery, Stamoudis, Irwin, and Greenough, 1996). They found that enriched animals exhibited an increase of about 60% in density of multiple-head spines on MSNs dendrites relatively to animals reared individually. Remarkably, this increase was considerably greater than the overall difference in spine density previously described (Comery et al., 1995). In this respect, spines added following an EE exposure either preferentially occurred on preexisting spines or preferentially formed multiple heads.

Studies on Models of Pathologies

Experience-dependent plastic rearrangements of the brain are heavily recruited in case of damage. A complex stimulation seems to be able to create a more effective neuronal network to better sustain complex functions. It has been demonstrated that animals reared from weaning in EE show less vulnerability to brain injury and exhibit better capability of functional recovery. Moreover, therapeutic exposition to EE after brain damage - even if of short duration - improves functional recovery. Structural changes associated to the functional improvement are supposed to support it. In particular, a number of studies investigated experience-dependent neostriatal plastic changes in several animal models of pathologies. In such studies, neuronal morphological changes were associated to an improved coping to the functional impairment. Such works were focused on diseases involving the neostriatum, inducing a number of motor dysfunctions (intracerebral hemorrhage, stereotyped behavior, Huntington's Disease, Parkinson's Disease).

Intrastriatal hemorrhage (ISH). Recent studies investigated in rodents the effects of therapeutic exposition to EE after ISH (Auriat, Wowk, and Colbourne, 2010; MacLellan, Plummer, Silasi, Auriat, and Colbourne, 2011). In humans, ISH is a cerebral vascular accident causing long-term impairments of motor function and activity of daily livings. In the cited studies, ISH was modeled in adult rats by the unilateral infusion of collagenase or autologous whole blood in the neostriatum. Both kinds of lesion induced motor impairment in behavioral testing (skilled reaching, walking). Two weeks of rehabilitative exposition to EE (starting one week after the lesion) provoked a significant improvement in motor deficits. In association, the effects of rehabilitation on dendritic morphology of MSNs of lesioned animals were assessed. In the first model of ISH, enriched animals showed a significant increase of MSN dendritic length in peri-hematoma and contralateral neostriatum, not accompanied by change in neurogenesis. So, the structural rearrangement contributing to functional recovery appears to be in this case synaptogenesis, and not replacement of lost cells (Auriat et al., 2010). Differently, after whole blood-induced ISH rehabilitative EE did not enhance MSN dendritic length. These different results may be related to insult severity, since collagenase model induces greater injury with consequent greater recruitment of contralateral structures in the recovery process (MacLellan et al., 2011).

Stereotyped behavior. EE-induced neostriatal plastic rearrangements have been studied in a mouse model of stereotyped behavior (Lewis, 2004; Turner, Lewis, and King, 2003; Turner, Yang, and Lewis, 2002; Turner and Lewis, 2003). Stereotypies are repetitive and rhythmical motor behaviors without any apparent purpose. These behaviors are an essential feature of autism and are frequently observed in subjects with mental retardation or other developmental disorders. Deer mice housed in standard laboratory conditions develop high rates of spontaneous and persistent stereotypies (e.g. jumping, backward flipping), providing a reliable experimental model. Exposition to EE from weaning onwards or in adulthood prevents the development of stereotyped behaviors in about 70% of deer mice. In mice reared in enriched environment for sixty days from weaning, this phenomenon was associated to increased neuronal metabolic activity in the neostriatum (Turner et al., 2002). Moreover, Turner and Lewis (2003) showed an increase in neostriatal level of brain-derived neurotrophic factor (BDNF), a neurotrophin highly promoting experience-dependent neuronal plasticity. In fact, EE was also found to induce increased spine density on neostriatal MSNs (Turner et al., 2003). The increase in synapse number appears to be the possible mechanism supporting the greater functional flexibility and adaptation of enriched nonstereotypic mice, through a more effective cortico-striatal circuitry.

Huntington's Disease (HD). EE effects on neostriatum have been investigated in transgenic HD mouse models (Spires et al., 2004a, 2004b). HD is a fatal inherited neurodegenerative disorder affecting neostriatum and cerebral cortex, characterized by progressive motor, cognitive and psychiatric symptoms. The R6 mouse model presents many of the features of human HD. These transgenic mice show a progressive behavioral deficit (hindlimb clasping on tail suspension, impaired performance on motor tests), hypoactivity, weight loss, cognitive decline and premature death. R6 mice exposed to EE from weaning have been found to show delayed onset and slowed progression of motor deficits in behavioral testing. As for molecular and morphological changes in the striatum, EE entirely rescued HD-induced reduction in neostriatal BDNF levels (Spires et al., 2004b). Nevertheless, no EE effects were found on HD-dependent reduction in MSNs dendritic spine density and dendritic spine length (Spires et al., 2004a). However, a different result was found in a set of studies regarding EE-effects on neostriatal graft morphology in another model of HD (Döbrössy and Dunnett, 2004, 2006). In this model, adult rats lesioned unilaterally in the lateral dorsal neostriatum with quinolinic acid received neostriatal grafts and were then exposed to EE. Enriched grafted animals showed a significantly better functional recovery when compared to the standard ones (Döbrössy and Dunnett, 2004). In association, enriched grafted animals exhibited greater spine density and larger cell volumes of MSNs (Döbrössy and Dunnett, 2006). Thus, EE is able to improve plastic integration of grafts in the damaged neostriatal circuitry.

Parkinson's Disease (PD). It is noteworthy that EE-dependent neostriatal rearrangements have been studied also in mouse models of PD (Bezard et al., 2003). PD is a progressive neurological disease inducing the loss of dopaminergic neurons in the substantia nigra pars compacta. The consequent impairment of the nigrostriatal system induces a variety of motor symptoms, including tremor, rigidity and dysfunctions in skilled movements. In mice, administration of 1-methyl-4-phenyl-1,2,3,6-tetradropyridine (MPTP) causes the same neuronal loss characterizing PD. In this model, previous exposition to EE has been found to protect against MPTP-induced neuronal loss (Bezard et al., 2003; Faherty, Raviie Shepherd, Herasimtschuk, and Smeyne, 2005). In association, an increase in neostriatal BDNF levels was found in EE-exposed animals (Bezard et al., 2003). This augment in neurotrophic expression indicates that presumably plastic rearrangements in neostriatal structure may be involved in the protective effect of EE against PD.

A Study on Extra-Striatal Pathology

As mentioned above, EE has beneficial rehabilitative and protective effects on symptoms of pathologies directly involving the neostriatum. However, our research group has recently demonstrated that EE evokes plastic rearrangements in the neostriatum also in the presence of cerebellar lesions. Many experimental and clinical studies have considered the cerebellum and the neostriatum as key structures in motor control that operate separately. In fact, their different role has been described in motor learning, timing, and order during execution of complex motor sequences. Unlike cerebellar regions, basal ganglia exhibit planning-related activity before, but not during, movement. We have demonstrated that these two structures are more interconnected than previously thought. In particular, our studies were aimed at investigating whether a unilateral cerebellar lesion – i.e. hemicerebellectomy (HCb) - evoked changes in the morphology of neostriatal FSIs and whether these morphological changes were modulated by different post-operative housing conditions. We focused on FSIs because of their functional relevance in the neostriatal circuitry. in the hypothesis of their specific involvement in the cerebellar-striatal interaction.

In standard housed hemicerebellectomized (HCbed) animals, the lesion did not affect FSIs density but progressively shrank dendritic branching in both sides of the neostriatum.

Namely, these plastic changes, already evident 15 days after the cerebellar ablation, became very marked 30 days after the lesion. This cerebellar effect on FSI morphology was completely abolished in the presence of post-operative enrichment. EE not only counteracted the shrinkage of FSI dendritic arborization but also provoked a progressive increase in dendritic length as the enrichment period lengthened. Due to this increase, arborization in enriched HCbed animals reached a length exceeding that of the control level (De Bartolo et al., 2011) (Fig. 1). It has been also demonstrated that rearing in EE from weaning on elicited a striking increase of FSI dendritic branching in comparison to naïve animals. This dendritic lengthening was maintained also in the presence of HCb, indicating that EE totally prevents effects of cerebellar lesion and suggesting a powerful neuro-protective action of the long-term exposure to environmental complexity (Cutuli et al., 2011) (Figure 1). We can hypothesize that HCb induces the described neostriatal responses by provoking changes in cortical circuitries. For example, the dendritic shrinkage of the FSI could be linked to cortical actions of opposite sign. A decrease in glutamatergic cortical drive could occur, leading to atrophy of dendritic FSI arborization. This effect on dendritic arborization has already been described in pyramidal cortical neurons as a consequence of decreased afferent activity from the cholinergic forebrain. Alternatively, an increase in glutamatergic cortical drive might occur, leading to excitotoxicity phenomena. Excitotoxicity induces either neuronal death through rapid necrosis or delayed apoptosis or dendrotoxicity, a reversible form of damage affecting only dendritic arborization. The shrinkage of FSi dendritic arborization may be a consequence of dendrotoxicity. Since experiential factors are able to improve both brain structure and function, the increased cortical synaptogenesis observed in these studies may represent an index of enhanced connectivity in the circuit regulating the modulation of voluntary motor activity and motor learning.

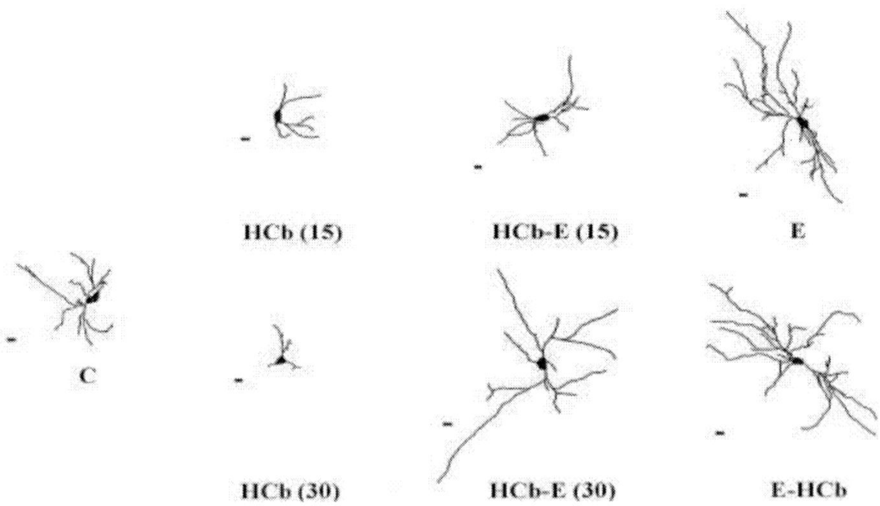

Figure 1. Camera lucida drawings of representative FSIs belonging to different experimental conditions. C: control animals; HCb (15): adult HCbed animals sacrificed after 15 post-operative days; HCb (30): adult HCbed animals sacrificed after 30 post-operative days; HCb-E (15): adult HCbed animals enriched for 15 post-operative days and then sacrificed; HCb-E (30): adult HCbed animals enriched for 30 post-operative days and then sacrificed; E: animals enriched from weaning to adulthood; E-HCb: animals enriched from weaning, HCbed and then sacrificed in adulthood. Scale bars: 10 μm. (Modified from Cutuli et al., 2011 and De Bartolo et al., 2011).

In fact, it has been demonstrated that these abilities require heavy neostriatal involvement. Thus, strengthened cortical networks seem to induce a strengthening of cortical projections on neostriatal target (so impinged by more powerful and tuned input). Exposure to EE after a cerebellar lesion could induce dendritic growth of neostriatal FSIs by means of this mechanism, allowing a more effective coping to cerebellar damage. In fact, HCb provokes postural and motor deficits that spontaneously recover in about one month. It has been demonstrated that exposure to EE both from weaning than in adulthood shortens this recovery time.

Conclusion

This chapter highlights that the neostriatum is a particularly plastic structure of the central nervous system. In fact, its projection neurons and interneurons exhibit marked plastic rearrangement in response to pathological events as well as to life experiences. In particular, a stimulant lifestyle is able to beneficially influence plastic neuronal changes elicited by several kinds of pathologies, striatal or extrastriatal. The positive influence of complex environments can act preventing or counteracting structural alterations that underlie functional impairments. Up to now, interventions aimed at compensate for the effects of diseases have been mainly based on the development of pharmacological compounds targeted against specific receptors associated with symptoms. The present chapter promotes the application of behavioral strategies such as exposition to complex environments and physical exercise to better cope with pathologies.

References

Auriat, A. M., Wowk, S., and Colbourne, F. (2010). Rehabilitation after intracerebral hemorrhage in rats improves recovery with enhanced dendritic complexity but no effect on cell proliferation. *Behavioural Brain Research*, *214*, 42-47.

Bezard, E., Dovero, S., Belin, D., Duconger, S., Jackson-Lewis, V., Przedborski, S., Piazza, P. V., Gross, C. E., and Jaber, M. (2003). Enriched environment confers resistance to 1-methyl-4-phenyl-1,2,3,6-tetrahydropyridine and cocaine: involvement of dopamine transporter and trophic factors. *Journal of Neuroscience*, *23*, 10999-11007.

Bolam, J.P., Hanley, J.J., Booth, P.A.C., and Bevan, M.D. (2000). Synaptic organization of basal ganglia. *Journal of Anatomy*, *196*, 527-542.

Bruel-Jungerman, E., La Roche, S., and Rampon, C. (2005). New neurons in the dentate gyrus are involved in the expression of enhanced long-term memory following environmental enrichment. *European Journal of Neuroscience, 21*, 513-521.

Comery, T. A., Shah, R., and Greenough, W. T. (1995). Differential rearing alters spine density on medium-sized spiny neurons in the rat corpus striatum: evidence for association of morphological plasticity with early response gene expression. *Neurobiology of Learning and Memory*, *63*, 217-219.

Comery, T. A., Stamoudis, C. X., Irwin, S. A., and Greenough, W. T. (1996). Increased density of multiple-head dendritic spines on medium-sized spiny neurons of the striatum in rats reared in a complex environment. *Neurobiology of Learning and Memory*, *66*, 93-96.

Cutuli, D., Rossi, S., Burello, L., Laricchiuta, D., De Chiara, V., Foti, F., De Bartolo, P., Musella, A., Gelfo, F., Centonze, D., and Petrosini, L. (2011). Before or after does it matter? Different protocols of environmental enrichment differently influence motor, synaptic and structural deficits of cerebellar origin. *Neurobiology of Disease, 42*, 9-20.

De Bartolo, P., Gelfo, F., Burello, L., De Giorgio, A., Petrosini, L., and Granato, A. (2011). Plastic changes in striatal fast-spiking interneurons following hemicerebellectomy and environmental enrichment. *The Cerebellum, 10*, 624-632.

De Bartolo, P., Leggio, M.G., Mandolesi, L., Foti, F., Gelfo, F., Ferlazzo, F., and Petrosini., L. (2008). Environmental enrichment mitigates the effects of basal forebrain lesions on cognitive flexibility. *Neuroscience, 154*, 444-453.

Döbrössy, M. D., and Dunnett, S. B. (2004). Environmental enrichment affects striatal graft morphology and functional recovery. *European Journal of Neuroscience*, *19*, 159-168.

Döbrössy, M. D., and Dunnett, S. B. (2006). Morphological and cellular changes within embryonic striatal grafts associated with enriched environment and involuntary exercise. *European Journal of Neuroscience*, *24*, 3223-3233.

Faherty, C. J., Kerley, D., and Smeyne, R. J. (2003). A Golgi-Cox morphological analysis of neuronal changes induced by environmental enrichment. *Brain Research. Developmental Brain Research*, *141*, 55-61.

Faherty, C. J., Raviie Shepherd, K., Herasimtschuk, A., Smeyne, R. J. (2005) Environmental enrichment in adulthood eliminates neuronal death in experimental Parkinsonism. *Brain Research. Molecular Brain Research*, *134*, 170-179.

Foti, F., Laricchiuta, D., Cutuli, D., De Bartolo, P., Gelfo, F., Angelucci, F., and Petrosini, L. (2011). Exposure to an enriched environment accelerates recovery from cerebellar lesion. *Cerebellum, 10*, 104-119.

Gelfo, F., Cutuli, D., Foti, F., Laricchiuta, D., De Bartolo, P., Caltagirone, C., Petrosini, L., and Angelucci, F. (2010). Enriched environment improves motor function and increases neurotrophins in hemicerebellar lesioned rats. *Neurorehabilitation and Neural Repair, 25*, 243-252.

Gelfo, F., De Bartolo, P., Giovine, A., Petrosini, L., and Leggio, M.G. (2010). Layer and regional effects of environmental enrichment on the pyramidal neuron morphology of the rat. *Neurobiology of Learning and Memory, 91*, 353-365.

Greenough, W.T., Black, J.E., and Wallace, C.S. (1987). Experience and brain development. *Child Development, 58*, 539-559.

Hebb, D.O. (1947). The effects of early experience on problem-solving at maturity. *American Psychology, 2*, 306-307.

Kawaguchi, Y. (1993). Physiological, morphological, and histochemical characterization of three classes of interneurons in rat neostriatum. *The Journal of Neuroscience*, *13*, 4908-4923.

Kawaguchi, Y. (1997). Neostriatal cell subtypes and their functional roles. *Neuroscience Research*, *27*, 1-8.

Kawaguchi, Y., Wilson, C.J., Augood, S.J., and Emson P.C. (1995). Striatal interneurons: chemical, physiological and morphological characterization. *Trends in Neuroscience, 18*, 527-535.

Kempermann, G., Kuhn, H.G., and Gage, F.H. (1997). More hippocampal neurons in adult mice living in an enriched environment. *Nature, 386*, 493-495.

Kolb, B., Forgie, M., Gibb, R., Gorny, G., and Rowntree, S. (1998). Age, experience and the changing brain. *Neuroscience and Biobehavioral Reviews, 22*, 143-15.

Koòs, T., and Tepper, J.M. (1999). Inibitory control of neostriatal projection neurons by GABAergic interneurons. *Nature Neuroscience, 2*, 467-472.

Lambert, T.J., Fernandez, F.M., and Frick, K.M. (2005). Different types of environmental enrichment have discrepant effects on spatial memory and synaptophysin level in female mice. *Neurobiology of Learning and Memory, 83*, 206-216.

Leggio, M.G., Mandolesi, L., Federico, F., Spirito, F., Ricci, B., Gelfo, F., and Petrosini, L. (2005). Environmental enrichment promotes improved spatial abilities and enhanced dendritic growth in the rat. *Behavioural Brain Research, 163*, 78-90.

Lewis, M. H. (2004). Environmental complexity and central nervous system development and function. *Mental Retardation and Developmental Disabilities Research Reviews*, *10*, 91-95.

MacLellan, C. L., Plummer, N., Silasi, G., Auriat, A. M., and Colbourne, F. (2011). Rehabilitation promotes recovery after whole blood-induced intracerebral hemorrhage in rats. *Neurorehabilitation and Neural Repair*, *25*, 477-483.

Mandolesi, L., De Bartolo, P., Foti, F., Gelfo, F., Federico, F., Leggio, M.G., and Petrosini, L. (2008). Environmental enrichment provides a cognitive reserve to be spent in the case of brain lesion. *Journal of Alzheimer Disease, 15*, 11-28.

Naka, F., Narita, N., Okado, N., and Narita, M. (2005). Modification of AMPA receptor properties following environmental enrichment. *Brain Development, 27*, 275-278.

Nithianantharajah, J., and Hannan, A.J. (2006). Enriched environments, experience-dependent plasticity and disorders of the nervous system. *Neuroscience, 7*, 697-709.

Petrosini, L., De Bartolo, P., Foti, F., Gelfo, F., Cutuli, D., Leggio, M.G., and Mandolesi, L. (2009). On whether the environmental enrichment may provide cognitive and brain reserves. *Brain Research Reviews, 61*, 221-239.

Pinaud, R., Penner, M. R., Robertson, H. A., and Currie, R. W. (2001). Upregulation of the immediate early gene arc in the brains of rats exposed to environmental enrichment: implications for molecular plasticity. *Brain Research. Molecular Brain Research*, *91*, 50-56.

Pinaud, R., Tremere, L. A., Penner, M. R., Hess, F. F., Robertson, H. A., and Currie, R. W. (2002). Complexity of sensory environment drives the expression of candidate-plasticity gene, nerve growth factor induced-A. *Neuroscience*, *112*, 573-582.

Plotkin, J.L., Wu, N., Chesselet, M-F., and Levine, M.S. (2005). Functional and molecular development of striatal fast-spiking GABAergic interneurons and their cortical inputs. *European Journal of Neuroscience, 22*, 1097-1108.

Rosenzweig, M.R. (1966). Environmental complexity, cerebral change and behaviour. *American Psychology, 21*, 3221-3232.

Rosenzweig, M.R., and Bennet, E.L. (1978). Experiential influences on brain anatomy and brain chemistry in rodents. In: Gottlieb, G. (Ed.), *Studies of the development of behaviour and the nervous system* (pp. 389-327). New York, San Francisco, London: Academic Press.

Rosenzweig, M.R., Krech, D., Bennet, E.L., and Diamond, M.C. (1962). Effects of environmental complexity and train on brain chemistry and anatomy. *Journal of Comparative Physiological Psychology, 55*, 429-437.

Sale, A., Berardi, N., and Maffei, L. (2009). Enrich the environment to empower the brain. *Trends in Neuroscience, 32*, 233-239.

Spires, T. L., Grote, H. E., Garry, S., Cordery, P. M., Van Dellen, A., Blakemore, C., and Hannan, A. J. (2004a). Dendritic spine pathology and deficits in experience-dependent dendritic plasticity in R6/1 Huntington's disease transgenic mice. *European Journal of Neuroscience, 19*, 2799-2807.

Spires, T. L., Grote, H. E., Varshney, N. K., Cordery, P. M., van Dellen, A., Blakemore, C., and Hannan, A. J. (2004b). Environmental enrichment rescues protein deficits in a mouse model of Huntington's disease, indicating a possible disease mechanism. *Journal of Neuroscience, 24*, 2270-2276.

Tepper, J.M., and Bolam, J.P. (2004). Functional diversity and specificity of neostriatal interneurons. *Current Opinion in Neurobiology, 14*, 685-692.

Tepper, J.M., Tecuapleta, F., Koòs T., and Ibàñez-Sandoval, O. (2010). Heterogeneity and diversity of striatal GABAergic interneurons. *Frontiers in Neuroanatomy, 4*, 1-18.

Tepper, J.M., Wilson, C.J., and Koòs, T. (2008). Feedforward and feedback inhibition in neostriatal GABAergic spiny neurons. *Brain Research Reviews, 58*, 272-281.

Thiriet, N., Amar, L., Toussay, X., Lardeux, V., Ladenheim, B., Becker, K. G., Cadet, J. L., Solinas, M., and Jaber, M. (2008). Environmental enrichment during adolescence regulates gene expression in the striatum of mice. *Brain Research, 41*, 1222-1231.

Turner, C. A., and Lewis, M. H. (2003). Environmental enrichment: effects on stereotyped behavior and neurotrophin levels. *Physiology and Behavior, 80*, 259-266.

Turner, C. A., Lewis, M. H., and King, M. A. (2003). Environmental enrichment: effects on stereotyped behavior and dendritic morphology. *Developmental Psychobiology, 43*, 20-27.

Turner, C. A., Yang, M. C., and Lewis, M. H. (2002). Environmental enrichment: effects on stereotyped behavior and regional neuronal metabolic activity. *Brain Research, 938*, 15-21.

Van Dellen, A., Cordery, P.M., Blakemore, C., and Hannan, A.J. (2008). Wheel running from a juvenile age delays onset of specific motor deficits but does not alter protein aggregate density in a mouse model of Huntington's disease. *BMC Neuroscience, 9*, 34.

Van Praag, H., Kempermann, G., and Gage, F.H. (2000). Neuronal consequences of environmental enrichment. *Nature Reviews of Neuroscience, 1*, 191-198.

In: Striatum: Anatomy, Functions and Role in Disease
Editors: Hugo T. Maldonado and Ignacio M. Ortega
ISBN 978-1-61942-384-8

Chapter VIII

Neuroimaging of Human Striatum in Cocaine Addiction

Alfonso Barrós-Loscertales, Juan Carlos Bustamante, Victor Costumero-Ramos, Paola Fuentes-Claramonte, Patricia Rosell-Negre, Juan José Llopis-Llacer and César Ávila

Neuropsychology and neuroimaging research group. Departamento de Psicología Básica, Clínica y Psicobiología. Universitat Jaume I de Castellón

Abstract

The striatum has been shown to play a critical role mediating cocaine addictive behavior. Functional and structural alterations in the striatum are a result of complex processes that are suggested to lead to drug craving and compulsive drug seeking in cocaine addicts. Single drug intake does not seem to produce stable structural or functional changes in the striatum, but the repetition of acute functional and behavioral drug-related effects produce later changes in brain structures linked to addiction until drug-taking transforms into a habit (Pierce and Vanderschuren 2010).

Three associated factors related to cocaine addiction are current topics of intense research interest: motivation, cognition and impulsivity. These three factors are functionally linked to the striatum, among other brain regions (Winstanley 2007). Within a neuropsychological perspective of cocaine addiction based on neuroimaging results, the functional and structural changes associated with cocaine addiction are reflected in addicts′ observable emotions, motivations, cognitions and their behavioral manifestations. Motivational changes in cocaine addiction directly involve or are mediated by the striatum (Childress et al., 1999; Garavan et al., 2000; Gu et al., 2010; Volkow et al., 2006; Wilcox et al. 2011). Although the research largely focused on understanding the reinforcing effects of cocaine, cognitive changes are also important to understand the generation and maintenance of addiction (Goldstein and Volkow 2002). Deficit in impulse control is a key feature of cocaine addiction and other psychiatric disorders (Baler and Volkow, 2006; Garavan et al., 2008). Likewise, individual differences in personality are suggested to modulate impulse control manifestation in cocaine addiction (Murray et al., 2003; Patkar et al., 2004; Winstanley, 2007). The review of neuroimaging literature regarding personality traits (Barrós-Loscertales et al., 2010; Hahn et al., 2009) and cocaine addiction (Barrós-Loscertales et al. 2011; Gu et al. 2010; Wilcox et al. 2011) suggests a common pattern of the striatum´s reduced structural volume and changing functionality underlying its cognitive manifestation.

In summary, the failure of control processes and the activation of implicit automatic ones by external and internal drug-related cues may be explained by the interaction between motivational and cognitive processes in cocaine addiction (Goldstein and Volkow 2002; Baler and Volkow 2006), taking into account modulating personality traits. For example, cocaine addicts under treatment may fail in their abstinence due to the lack of cognitive control over behavior, but this lack of control is probably caused by drug cues and the presence of the drug itself. Thus, given the reviewed literature, the striatum is suggested to be an important part of the neurobiological mechanism underlying the cognitive and motivational interactions in human cocaine addiction. The aim of this chapter is to review neuroimaging evidence regarding the human phenomenon of cocaine addiction within the striatum.

Introduction

Cocaine addiction implicates behaviors that relate to loss of cognitive control and alteration of reward and motivational processes (Goldstein and Volkow 2002). The striatum has been shown to play a critical role in mediating cocaine addiction within the dopamine circuitry. Specifically, long term cocaine effects in the striatum involve changes in the control of cognition, motivation, movement and reward. While other neurotransmitters are also considered, dopamine is considered a main neurotransmitter involved in these effects (Volkow et al. 2008). However, dopamine´s role in human cocaine addiction, as well as those structures in the dopamine circuit such as the striatum, is not fully understood. Tracing neurotransmitters within the human brain by means of positron emission tomography (PET) and single photon emission computed tomography (SPECT) radiotracers are used for studying dopamine receptors in the brain and, indirectly, image effects of cocaine at the levels of neurotransmitters (see Martinez and Narendran, 2011 for a review). PET and SPECT techniques reveal acute, transient and sustained changes in the brain of cocaine users, particularly in the striatum (Nora D Volkow et al. 2006; Cox et al. 2009). The time persistence of these effects is unknown but dopamine D2 receptor decreases have been shown to be persistent after 3 months of inpatient treatment in humans (Volkow et al. 1993) and one year in some monkeys (M. A. Nader et al. 2006). The analysis of structures and brain processes linked to cocaine addiction has also been conducted by means of structural and functional Magnetic Resonance Imaging (MRI). MRI techniques are showing the involvement of cortical brain regions in cocaine addiction but the striatum´s role is not as clearly manifested in these studies with human subjects as in PET/SPECT studies (Martinez and Narendran 2010) and animal research (Bradberry 2008). In the following, we will review the anatomical and functional studies that yielded the involvement of the striatum in cognitive and motivational processes, trying to specify a spatial distinction between ventral striatum (VST) and dorsal striatum (DST) and within them as caudate, putamen and nucleus accubens (NAcc) when possible.

The nucleus accumbens at the VST is directly or indirectly triggered by all addictive drugs producing transient increases in extracellular DA. From social use to compulsive use of cocaine, it is suggested that a spatial change, from a former main role of the VST and cocaine enthusiastic effects to a later DST main role, occurs once the drug intakes become habitual (Porrino et al. 2007). In this sense, Breiter et al. (1997) showed an increased hemodynamic response in the VST and DST (NAcc, caudate and putamen) after acute cocaine infusion by means of functional MRI. Moreover, DST (caudate) showed its correlation with rush and the VST (NAcc) showed a higher correlation with craving than with rush (Breiter et al. 1997). On the other hand, Risinger et al. (2006) found that VST (NAcc) showed a reduced activation related with "high" effects of acute cocaine self-administration, but a positive correlation with craving and was not associated with rush. Furthermore, this same research group showed that VST activation during acute cocaine administration was independent of cocaine expectations (Kufahl et al. 2008). Regarding these acute hemodynamic changes in the ventral striatum, early reports on brain blood functioning informed that regional cerebral blood flow used to increase after cocaine abuse in the striatum, even after 7 days, and reversed to baseline levels after longer periods of abstinence (Bell et al. 1994). Thus, VST and DST are suggested to be differently involved in reward and motivation circuits underlying addiction (Volkow et al. 2010b). These acute and latterly sustained effects of cocaine might have important implications for functional studies and the need to control their effects.

In summary, VST and DST are known to be functionally responsible for cocaine effects after its acute administration. The aim of this chapter is to review neuroimaging evidence regarding the human phenomenon of cocaine addiction within the striatum. Striatum involvement in cocaine addiction is clearly reported in animal studies, but its role in human addiction is far from understood. In the next pages, we will review the results of functional studies that yielded the striatum as a region involved in the phenomenon of cocaine addiction in humans. First, we will review those studies that showed functional changes in the striatum associated with cognitive control processes. Second, we will review studies that analyzed functional response to motivational stimuli, including natural rewarding stimuli as well as drug related stimuli. Finally, we will review those results that involved a change in the striatum of cocaine addicts linked to cognitive-motivational interactions and impulsivity.

Cognitive Control

Cognitive control has been defined as the series of processes by which the human cognitive system is able to configure itself for the performance of specific tasks through appropriate adjustments in perceptual selection, response biasing and the on-line maintenance of contextual information (Botvinick et al. 2001). The striatum is known to be involved in cognitive control processes (McClure et al. 2003). This structure is suggested to contribute to flexible behavior such that cortically initiated operations are communicated via the striatum to other parts of the corticostriatal circuitry (Kübler et al., 2010). In this sense, the lack of flexibility in cocaine addicts′ behavior would involve the brain function of the striatum.

Stroop task is a paradigmatic task for the study of cognitive control – inhibitory control processes (Nigg 2000). Brain activation during Stroop task performance has been related to treatment outcome of cocaine addicts (Brewer et al. 2008). Brewer et al. (2008) analyzed the association between pre-treatment brain activation during a Stroop task and treatment outcomes in treatment-seeking cocaine dependents. Task-related activation was found in the bilateral DST (putamen/globus pallidum). Striatum (right putamen) activation was related to self-reported abstinence and number of negative urine tests (Brewer et al. 2008). On the other hand, Ersche et al. (2009) and Barrós-Loscertales et al. (2011) found striatum involvement in neither a color-word Stroop task (Ersche et al. 2010) nor counting-Stroop task performance (Barrós-Loscertales et al., 2011). Both task related activations in the striatum were not different between groups, stimulant dependent/cocaine dependent patients and healthy controls, in either study. Therefore, brain activation regarding inhibitory control function during Stroop-task performance did not show differential activation for cocaine addicts but was associated with later treatment outcomes.

Regarding working memory, DST (caudate) contributions have been specifically involved in manipulating and maintaining information in WM (Lewis et al. 2004; Landau et al. 2009). Working memory function in cocaine addiction has been already studied. Moeller et al. (2010) found a reduced activation in the left DST (caudate) of cocaine-dependent patients. In this case they also studied the associated activation of the striatum during task performance with treatment effects, but they did not find the association in the striatum (Moeller et al. 2010) as was reported by Breiter et al. (2009) during a color-word Stroop task. Tomasi et al. (2007) showed a reduced activation in the DST (putamen) in cocaine dependent patients, with a reduced effect on working memory load, particularly for those participants with positive urine tests (Tomasi et al. 2007). Otherwise, Bustamante et al. (2010) showed neither functional involvement of the striatum in a working memory task, nor functional differences in cocaine addicts compared to a control group. Likely, task performance differences in each group between studies and methodological changes may explain the lack of agreement in striatum involvement in working memory. Deficits in working memory related activation in cocaine dependence have been suggested to be associated with poor attentional switching (Kübler et al. 2005). Kübler et al. (2005) found reduced activation in the DST (putamen) during attentional switching in a working memory task. Other studies have not found the involvement of the striatum in visual attentional tasks (Tomasi et al. 2007) or in a response inhibition task with varying working memory demands (Hester and Hugh Garavan 2004). The involvement of the striatum during attentional switching in cocaine dependence was also identified by Kaufman et al. (2003) in the DST (putamen) during successful (bilateral DST) and failed (right DST) inhibitions, but they were not different in cocaine addicts when compared to healthy controls. Likewise, although the striatum was involved in correct inhibitions in a STOP task, its response did not show to be different between groups of cocaine abstinent patients and controls and was shown to be independent of the time of abstinence in a study of Connoly et al. (2011) (Connolly et al. 2011). Thus, the striatum´s role subserving executive processes such as working memory and attentional switching seems to be affected in the former by cocaine effects. It is suggested that cognitive inflexibility in cocaine addiction may be related to other regions, like the OFC and the basolateral amygdala, rather than the striatum (Stalnaker et al. 2009); however, all of them are closely inter-connected.

In summary, cognitive tasks regarding inhibitory control, attentional switching and working memory involve the striatum. Working memory and attentional switching studies report reduced functionality in the striatum of cocaine addicts. On the other hand, the importance of cognitive-related activation for prospective studies on treatment effects seems to be independent of dysfunctions identified by group differences between cocaine addicts and matched controls. Future research would benefit from the identification of the cognitive processes that are affected by a dysfunction in the striatum

Motivational Control

The neural basis of motivation, reward and saliency processes behind cocaine addiction seems to be identified but poorly understood. Learning from positive and negative feedback seems to be mediated by dopamine neurotransmitter (Schultz 2006). It has been suggested that the insensitiveness to negative consequences of an action may be a characteristic of cocaine addictions, as well as for other addictive behaviors (Klein et al. 2007). Likewise, the dopamine neuroadaptations produced by chronic cocaine intake are suggested to contribute to reducing reward sensitivity and executive cognitive dysfunction (Volkow et al. 1997; Hester and Garavan 2004). Hypodopaminergic state after chronic cocaine administration seems to explain an addict's decreased sensitivity to natural rewards (Volkow et al. 2010b). Therefore, cocaine leads addicts′ behavior, changing sensitivity to positive and negative consequences of drug taking and other natural reinforcing stimuli.

Drug cues are suggested to play a main role in cocaine addiction by perpetuating drug abuse by inducing craving, which prompts drug-seeking behavior. It is suggested that a wide network of brain structures that involve cognitive and emotional processes participates in the production of subjective craving (Garavan et al., 2000). Exposure to cocaine-related cues activates a wide range of brain areas including the striatum (Garavan et al. 2000; Childress et al. 1999; Kilts et al. 2001; Kilts et al. 2004; Wexler 2001), although other studies failed to show such activation (Maas et al. 1998; Bonson et al. 2002). Studies that analyzed striatum-related response to craving found that the left DST (caudate) response to cocaine cues was specific compared with nature films within cocaine users, and when cocaine users were compared to healthy controls, the former showed a higher activation by means of fMRI (Garavan et al. 2000). Furthermore, craving produced by cocaine-related cues correlated with the occupancy of dopamine receptors in the DST (putamen) during its view in a PET study (Wong et al. 2006; Volkow et al. 2006). Kilts et al. (2001) showed that male cocaine addicts show the activation of the VST (NAcc) during cue-induced cocaine craving, and posterior DST (caudate) activation negatively correlated with the subjective reported craving. Another cue-induced cocaine craving study conducted in a sample of women (Kilts et al. 2004) based on an imagery paradigm showed that a woman′s striatum activation to cocaine-related scripts involved the VST (NAcc), but it was not different from male cocaine addicts; while men activated the DST more than women. However, a similar paradigm in fMRI failed to involve the striatum, likely due to differences in craving reported by the sample and timing parameters in the paradigm, and, ultimately, did not find interaction between stress response and craving activation (Duncan et al. 2009). On the other hand, Wexler et al. (2001) showed striatum involvement in drug-related tapes and other emotional conditions in cocaine dependent patients, but left VST (NAcc) showed reduced activation in cocaine dependent patients during the final period of a tape viewing than during the post-tape baseline. This last result contrasts with previous reports, although the analysis was restricted to the specified condition. Otherwise, although striatum metabolism has shown to be usually increased by craving, it has been shown to be decreased when craving is inhibited. Volkow et al. (2010) showed a reduction in the glucose metabolism of the bilateral VST (NAcc) when cocaine subjects were instructed to inhibit/ignore their craving while watching cocaine-related videos. Likewise, this difference was true for the right VST (NAcc) when comparing the inhibit/ ignore condition to the passive watching condition. Striatum activation was interpreted in terms of connectivity with the right inferior frontal gyrus (BA44) and also maybe the ventral tegmental areas and amygdale (Volkow et al. 2010).

Lower and higher striatum functionality maybe hypothesized from cocaine addiction depending on the theories under different conditions. Low reward responsiveness is commonly hypothesized in cocaine addicts from the theory of reward deficiency syndrome of addiction (Blum et al. 2000), but the opposite may be suggested from the incentive salience and impulsivity theories (Robinson and Berridge 2008; Hommer et al. 2011). Bjork et al. (2008) and Jia et al. (2011) analyzed brain response in cocaine addicts to rewards different from cocaine and drug-related cues. Bjork et al. (2008) reported striatal hypersensitivity to reward in substance dependent patients characterized by comorbidity to cocaine and alcohol dependence. Jia et al. (2011) showed that treatment-seeking cocaine addicts, when compared with healthy controls, had a higher activation during notification of reward outcome in bilateral VST (NAcc) and right DST (caudate). Furthermore, right DST (caudate) activation correlated negatively with cocaine-negative urine tests during reward anticipation, while right VST correlated negatively with abstinence and negative urine tests. Otherwise, Asensio et al. (2010) found reduced functional activation in the VST and DST in response to appetitive (erotic) pictures, pointing out that its activation could be more related to arousal rather than valence. If striatum responsiveness to reward is altered in cocaine addicts, it will suggest a change in striatum functional association with other brain regions. Wilcox et al. (2011) found increased resting state correlation between the VST and the OFC, regions that showed to be responsive to drug cues-processing. Otherwise, striatum involvement in a reward processing task is dependent on task design. Goldstein et al. (2007a,b) studied cocaine addicts in a go/no-go task under different reward conditions (Goldstein et al. 2007a) and gradients (Goldstein et al. 2007b) under which the striatum was neither involved nor showed differential activations between groups. Therefore, the results on striatum role in reward responsiveness of cocaine addicts are dependent on the reinforcement (e.g., natural stimuli, money), experimental design and reward contingencies.

The role played by aversive affective states in cocaine addiction is not usually studied in neuroimaging of cocaine addiction. From animal studies, it has been suggested that cocaine cues evoke representations in the brain linked to aversive outcomes (Wheeler et al. 2008). Wheeler et al. (2008) showed that a cocaine related cue produced behavior related to aversion in rats, suggesting the involvement of the VST (NAcc) for processing of positive and negative outcomes during drug addiction process. Furthermore, the intensity of behavioral aversion was predictive of subsequent cocaine self administration. Wexler et al. (2001) suggested the association between craving and normal dysphoric states from the parallelism of the activation in other regions, different from the striatum, of cocaine dependent patients when watching drug-cues and sad stimuli. Thus, cocaine-cues related aversive states are proposed to trigger drug-seeking behavior. Dopaminergic function seems to be independent of subjective effects of stimulants (Martinez and Narendran 2010; Volkow et al. 1997). Metabolic reduction in the striatum induced by cocaine-cues was shown to be reduced by methylphenidate effects, that is, cocaine cues decreased VST metabolism to a lower extent under the effects of higher tonic dopamine level after having oral methylphenidate. The decrease in metabolism in the striatum after methylphenidate was not associated with craving, but striatum metabolism without methylphenidate was related to craving. Volkow et al. (2010) suggest that methylphenidate´s attenuation of brain reactivity to cocaine cues is distinct from that involved in craving since under both conditions cocaine cues produced craving to the same extent but were differently related to striatum metabolism of dopamine. Likewise, an earlier study showed that craving was positively correlated with the increase in dopamine receptor occupancy in the putamen, presumably because of the release of intrasynaptic dopamine (Wong et al. 2006). Thus, the reinforcing effects of cocaine are associated with increased dopamine in the nucleus accumbens (Kufahl et al. 2005), which underlies their reinforcing effects (Volkow et al. 2006), as well as cue induced craving. However, dopamine increase in the striatum does not elicit craving by itself, but does when cocaine cues are present (Volkow et al. 2008). Finally, other studies have shown the striatum of cocaine patients reduced activation during emotional processing of sad tapes (Wexler 2001), stress and stress related craving (Sinha et al. 2005)

The power of drug associated cues to trigger craving is suggested to implicate memory and learning circuits (Volkow et al. 2010b) once drug-cue conditioned reinforcing effects are established, that is, once addiction is a fact . Physiological measures such as brain activation changes due to drug cues have shown stronger correlation with relapses and treatment outcomes than craving scores(Brewer et al. 2008; Kosten et al. 2006). However, treatment outcome has been related to striatum activation only in changes regarding cognitive processes (Brewer et al. 2008). The use of virtual environments, which have shown to produce craving (Saladin et al., 2010), may help to develop more controlled contexts in which associations between cocaine cues, craving and treatment effects may offer new answers to the phenomenon of cocaine addiction, particularly regarding the striatum´s role. Otherwise, brain activation related to cocaine craving involved motivational and cognitive areas, which involves both processes in the cocaine addiction phenomenon (Garavan et al. 2000). Cognitive-motivational interactions may better show functional involvement of the striatum in cocaine addiction.

In summary, the processing of drug cues involves the striatum. Likewise, other more common rewards, such us money and erotic pictures, involve the striatum of cocaine addicts. When comparing drug cues with other commonly identified rewarding stimuli, such as money and erotic pictures, in fMRI experiments, drug cues seems to have a more consistent and stronger involvement of the striatum. Otherwise, it seems that fMRI experiments report a consistent, greater response of the striatum to monetary rewards, while striatum response to erotic stimuli seems to be reduced in cocaine addicts. Further research will clarify the different response of the striatum to each kind of reward in cocaine addicts, as well as the competition between them within their brains. The importance of these results will rely on the development of strategies for future psychological and pharmacological treatments.

Cognitive-Motivational Interactions: Impulsivity and Personality-Related Traits

The capacity to exert control is challenged when required to suppress thoughts and actions toward appetitive cues (Somerville and Casey 2010). The capacity or the effort needed to exert control depends on the sensitivity to environmental cues, especially reward-based cues. Theoretical models from different ambits explain how the capacity of control over environmental motivational cues target the striatum (Somerville and Casey 2010). By introducing monetary manipulations in an executive task, cognitive-motivational interactions are easily introduced. The striatum has been shown to be involved in cognitive-motivational interactions (Simões-Franklin et al. 2010). One of the simplest paradigms that involve cognitive-motivational interactions in cocaine addiction is the drug-word Stroop task. A couple of studies have used this paradigm in fMRI. The drug-word Stroop task has shown to involve the DST (caudate) in task performance (Goldstein et al. 2007; Ersche et al. 2010). However, contrast between groups has yielded neither functional differences within the striatum in drug-word Stroop task (Ersche et al. 2011), nor correlation between its activation with impulsivity, compulsivity, word′s valence or task performance in cocaine addicts or stimulant substance dependent individuals (Ersche et al. 2010; Goldstein et al. 2007).

Decision making involves the striatum in cognitive-motivational interaction tasks. Bolla et al. (2000) found an increased activation in DST (left putamen) for cocaine participants compared to controls during an Iowa Gambling task (IGT), although task performance was poorer in cocaine addicts but not statistically significant compared to other behavioral studies (Grant et al. 2000). Bjork et al. (2008) found activation in the DST (caudate) during reward decision making without risk in substance dependent subjects with history of cocaine dependence or abuse, but not in controls. Left DST was shown to be related to a lower activation in the control-motor condition and right DST to a higher increased activation under no risk reward conditions (Bjork et al. 2008). On the other hand, resting state functioning of the striatum by means of PET (Adinoff et al. 2003) and SPECT (Tucker et al. 2004) in cocaine addicts has not been related to decision making tasks such as the IGT. Therefore, the sum of these results may indicate that the striatum's role in decision making tasks seems dependent on task involvement rather than a general condition of brain functionality.

Dopamine D2 receptor density reduction is linked to multiple addictive and compulsive behaviors (Noble 2003; Bowirrat and Oscar-Berman 2005). Reduced protection against addiction is suggested to characterize individuals with low binding potentials in DA striatum. Likewise, impulsivity and personality related measures, such as sensation seeking (Zuckerman, 2005), are related to reduced binding potentials within the VST (NAcc/putamen) and with nonlinear concentrations of DA (Gjedde et al. 2010). Impulsivity and personality related measures define a stable condition that predisposes subjects to behave according to their cognitive control capabilities and reward sensitivity. Therefore, these measures involve the interaction of cognitive-motivational processing as a pre-existing condition in the subject. Thus, impulsivity as a behavioral stable trait is suggested to be related to chronic drug use. Clark et al. (2006) found that amphetamines and opiate users poorly performed the information sampling task. Addicts sampled less information and had a lower probability of responding correctly (Clark et al. 2006). However, the behavioral performance was not related to impulsivity (as measured by the Barrat Impulsiveness Scale, BIS) in these samples.

In animal studies, low D2 receptors in the striatum is related to impulsivity (Dalley et al. 2007) and drug self administration (Belin et al. 2008). Thus, it is suggested that low levels of D2 receptors in the striatum could promote drug abuse and addiction by exacerbated impulsivity (Volkow et al. 2010b). Impulsivity and addiction show parallels in decreased inhibitory control, intolerance to delay to reward and quick decision making due to lack of consideration. Personality traits related to reward sensitivity showed reduced volume in the striatum (Barrós-Loscertales et al. 2006), as well as in cocaine addiction (Barrós-Loscertales et al. 2011). Lesions in the VST (NAcc) increases impulsive choice dramatically (Cardinal et al. 2001). In alcohol addiction, Beck et al. (2009) showed that reduced striatum response to reward anticipation was related to increased impulsivity of alcohol addicts. Leland et al. (2006) conducted a study in young adults (age range 18-25) who used stimulants (e.g., cocaine, amphetamine) to analyze brain response to uncertainty and its association with impulsivity. The study showed that consumers showed a higher activation in the left DST (caudate), which was associated with impulsivity (Barrat Impulsivity Scale, BIS). Furthermore, impulsivity was higher in stimulant users than matched controls. Sample characteristics in Leland´s study, such as the reduced stimulant exposure, lack of dependency and non-treatment-seeking participants suggest that impulsivity is a pre-existing trait rather than an effect of chronic drug use(Leland et al. 2006). Therefore, impulsivity, personality-related traits and addiction seem to show parallels in neurochemical systems, brain circuitry and behavioral manifestation involving the striatum in a particular behavioral tendency under several cognitive and motivational conditions.

Conclusion

In conclusion, cognitive control and motivational processes are behind cocaine addiction. The striatum seems to be subserving these processes at different degrees for each of them. Previous results show that striatum is affected by cocaine in cognitive control (e.g., inhibitory control, error monitoring, working memory), reward and motivation. However, its role seems to be minimized when compared to animal studies. On the other hand, human research on cocaine addiction with PET show target results in the striatum, but it is not the case of most MRI studies. Likely, brain development, in the case of comparing animal and human research, gives rise to a major role of cortical brain regions (e.g., orbitofrontal cortex, anterior cingulate cortex) in human addiction when compared to the striatum. On the other hand, PET studies target neurochemical changes in addiction compared to hemodynamic changes related to fMRI studies. Likely, given the chemical nature of cocaine effects in the striatum, the indirect measure of function of MRI studies might explain the different results offered by one and the other. Finally, others explicitly noticed that a pure dopaminergic dysfunction in the striatum fails to account for the traits that characterize addictive behaviors such as craving and relapse (Volkow et al. 2010b). Likewise, a pure cognitive or motivational dysfunction is abandoned when trying to understand the phenomenon of cocaine addiction. Cocaine addiction is a phenomenon in which cognitive-motivational, chemical-functional, striato-cortico-limbic, and genetic-ambient interactions will draw a more precise picture of effective psychological and pharmachological treatments.

References

Adinoff, B. et al., 2003. Resting regional cerebral blood flow and gambling task performance in cocaine-dependent subjects and healthy comparison subjects. *The American Journal of Psychiatry*, 160(10), pp.1892-1894.

Baler, R.D. and Volkow, Nora D, 2006. Drug addiction: the neurobiology of disrupted self-control. *Trends in molecular medicine*, 12(12), pp.559-66.

Barrós-Loscertales, A et al., 2006. Striatum gray matter reduction in males with an overactive behavioral activation system. *European Journal of Neuroscience*, 24(7), pp.2071-2074.

Barrós-Loscertales, Alfonso et al., 2011. Reduced striatal volume in cocaine-dependent patients. *NeuroImage*, 56(3), pp.1021-1026.

Belin, D. et al., 2008. High impulsivity predicts the switch to compulsive cocaine-taking. *Science* (New York, N.Y.), 320(5881), pp.1352-5.

Bell, K.M., Milne, N. and Lyons, K.P., 1994. Regional cerebral blood flow and cocaine abuse. *The Western journal of medicine*, 161(4), pp.412-3.

Bjork, J.M. et al., 2008. Reduced posterior mesofrontal cortex activation by risky rewards in substance-dependent patients. *Drug and Alcohol Dependence*, 95(1-2), pp.115-128.

Blum, K. et al., 2000. Reward deficiency syndrome: a biogenetic model for the diagnosis and treatment of impulsive, addictive, and compulsive behaviors. *Journal Of Psychoactive Drugs*, 32 Suppl, pp.i-iv, 1-112.

Bonson, K.R. et al., 2002. Neural systems and cue-induced cocaine craving. *Neuropsychopharmacology□ : official publication of the American College of Neuropsychopharmacology*, 26(3), pp.376-86.

Botvinick, M.M. et al., 2001. Conflict monitoring and cognitive control. *Psychological review*, 108(3), pp.624-52.

Bowirrat, A. and Oscar-Berman, M., 2005. Relationship between dopaminergic neurotransmission, alcoholism, and Reward Deficiency syndrome. *American journal of medical genetics.* Part B, Neuropsychiatric genetics□ : the official publication of the International Society of Psychiatric Genetics, 132B(1), pp.29-37.

Bradberry, C.W., 2008. Comparison of acute and chronic neurochemical effects of cocaine and cocaine cues in rhesus monkeys and rodents: focus on striatal and cortical dopamine systems. *Reviews in the neurosciences*, 19(2-3), pp.113-28.

Breiter, H.C. et al., 1997. Acute effects of cocaine on human brain activity and emotion. *Neuron*, 19(3), pp.591-611.

Brewer, J.A. et al., 2008. Pretreatment brain activation during stroop task is associated with outcomes in cocaine-dependent patients. *Biological Psychiatry*, 64(11), pp.998-1004.

Bustamante, J.C., et al., 2010. Right parietal hypoactivation in a cocaine-dependent group during a verbal working memory task. *Brain Res*, 1375: 111-119.

Cardinal, R.N. et al., 2001. Impulsive choice induced in rats by lesions of the nucleus accumbens core. *Science* (New York, N.Y.), 292(5526), pp.2499-501.

Childress, A.R. et al., 1999. Limbic activation during cue-induced cocaine craving. *The American Journal of Psychiatry*, 156(1), pp.11-18.

Clark, L. et al., 2006. Reflection impulsivity in current and former substance users. *Biological Psychiatry*, 60(5), pp.515-522.

Connolly, C.G. et al., 2011. The neurobiology of cognitive control in successful cocaine abstinence. *Drug and alcohol dependence*. In press.

Cox, S.M.L. et al., 2009. Striatal dopamine responses to intranasal cocaine self-administration in humans. *Biological Psychiatry*, 65(10), pp.846-850.

Dalley, J.W. et al., 2007. Nucleus accumbens D2/3 receptors predict trait impulsivity and cocaine reinforcement. *Science* (New York, N.Y.), 315(5816), pp.1267-70.

Duncan, E. et al., 2009. An fMRI study of the interaction of stress and cocaine cues on cocaine craving in cocaine-dependent men. *The American journal on addictions / American Academy of Psychiatrists in Alcoholism and Addictions*, 16(3), pp.174-82.

Ersche, K.D. et al., 2011. Abnormal structure of frontostriatal brain systems is associated with aspects of impulsivity and compulsivity in cocaine dependence. *Brain: A journal of neurology*, 134(Pt 7), pp.2013-24.

Ersche, K.D. et al., 2010. Influence of compulsivity of drug abuse on dopaminergic modulation of attentional bias in stimulant dependence. *Archives of general psychiatry*, 67(6), pp.632-44.

Garavan, H et al., 2000. Cue-induced cocaine craving: neuroanatomical specificity for drug users and drug stimuli. *The American journal of psychiatry*, 157(11), pp.1789-98.

Gjedde, A. et al., 2010. Inverted-U-shaped correlation between dopamine receptor availability in striatum and sensation seeking. *Proceedings of the National Academy of Sciences of the United States of America*, 107(8), pp.3870-3875.

Goldstein, R Z et al., 2007. Role of the anterior cingulate and medial orbitofrontal cortex in processing drug cues in cocaine addiction. *Neuroscience*, 144(4), pp.1153-9.

Goldstein, Rita Z and Volkow, Nora D, 2002. Drug addiction and its underlying neurobiological basis: neuroimaging evidence for the involvement of the frontal cortex. *The American Journal of Psychiatry*, 159(10), pp.1642-1652.

Goldstein, Rita Z, Alia-Klein, Nelly, Tomasi, Dardo, et al., 2007. Is decreased prefrontal cortical sensitivity to monetary reward associated with impaired motivation and self-control in cocaine addiction? *The American Journal of Psychiatry*, 164(1), pp.43-51.

Goldstein, Rita Z, Tomasi, Dardo, et al., 2007. Subjective sensitivity to monetary gradients is associated with frontolimbic activation to reward in cocaine abusers. *Drug and Alcohol Dependence*, 87(2-3), pp.233-240.

Grant, S., Contoreggi, C and London, E D, 2000. Drug abusers show impaired performance in a laboratory test of decision making. *Neuropsychologia*, 38(8), pp.1180-1187.

Gu, H. et al., 2010. Mesocorticolimbic circuits are impaired in chronic cocaine users as demonstrated by resting state functional connectivity. *NeuroImage*, 53(2), pp.593-601.

Hester, R. and Garavan, Hugh, 2004. Executive dysfunction in cocaine addiction: evidence for discordant frontal, cingulate, and cerebellar activity. *Journal of Neuroscience*, 24(49), pp.11017-11022.

Hommer, D.W., Bjork, J.M. and Gilman, J.M., 2011. Imaging brain response to reward in addictive disorders. *New York*, 1216, pp.50-61.

Kilts, C D et al., 2001. Neural activity related to drug craving in cocaine addiction. *Archives of general psychiatry*, 58(4), pp.334-41.

Kilts, Clinton D et al., 2004. The neural correlates of cue-induced craving in cocaine-dependent women. *The American journal of psychiatry*, 161(2), pp.233-41.

Klein, T.A. et al., 2007. Genetically determined differences in learning from errors. *Science*, 318(5856), pp.1642-1645.

Kosten, T.R. et al., 2006. Cue-induced brain activity changes and relapse in cocaine-dependent patients. *Neuropsychopharmacology□ : official publication of the American College of Neuropsychopharmacology*, 31(3), pp.644-50.

Kufahl, P. et al., 2008. Expectation modulates human brain responses to acute cocaine: a functional magnetic resonance imaging study. *Biological psychiatry*, 63(2), pp.222-30.

Kufahl, P.R. et al., 2005. Neural responses to acute cocaine administration in the human brain detected by fMRI. *NeuroImage*, 28(4), pp. 904-914.

Kübler, A., Murphy, K. and Garavan, H, 2005. Cocaine dependence and attention switching within and between verbal and visuospatial working memory. *The European journal of neuroscience*, 21(7), pp.1984-92.

Landau, S.M. et al., 2009. Striatal Dopamine and Working Memory. *Cerebral Cortex*, 19(2), pp.445-454.

Leland, D.S. et al., 2006. Young adult stimulant users' increased striatal activation during uncertainty is related to impulsivity. *NeuroImage*, 33(2), pp.725-31.

Lewis, S.J.G. et al., 2004. Striatal contributions to working memory: a functional magnetic resonance imaging study in humans. *European Journal of Neuroscience*, 19(3), pp.755-760.

Maas, L.C. et al., 1998. Functional magnetic resonance imaging of human brain activation during cue-induced cocaine craving. *The American Journal of Psychiatry*, 155(1), pp.124-126.

Martinez, D. and Narendran, R., 2010. Imaging neurotransmitter release by drugs of abuse. *Current topics in behavioral neurosciences*, 3, pp.219-245.

McClure, S.M., Berns, G.S. and Montague, P.R., 2003. Temporal prediction errors in a passive learning task activate human striatum. *Neuron*, 38(2), pp.339-46.

Moeller, F.G. et al., 2010. Working memory fMRI activation in cocaine-dependent subjects: association with treatment response. *Psychiatry research*, 181(3), pp.174-82.

Murray, Heather W et al., 2003. Relationship of Aggression, Sensation Seeking, and Impulsivity, With Severity of Cocaine Use. *Addictive Disorders Their Treatment*, 2(4), pp.113-121.

Nader, M.A. et al., 2006. PET imaging of dopamine D2 receptors during chronic cocaine self-administration in monkeys. *Nature Neuroscience*, 9(8), pp.1050-1056.

Nigg, J.T., 2000. On Inhibition / Disinhibition in Developmental Psychopathology□ : Views From Cognitive and Personality Psychology and a Working Inhibition Taxonomy. *Psychological Bulletin*, 126(2), pp.220-246.

Noble, E.P., 2003. D2 dopamine receptor gene in psychiatric and neurologic disorders and its phenotypes. *American journal of medical genetics.* Part B, Neuropsychiatric genetics□ : the official publication of the International Society of Psychiatric Genetics, 116B(1), pp.103-25.

Patkar, A A et al., 2004. Pre-treatment measures of impulsivity, aggression and sensation seeking are associated with treatment outcome for African-American cocaine-dependent patients. *Journal of addictive diseases the official journal of the ASAM American Society of Addiction Medicine*, 23(2), pp.109-122.

Pierce, R.C. and Vanderschuren, L.J.M.J., 2010. Kicking the habit: the neural basis of ingrained behaviors in cocaine addiction. *Neuroscience and Biobehavioral Reviews*, 35(2), pp.212-219.

Porrino, L.J. et al., 2007. The effects of cocaine: a shifting target over the course of addiction. *Progress in neuropsychopharmacology biological psychiatry*, 31(8), pp.1593-1600.

Robinson, T.E. and Berridge, K.C., 2008. Review. The incentive sensitization theory of addiction: some current issues. Philosophical transactions of the Royal Society of London. *Series B, Biological sciences*, 363(1507), pp.3137-46.

Schultz, W., 2006. Behavioral theories and the neurophysiology of reward. *Annual review of psychology*, 57, pp.87-115.

Simões-Franklin, C. et al., 2010. Executive function and error detection: The effect of motivation on cingulate and ventral striatum activity. *Human brain mapping*, 31(3), pp.458-69.

Sinha, R. et al., 2005. Neural activity associated with stress-induced cocaine craving: a functional magnetic resonance imaging study. *Psychopharmacology*, 183(2), pp.171-80.

Somerville, L.H. and Casey, B., 2010. Developmental neurobiology of cognitive control and motivational systems. *Current opinion in neurobiology*, 20(2), pp.236-241.

Stalnaker, T.A. et al., 2009. Neural substrates of cognitive inflexibility after chronic cocaine exposure. *Neuropharmacology*, 56 Suppl 1(1), pp.63-72.

Tomasi, D, Goldstein, R Z, et al., 2007. Widespread disruption in brain activation patterns to a working memory task during cocaine abstinence. *Brain research*, 1171, pp.83-92.

Tomasi, Dardo, Goldstein, Rita Z, et al., 2007. Thalamo-cortical dysfunction in cocaine abusers: implications in attention and perception. *Psychiatry Research*, 155(3), pp.189-201.

Tucker, K.A. et al., 2004. Perfusion abnormalities and decision making in cocaine dependence.*Biol Psychiatry*,56(7): pp. 527-530.

Volkow, N D et al., 1993. Decreased dopamine D2 receptor availability is associated with reduced frontal metabolism in cocaine abusers. *Synapse* (New York, N.Y.), 14(2), pp.169-77.

Volkow, N D et al., 1997. Decreased striatal dopaminergic responsiveness in detoxified cocaine-dependent subjects. *Nature*, 386(6627), pp.830-833.

Volkow, Nora D, Wang, G.-J., Fowler, Joanna S, Tomasi, Dardo, Telang, Frank and Baler, R., 2010a. Addiction: decreased reward sensitivity and increased expectation sensitivity conspire to overwhelm the brain's control circuit. *BioEssays□ : news and reviews in molecular, cellular and developmental biology*, 32(9), pp.748-55.

Volkow, Nora D et al., 2006. Cocaine cues and dopamine in dorsal striatum: mechanism of craving in cocaine addiction. *Journal of Neuroscience*, 26(24), pp.6583-6588.

Volkow, Nora D, Fowler, Joanna S, et al., 2010. Cognitive control of drug craving inhibits brain reward regions in cocaine abusers. *NeuroImage*, 49(3), pp.2536-2543.

Volkow, Nora D, Wang, G.-J., Fowler, Joanna S, Tomasi, Dardo, Telang, Frank and Baler, R., 2010b. Addiction: decreased reward sensitivity and increased expectation sensitivity conspire to overwhelm the brain's control circuit. *BioEssays news and reviews in molecular cellular and developmental biology*, 32(9), pp.748-755.

Volkow, Nora D et al., 2008. Dopamine increases in striatum do not elicit craving in cocaine abusers unless they are coupled with cocaine cues. *NeuroImage*, 39(3), pp.1266-1273.

Wexler, B. E., 2001. Functional Magnetic Resonance Imaging of Cocaine Craving. *American Journal of Psychiatry*, 158(1), pp.86-95.

Wheeler, R. a et al., 2008. Behavioral and electrophysiological indices of negative affect predict cocaine self-administration. *Neuron*, 57(5), pp.774-85.

Wilcox, C.E. et al., 2011. Enhanced cue reactivity and fronto-striatal functional connectivity in cocaine use disorders. *Drug and alcohol dependence*, 115(1-2), pp.137-44.

Williams, M.J. and Adinoff, B., 2008. The role of acetylcholine in cocaine addiction. *Neuropsychopharmacology*, 33(8), pp.1779-1797.

Winstanley, C.A., 2007. The orbitofrontal cortex, impulsivity, and addiction: probing orbitofrontal dysfunction at the neural, neurochemical, and molecular level. *Annals Of The New York Academy Of Sciences*, 1121(604), pp.639-655.

Wong, D.F. et al., 2006. Increased occupancy of dopamine receptors in human striatum during cue-elicited cocaine craving. *Neuropsychopharmacology*, 31(12), pp.2716-2727.

In: Striatum: Anatomy, Functions and Role in Disease
Editors: Hugo T. Maldonado and Ignacio M. Ortega
ISBN 978-1-61942-384-8

Chapter IX

Roles of the Striatum in Speech and Language Disorders: Perspectives from the Genetics of Language

Hiroshi Takahashi*[*1], Kaoru Takahashi[2] and Fu-Chin Liu[3]
[1]Department of Neurology, National Hospital Organization, Tottori Medical Center, Tottori, Japan
[2]Department of Integrated Pathology, Tokyo Medical and Dental University, Bunkyo-ku, Tokyo, Japan
[3]Institute of Neuroscience, National Yang-Ming University, Taipei, Taiwan, Republic of China

Abstract

The basal ganglia, generally accepted to be a motor control center, are not considered to be related to language function. However, recent detailed analyses of language in patients suffering from Parkinson's disease and Huntington's disease suggested that the basal ganglia circuitry might underlie the neural processing for language.

Recent human molecular genetic approaches have identified FOXP2, encoding a transcription factor, as a disease-causing gene for a rare inherited form of a speech and language disorder. More recently, mutations in FOXP1, another gene from the same subfamily, were found in individuals with autism spectrum disorders with speech and language deficits.

FOXP1 and FOXP2 are expressed in distinct but overlapping regions of the developing mouse, bird, non-human primate and human. Of importance, the expression of both genes is quite remarkable in the developing striatum, and to a lesser extent in the cerebral cortex. Thus, the spatio-temporal pattern of FOXP2 and FOXP1 expression suggests that the basic neural network underlying speech and language may include the cortico-striatal circuit. Moreover, morphometric and functional imaging studies in

* Correspondence to: H. Takahashi, Department of Neurology, National Hospital Organization, Tottori Medical Center, Tottori, Tottori 689-0203,Japan, Tel: +81-857-59-1111, ext 245; fax: +81-857-59-1589, E-mail address: hiroshi@tottori-iryo.hosp.go.jp (H. Takahashi).

patients with FOXP2 mutations support this assumption. The fact that mice carrying mutations in Foxp2 show morphological and functional alterations in the striatum and a significant phenotypic change in ultrasonic vocalization also supports the importance of cortico-striatal circuits.

A better understanding of the role of the striatum in language may help the development of novel therapeutics for speech and language disturbances in various diseases.

Introduction

The basal ganglia are not generally considered to be a brain region that is necessary for language function, although there are many reports on the relationship between the basal ganglia and language.

Since Broca's description of non-fluent aphasia resulting from damage to the left frontal lobe, morphometric and imaging studies of patients suffering from cortical damage, and functional brain imaging studies of healthy subjects performing language tasks, have repeatedly suggested that specific cortical regions are involved in various aspects of language processing. The left inferior frontal gyrus (Broca's area) and superior temporal gyrus (Wernicke's area) are considered to be the language centers as proposed by Lichtheim's diagram (or its modifications) at the end of the nineteenth century [1]. This classical diagram is not conceptually different from the current model for language processing. The current model attempts to provide a topographic map of the brain modules that mediate speech and language and to relate this topographic map to the anatomic regions of the brain; that is, Broca's area, the angular gyrus and Wernicke's area correspond to syntax, semantics and phonology, respectively [2].

Recent detailed analyses of language in patients suggested that the basal ganglia circuitry might underlie the neural processing for language. Aphasic syndromes usually occur following damage to the cerebral cortex. However, atypical aphasia has been reported following cerebrovascular damages to the basal ganglia. Damasio and Damasio hypothesized that the basal ganglia circuitry contributes to grammatical rule processing in conjunction with the frontal lobe [3]. Ullman and colleagues found that grammatical mistakes occurred in patients suffering from Parkinson's disease and Huntington's disease, in which the basal ganglia are damaged, and that these patients developed a declarative/procedural model of language [4,5]. According to the model, the mental grammar involves procedural memory-like skills and habits, and is rooted in the frontal lobe-basal ganglia, whereas the mental lexicon depends on declarative memory and is rooted in the temporal lobe.

Here, we introduce the recently discovered language genes *FOXP2* and *FOXP1* as disease-causing genes for speech and language disorders, and discuss their expression in the basal ganglia as well as their relation to the cognitive functions of speech and language.

Genetics of Language

Heredity in Speech and Language Disorders

Speech and language disorders are common in childhood. Among them, specific language impairment (SLI) is defined by the state when only language development is deficient for no obvious reason. An epidemiological study of pre-school children in the United States estimated its prevalence as ≤7% [6]. SLI is not caused by environmental factors such as brain damage around the time of birth, poor parenting or hearing loss. Alternatively, SLI is considered to be strongly influenced by heritable factors for the following reasons. SLI tends to run in families (20–40%); twin studies indicated that concordance for monozygotic twins (who are genetically identical) is close to 100%, and that for dizygotic twins is ~50% in terms of SLI diagnosis [7,8]. Although twin studies have shown that genetic factors play an important role in the etiology of such a disorder, a gene that predisposes individuals to speech and language disorders had not been identified until *FOXP2* was discovered as a causative gene for a very rare speech and language disorder.

The KE Family: A Unique Family Case of Speech and Language Disorder

In 1990, a unique case of a large three-generation pedigree, half of whose family members have a developmental verbal dyspraxia, was reported [9]. Verbal dyspraxia is inherited in a pattern consistent with an autosomal dominant penetrance. The patients in the family (called the KE family) have no hearing loss or neurological deficits that affect swallowing or limb movements. Nor do they have any abnormality of other organs. Therefore, the disease observed in the affected members of the KE family is truly regarded as a very distinctive speech and language disorder.

Although many neuropsychologists have extensively analyzed the results of behavioral tests in members of the KE family, there have been inconsistencies in the analyses, and it is still unclear how many core deficits there are. However, it is considered that there is at least one core deficit, verbal dyspraxia, underlying their speech and language disorders. In several studies, deficit patterns in language tests in the affected members resemble 'Broca's aphasia', which is usually seen in patients suffering from brain damage in the 'Broca's language center' located in the left inferior frontal lobe [10].

Discovery of FOXP2 as a 'Language Gene'

Fisher and colleagues at the University of Oxford performed a genome-wide screen of candidate genes underlying the speech and language disorders in the KE family using standard positional cloning techniques in combination with bioinformatics. In 1998, they successfully mapped the gene locus to the long arm of chromosome 7 [11]. Three years later, they identified *FOXP2* as the causative gene for the speech and language disorder [12].

The *FOX* gene family encodes a large group of transcription factors that share a common DNA binding domain of sequences called the forkhead [13]. Within the *FOX* family, the *FOXP* subfamily consists of four members characterized by a zinc finger domain and a leucine zipper motif in addition to a forkhead domain [14].

In the affected KE family members, one point mutation predicted to result in an arginine-to-histidine substitution (R553H) was found in the forkhead domain in the *FOXP2* gene [12]. R553 is invariant among all FOX proteins in species ranging from yeast to humans. This mutation was found in every affected member, but not in unaffected family members or in unrelated control subjects.

There has also been a report of a patient (initials CS) with a translocation between chromosomes 5 and 7 and similar symptoms to the affected members of the KE family [12]. The translocation breakpoint in CS disrupted the gene structure of *FOXP2*. Furthermore, a nonsense mutation at arginine 328 (R328X) was identified in a family, whose affected members had verbal dyspraxia [15]. Therefore, it is likely that the amino acid substitution in the FOXP2 protein leads to a loss of function of one copy of the *FOXP2* gene and that the remaining copy is insufficient to fulfill the normal function of FOXP2 (that is, haploinsufficiency).

Discovery of FOXP1 as another Language Gene

By analogy with *FOXP2*, other *FOXP* subfamily genes are suggested to be good candidates for involvement in speech and language disorders.

In 2009, a patient with a large deletion on chromosome 3, including *FOXP1* and three other genes, was reported [16]. The patient had speech and language deficits and other symptoms such as blepharophimosis and contractures of the hands and feet. In 2010, *FOXP1* deletions were identified in three unrelated patients with speech and language deficits and moderate mental retardation [17]. *De novo* mutations in *FOXP1* were also identified in patients with speech and language deficits and autism [18,19]. These patients with *FOXP1* mutations have broader developmental deficits than the restricted speech and language deficits seen with *FOXP2* mutations. This could be explained by the possibility that *FOXP1* disruption might have a more global impact on brain development than *FOXP2* disruption.

Expression of Foxp/FOXP Subfamily Members

Because *FOXP2* and *FOXP1* are causative for speech and language disorders, the expression of these genes in the brain is of particular interest. The expression patterns of *Foxp1, 2* and *4* mRNAs or proteins in rodent, nonhuman primate and human brains have been reported by several groups [20-27]. Overall, the expression patterns in fetal mouse, rat, nonhuman primate and human brains show striking similarities at comparative developmental stages. Therefore, we first describe the data on the expression pattern of *Foxp1, 2* and *4* in rodents. Thereafter, specific comments on the expression of *FOXP2* and *FOXP1* genes in nonhuman primates and humans will be added.

Foxp1, Foxp2 and *Foxp4* are expressed in several structures of the central nervous system during development, including the cerebral cortex, striatum, thalamus, cerebellum and spinal cord. Their expression patterns overlap considerably. However, detailed analysis revealed a distinct pattern of expression for each member in some neuronal types, even though they are expressed in the same anatomical regions. Biochemical analyses have revealed that homo- or heterodimerization of Foxp1, Foxp2 and Foxp4 proteins is required for DNA binding and their transcriptional activities [28]. Thus, the precise combination of homodimers and heterodimers of different Foxp proteins in the same neurons may regulate the transcription of downstream target genes during brain development and control the patterning of brain structures.

Here we focus on the expression patterns of *Foxp1, 2,* and *4* in the developing and adult basal ganglia where they are highly expressed.

Basal Ganglia

Foxp1, Foxp2 and *Foxp4* share partially overlapping and yet differentially regulated expression patterns during striatal development [20-27]. In embryonic stages, all three are expressed in the striatal primordia (lateral ganglionic eminence, LGE). Expression of *Foxp2* and *Foxp1* is persistent in adulthood, whereas expression of *Foxp4* is developmentally down-regulated in the postnatal stage.

These three genes have a common character in that all are expressed only in the LGE, but not in the MGE (medial ganglionic eminence). However, there were subtle differences among their expression patterns within the LGE. It has been revealed that the LGE can be divided into a large ventral domain (ventral LGE) giving rise to the striatum and a smaller dorsal domain (dorsal LGE) giving rise to the interneurons that migrate in the rostral migratory stream to populate the olfactory bulb [29]. Both *Foxp2* and *Foxp4* are expressed in the subventricular zone (SVZ) and the mantle zone of the dorsal and ventral LGE, while *Foxp1* is only expressed in the SVZ and the mantle zone of the ventral LGE, but not in the dorsal LGE [23].

The ontogenic expression patterns of *Foxp* members are distinct between striatal compartments [22, 23]. The striatum comprises two distinct neurochemical compartments, striosomes and the matrix [30-32]. The expression levels of various neurochemicals, neurogenesis and neural connectivity are all different in these two compartments.

In the early embryonic stage, expression of *Foxp1* starts later than that of *Foxp2* and *Foxp4*. *Foxp1* expression is observed in both the striosomal and matrix compartments until adulthood. Expression of *Foxp2* and *Foxp4* in the striatum starts during the same early embryonic stage, and similar and homogeneous expression patterns continue until the late embryonic stage. Thereafter, *Foxp2* expression becomes restricted to the striosomal compartment and continues until adulthood. By contrast, *Foxp4* expression declines in compartmental order: first in the striosomes and later in the matrix, from the late embryonic to the early postnatal stages. The differential expression of *Foxp1, Foxp2* and *Foxp4* may play an important role in establishing the specific types of neurons in each compartment of the striatum.

In the fetal human brain, *FOXP2* and *FOXP1* mRNAs are also expressed in the striatal primordia [21,25]. The expression of *FOXP2* is developmentally regulated: the expression is quite low in the adult according to northern blot analysis [12]. *FOXP2* and *FOXP1* expression patterns in the human brain have not been examined in the perinatal stages because of the limited amount of human brain material and for ethical reasons. Expression data for *FoxP2* and *FoxP1* at this stage are available in non-human primates.

In developing nonhuman primates, *FoxP2* is selectively expressed in the striosomal compartment of the basal ganglia during the perinatal period [24]. Thus, the *Foxp2/FOXP2* expression pattern in the striatum seems to be conserved in rodents and primates. Nevertheless, there are several aspects in which *Foxp2/FoxP2* striatal expression differs between primates and rodents. First, striosomal *FoxP2* expression in the monkey striatum is only detected during the perinatal and early postnatal periods, and the expression level declines postnatally. In contrast, *Foxp2* striosomal expression in the rodent striatum persists into adulthood. Second, regional differences in *FoxP2* mRNA expression exist within the striatum. The primate striatum comprises the caudate nucleus and the putamen. In the monkey brain, the *FoxP2* mRNA expression level in the striosomal compartment is different between the caudate nucleus and the putamen; specifically, *FoxP2* expression in the caudate nucleus is higher than that in the putamen in the perinatal stage and barely detectable in the putamen in the postnatal stage. In contrast to *FoxP2* expression, *FoxP1* expression is homogeneous in the caudate nucleus and the putamen during the prenatal and postnatal periods in monkeys [24]. Thereafter, *FoxP1* expression declines in both the caudate nucleus and the putamen.

Imaging Studies on KE Family Members

No autopsy records of affected members of the KE family have been reported. Therefore, we have to wait for the detailed neuropathological analyses in the future. However, neuroimaging techniques have enabled us to investigate the gross structural and functional abnormalities in the brains of the affected members of the KE family [33,34]. Investigations using voxel-based morphometric (VBM) methods of MRI analysis have revealed the structural brain abnormalities in the affected members. The VBM analyses showed bilateral abnormalities in the caudate nucleus, the inferior frontal gyrus (Broca's area), the precentral gyrus, the temporal pole and the cerebellum in affected members compared with unaffected members and age-matched controls. In addition, the reduction in volume was significantly correlated with the performance of the affected members on several language tasks. A functional abnormality in the caudate nucleus was also found in a positron emission tomography (PET) study [35]. Further analyses have been conducted using functional MRI [36]. An atypical brain activation pattern was observed in the affected members when performing both silent and spoken verb generation tasks, as well as word repetition tasks. That is, unaffected members showed a typical left-dominant activation in the inferior frontal gyrus, including Broca's area, in both generation tasks, and a more bilateral activation in the repetition tasks, whereas the affected members showed significant underactivation of Broca's area and its right homolog, as well as of language-related cortical regions and the putamen. Moreover, only in the affected members was paradoxical activation observed in cortical regions that are not usually involved in language tasks. The underactivation of Broca's area in affected members reminds us of patients suffering from motor aphasia caused by cerebrovascular brain damage. The language deficits in both cases are very similar. The functional abnormality in the putamen suggests dysfunction of the striatum.

Phenotypes in Foxp2 Mutant Mice and "Humanized" Foxp2 Mice

Foxp2 mutant mice have been generated and analyzed by several groups [37-40]. Homozygotes deficient for both *Foxp2* alleles (null mutant) show severe motor impairment, premature death and an absence of ultrasonic vocalization when pups are isolated from their mothers. Shu and colleagues reported abnormalities in the cerebella of homozygotes; specifically, the alignment of Purkinje cells was irregular [39]. Other groups have generated knock-in mice with a point mutation in the *Foxp2* gene to give rise to an R552H mutation (corresponding to the human FOXP2 R553H mutation) [37,38]. Homozygous R552H mice reported by Fujita and colleagues showed largely similar phenotypes to the KO mice reported by Shu [37,39]. There were some different phenotypes and interpretations in another line of mutant mice with the same R552H mutation [38]. Homozygous R552H mice were able to produce complex ultrasonic vocalization in response to isolation. Heterozygous R552H mice were overtly normal in terms of brain structure and development. The most interesting findings in their study were that heterozygous R552H mice show significant deficits in motor-skill learning and abnormal synaptic plasticity is observed in striatal and cerebellar brain slices by electrophysiological analysis.

DNA sequence comparison of the *Foxp2* genes among many species has revealed that the *Foxp2*-encoded protein is extraordinarily conserved among mammals. There are only two amino acids (out of 715 amino acid residues) that differ between humans and chimpanzees, and three that differ between humans and mice. Surprisingly, the amino acid sequence of the forkhead domain is completely identical among rodents, nonhuman primates and humans. To clarify the role of the substitutions in FOXP2, mice with a humanized version of Foxp2 were generated by homologous recombination techniques [40]. These mice had qualitatively different ultrasonic vocalizations, decreased exploratory behavior and decreased dopamine concentrations in the brain. Moreover, medium spiny neurons, which make up more than 90% of striatal neurons, had increased dendrite lengths and increased synaptic plasticity in the "humanized" Foxp2 mice. Mice carrying one nonfunctional *Foxp2* allele showed the opposite effects. These results may partly explain the enhanced capability of cortico-striatal circuits in the human brain that regulate critical aspects of language and a possible involvement of cortico-striatal circuits in the brains of FOXP2-mutated KE family members.

The FOXP2 Expression Pattern in the Brain and its Relation to the Cognitive Functions of Speech and Language

FOXP2 is highly expressed in the developing human brain, and its expression is down-regulated in the adult. This suggests that the speech and language impairments in the affected members of the KE family might be due to the developmental defects of the neural network critically involved in speech and language functions, and that formation of the network is dependent upon a gene network via FOXP2. The spatiotemporal *FOXP2* expression pattern suggests that the basic neural network that underlies speech and language may include motor-related circuits, including cortico-striatal circuits.

This assumption is supported by brain imaging studies on KE family members. Morphometric analysis using MRI and functional anatomical studies using PET and fMRI have revealed a bilateral abnormality in the inferior frontal cortex, caudate-putamen and cerebellum [33-36]. In particular, preferential expression of FOXP2 in the striosomes of the caudate nucleus seems to be well correlated with the brain abnormalities in FOXP2-mutated KE family patients.

The affected members of the KE family show impaired movement of mouth, lips and tongue during speech. Canales and Graybiel have shown that a striosome-dominant activation could occur under conditions in which repetitive behaviors are induced by dopamine agonists [41]. Moreover, dopamine agonist-induced dyskinesia of repetitive movements is present in experimental parkinsonism [42,43]. Therefore, we hypothesized that the symptoms of orofacial dyspraxia in KE family patients may be related to dysfunction of the striosomal system in the striatum.

As described above, language impairments in the affected members of the KE family resemble those in Broca's aphasia, which usually involves the inferior frontal lobe. Although the basal ganglia are not generally considered to be necessary for language acquisition, several reports suggest that the caudate nucleus, in particular, may be involved in language processing [4,5]. Using fMRI, Crinion and colleagues demonstrated that neuronal responses within the left caudate are sensitive to changes in language or the meaning of words in German–English and Japanese–English bilingual individuals. It was therefore suggested that the left caudate plays a universal role in monitoring and controlling the language in use [44].

Hypothesis for the Role of the Cortico-Striatal Circuit in Language Acquisition

Preferential expression of *FOXP2/FOXP1* in the striatum and morphometric and functional changes in the striatums of *FOXP2*-mutated patients suggest some roles of the striatum in language functions. On the other hand, as shown in the classical Lichtheim's diagram, several regions of the cerebral cortex have long been considered to be involved in language functions. So how is this striatal involvement in language related to the classical model of language processing? The following interpretation might be possible.

Considering that both *FOXP2* and *FOXP1* are highly expressed in the immature brain, but not in the adult one, a neural network critical for language acquisition may be formed very early in development, and its formation may be dependent upon a gene network including *FOXP2* and *FOXP1*. Therefore, *FOXP2* (or *FOXP1*) mutations cause disorganization of the formation of this network that is critical for language acquisition, resulting in speech and language disorders. Thus, the language disorder caused by *FOXP2* mutations can be recognized as a kind of congenital anomaly.

Many animals have cortico-striatal circuits that are necessary for working memory. Human beings might apply part of these cortico-striatal circuits to the basis of information processing in language. Dysfunction in these circuits may result in speech and language disorders. If the role of the striatum in language function decreases during brain maturation and the cerebral cortex is the main structure underlying language processing in the adult, language disturbances may not be so severe when the striatum is damaged in the adult.

This scheme is true for song learning in songbirds. Birdsong is a complex learned vocal behavior, with similarities to human speech. Song learning involves two distinct phases—sensory learning and sensori-motor learning [45]. During sensory learning, a young bird listens to and memorizes tutor songs. In the ensuing phase of sensori-motor learning, the bird relies on auditory feedback to match its song to the memorized song.

If basal ganglia are damaged during sensory learning, the bird cannot sing properly as an adult. However, damage to the basal ganglia in adult birds has little effect on previously learned behavior. Thus, the basal ganglia are required for song learning in the first phase, but not for song production in the second phase when the song has already been learned. The cerebral cortex is necessary for song production.

Perspectives

The discovery of *FOXP2* and *FOXP1* genes as 'Language Genes' sheds light on the role of the striatum and cortico-striatal circuits in language acquisition.

Identification of genes downstream of *FOXP2/Foxp2* may provide insights into the molecular mechanisms underlying neural development such as striatal compartmentalization and the formation of the cortico-striatal neural network potentially related to language acquisition. The identification of genes downstream of *FOXP2/Foxp2* might also lead to the discovery of susceptibility genes for SLI and autism. Further understanding of the gene network may be valuable for the development of therapeutics for SLI and autism.

References

[1] Heilman KM. *J Clin Neurol* (2006) 2:149-162.

[2] Grabowski TJ, Damasio AR. Investigating language with functional neuroimaging In: Toga AW and Mazziotta JC eds. *Brain Mapping The Systems*. San Diego: Academic Press (2000) 425-461.

[3] Damasio AR, Damasio H. *Sci Am* (1992) 267: 88-95.

[4] Ullman MT, Corkin S, Coppola M et al. *J Cogn Neurosci* (1997) 9: 266-276.

[5] Ullman MT. *Nature Rev Neurosci* (2001) 2: 717-726.

[6] Tomblin JB, Records NL, Buckwalter P et al. *J Speech Lang Hear Res* (1997) 40: 1245-1260.

[7] Bishop DVM, North T, Donlan C. *Dev Med Child Neurol* (1995) 37:56-71.

[8] Choudhury N, Benasich AA . *J Speech Lang Hear Res* (2003) 46: 261-272.

[9] Hurst JA, Baraitser M, Auger E et al. *Dev Med Child Neurol* (1990) 32: 352-355.

[10] Watkins KE, Dronkers NF, Vargha-Khadem F, et al. *Brain* (2002)125: 452-464.

[11] Fisher SE, Vargha-Khadem F, Watkins KE et al. *Nature Genet* (1998) 18: 168-170.
[12] Lai CSL, Fisher SE, Hurst JA et al. *Nature* (2001) 413: 519-523.
[13] Carlsson P, Mahlapuu M. *Dev Biol* (2002) 250: 1-23.
[14] Shu W, Yang H, Zhang L et al. *J Biol Chem* (2001) 276: 27488-27497.
[15] MacDermot KD, Bonora E, Sykes N et al. *Am J Hum Genet* (2005) 76: 1074-1080.
[16] Pariani MJ, Spencer A, Graham JM et al. *Eur J Med Genet* (2009) 52: 123-127.
[17] Horn D, Kapeller J, Rivera-Brugues N et al.*Hum Mut* (2010) 31: E1851-1860.
[18] Hamdan FF, Daoud H, Rochefort D et al. *Am J Hum Genet* (2010) 87: 671-678
[19] O'Roak BJ, Deriziotis P, Lee C et al. *Nat Genet* (2001) 43: 585-589.
[20] Ferland RJ, Cherry TJ, Preware PO et al. *J Comp Neurol* (2003) 460: 266-279.
[21] Lai CS, Gerrelli D, Monaco AP et al. *Brain* (2003) 126:2455-2462.
[22] Takahashi K, Liu F-C, Hirokawa K et al. *J Neurosci Res* (2003) 73:61-72.
[23] Takahashi K, Liu FC, Hirokawa K et al. *J Neurosci Res* (2008) 86:3106-3116.
[24] Takahashi K, Liu FC, Oishi T et al. *J Comp Neurol* (2008) 509:180-189.
[25] Teramitsu I, Kudo LC, London SE et al. *J Neurosci* (2004) 24:3152-3163.
[26] Tamura S, Morikawa Y, Iwanishi H et al. *Gene Expression Patterns* (2003) 3:193-197.
[27] Tamura S, Morikawa Y, Iwanishi H et al. *Neuroscience* (2004) 124:261-267.
[28] Li S, Weidenfeld J, Morrisey EE. *Mol Cell Biol* (2004) 24:809-822.
[29] Campbell K. *Curr Opin Neurobiol* (2003)13:50-56.
[30] Graybiel AM. *Trends In Neuroscience* (1990) 15:244-254.
[31] Graybiel AM, Penney JB. Chemical architecture of the basal ganglia. In: Bloom FE, Björklund A, Hökfelt T,eds. *Handbook of Chemical Neuroanatomy. The Primate Nervous System. Part III.* Amsterdam: Elsevier Science (1999) 15: 227-284.
[32] Gerfen CR, Wilson CJ. The basal ganglia. In: Swanson LW, Björklund A, Hökfelt T, eds. *Handbook of Chemical Neuroanatomy. Integrated Systems of the CNS. Part III.* Amsterdam: Elsevier Science (1996)12:371-468.
[33] Belton E, Salmond CH, Watkins KE et al. *Hum Brain Mapp* (2003)18: 194-200.
[34] Watkins KE, Vargha-Khadem F, Ashburner J et al. *Brain* (2002)125:465-478.
[35] Vargha-Khadem F, Watkins KE, Price CJ et al. *Proc Natl Acad Sci USA* (1998) 95:12695-12700.
[36] Liégeois F, Baldeweg T, Connelly A et al. *Nat Neurosci* (2003) 6:1230-1237.
[37] Fujita E, Tanabe Y, Shiota A et al. *Proc Natl Acad Sci USA* (2008)105: 3117-3122.
[38] Groszer M, Keays DA, Deacon RM et al. *Curr Biol* (2008) 18:354-362.
[39] Shu W, Cho JY, Jiang Y et al. *Proc Natl Acad Sci USA* (2005) 102: 9643-9648.
[40] Enard W, Gehre S, Hammerschmidt K et al. *Cell* (2009)137:961-971.
[41] Canales JJ, Graybiel AM. *Nat Neurosci (*2000) 3:377-383.
[42] Cenci MA, Tranberg A, Andersson M et al. *Neuroscience* (1999) 94:515-527.
[43] Saka E, Elibol B, Erdem S et al. *Brain Res* (1999) 825:104-114.
[44] Crinion J, Turner R, Grogan A et al. *Science* (2006) 312:1537-1540.
[45] Brainard MS, Doupe AJ. *Nat Rev Neurosci* (2000) 1: 31-40.

In: Striatum: Anatomy, Functions and Role in Disease
Editors: Hugo T. Maldonado and Ignacio M. Ortega
ISBN 978-1-61942-384-8

Chapter X

Iron-Dextran Infusion into the Substantia Nigra: Effects on the Striatal Dopamine

Alfonso Alfaro-Rodríguez[ac3]***, Rigoberto Gonzalez-Pina***[b] ***and Antonio Bueno-Nava***[ac]

[a]Departamento de Neurofisiología-Laboratorio de Cromatografia y Microdiálisis, Instituto Nacional de Rehabilitación, SSA, MexicoCity D.F., Mexico

[b]Departamento de Neurofisiología-Laboratorio de Neuroplasticidad, Instituto Nacional de Rehabilitación, SSA, Mexico City D.F., Mexico

[c]Departamento de Neurofisiología-Laboratorio de Neuroquímica, Instituto Nacional de Rehabilitación, SSA, Mexico City D.F., Mexico

Abstract

Iron is essential for the normal central nervous system (CNS) growth and development. Now a lot of evidences point out that the iron levels in basal ganglia and substantia nigra are higher in PD brains than in normal brains. As a long term effect, iron chloride infusions into the rat SNc can decrease striatal dopamine (DA) levels. However, the striatal dopamine content after iron-dextran infusion into the rat SNc has not been completely elucidated. Thus, the aim of this work was to measure the striatal DA concentration after iron-dextran infusion into the SNc. 40 male Wistar rats that were used and divided into five groups to determine the striatal DA content. The groups consisted of control, saline infused at 7 and 30 days, and iron-dextran infused at 7 and 30 days. Motor performance was assessed in iron-dextran and saline infused groups at 30 days. The striatal DA levels were determined with HPLC. There was a significant ($P < 0.05$) decrease in DA concentrations in the striatum ipsilateral to the injury site. In contrast, there were no significant differences in DA concentration between the sham-operated and

[3] Corresponding author. A. Alfaro-Rodriguez, Departamento de Neurofisiologia-Laboratorio de Neuroquimica, Torre de Investigacion, Instituto Nacional de Rehabilitacion, SSA, Calz. México-Xochimilco 289, Col. Arenal de Guadalupe Deleg. Tlalpan C.P. 14389 Mexico City, MEXICO. E-mail: alfa1360@yahoo.com.mx.

control groups. We also observed increased motor deficit in iron-dextran infused rats. In conclusion, the striatal DA reduction observed after iron-dextran infusion could be associated with oxidative injury in the SNc. On the other hand, the motor deficit could be a result of disturbances in striatal and cortical dopaminergic neuromodulation.

Introduction

Iron is essential for the normal central nervous system (CNS) growth and development. In the brain, iron overload and iron-induced oxidative stress constitute a common mechanism that is involved in the development of neurodegenerations such as Parkinson's disease (PD) and Alzheimer's disease. Now a lot of evidences point out that the iron levels in basal ganglia and substantia nigra are higher in PD brains than in normal brains. Therefore, iron metabolism needs to be tightly regulated by various proteins that transport, sequester, and mobilize iron.

The basal ganglia are associated with the executive and motor functions of the sensorimotor cortex [1]. In rats, the basal ganglia include the striatum and the substantia nigra pars compacta (SNc). The striatum receives afferent input from the sensorimotor cortex and SNc [2]. The SNc contains dopaminergic neurons, and most studies have indicated that stimulation of dopamine receptors produce effects on striatal glutamatergic and GABAergic signaling [3,4]. In this context, SNc damage or drug treatments may interfere with the signal transduction process that is modulated by dopamine receptors [5]. Iron is a catalyst for such oxygen radicals as hydroxyl radicals, which react readily with unsuturated fatty acids, proteins, carbohydrates, DNA and RNA [6]. Many previous studies have shown that damage to and degeneration of the SNc, which lead to a loss of dopaminergic neurons in animal models of parkinsonism, are associated with oxidative stress [7,8]. Numerous studies have also indicated that intranigral infusion of iron can induce oxidative injury in the rat brain [9,10]. This can subsequently lead to degeneration of the dopaminergic neurons [11,12] since the nigrostriatal afferent connections from SNc are highly circumscribed.

Iron-dextran is used in anemic patients, and it is a stable parenteral iron product [13]. Furthermore, ferric chloride infusions into the rat SNc can decrease the long term levels of striatal dopamine (DA) [11]. However, other reports have also shown that the sequelae from cortical injuries could be short-term [14]. However, the striatal dopaminergic content after iron-dextran infusion into the rat SNc has not been evaluated. The metabolism of iron-dextran in the central nervous system and in other systems is slower than the metabolism rate for ferrous/ferric forms [15]. Since it is known that iron could induce free radicals through the Fenton's reaction in the brain, we hypothesized that iron-dextran could also induce chronic injuries with prolonged effect in the brain through gradual increases in free radical formation. Such a model for inducing neurodegeneration would allow future studies on the mechanisms of free radical-mediated loss of dopaminergic neurons in the SNc.

Material and Method

We used 40 male Wistar rats (260-310 g) provided by the vivarium of the Instituto Nacional de Rehabilitacion. Rats were maintained on a 12-h/12-h light/darkness schedule, and they were treated according to the Guide for the Care and Use of Experimental Animals [16]. These animals were allocated into five groups: control (C, n = 8), sham-operated and sacrificed at 7 days (S7; infusion of saline solution in SNc, n = 8), sham-operated and sacrificed at 30 days (S30; infusion of saline solution in SNc, n=8), injured and sacrificed at 7 days (I7; iron-dextran infusion in SNc, n = 8) and injured and sacrificed at 30 days (I30; iron-dextran infusion in SNc, n = 8). Before surgeries, these animals were anesthetized with Ketamine-Xylazine (80 mg/Kg-5 mg/Kg) and were mounted on a stereotaxic frame (Stoelting Corp., Wood Dale, IL). The skulls of the animals were exposed with an incision on the scalp, and a trephine hole was made (1 mm diameter, approximately) for intranigral infusion of iron-dextran (1 mg in 10 uL) or saline solution (10 uL) in the following coordinates: AP = -5.3, L = 2.3, DV = 7.7 with respect to bregma [17]. The solutions were infused at a rate of 1 uL/min using a microinjection pump (MA/Microdialysis AB, Sweden: Mod CMA/400). After the injections, the scalps were sutured. Post-operative care of the animals was consistent with the methods described by Bueno-Nava et al [14]. Given that this type of injury can lead to a permanent loss of neurons, we expected that any sequelae from the surgery would remain for a long time. Thus, the behavioral sequelae of the S30 and I30 animals were evaluated using a motor evaluation protocol as described in the sensorimotor assessment by Garcia et al. [18] and Gonzalez-Pina et al [19]. The sensitivity and reliability of these methods were previously described by Pantoni et al [20].

Animals were decapitated at different times (7 and 30 days) between 18:00 h and 19:00 h in order to eliminate the variations in DA levels that are due to circadian rhythms. The procedure for the extraction and analysis of DA was performed according to Gonzalez-Pina and Paz [21]. The brains were extracted and placed on a cool plate to isolate both sides of the striatum. Tissue was collected in Teflon tubes, and a solution of 0.5 ml of perchloric acid 0.4 N containing 0.1% w/v of sodium metabisulfite was added. The tissues were then homogenized and centrifuged at 15,000 rpm for 20 min in 4°C. The supernatant was filtered and stored at -70°C for chromatographic analysis. DA content was analyzed by high performance liquid chromatography (Alltech, HPLC Pump, Model: 626) coupled to a coulometric electrochemical detector (ESA, Model: Coulochem III). Detection conditions were as follows: analytical cell (ESA 5011A) with the potentials = +350 mV, E_1 = +200 mV and E_2 = -200 mV. The peaks were sent to a computer with an EZCrom SI (version 3.2.1) program. In order to determine the concentrations of DA, the chromatograms of the samples were interpolated with the chromatogram obtained from five standard samples whose DA concentrations were known. An analytical column for catecholamines was used (Alltech, Adsorbosphere Catecholamine, 100 x 4.6 mm, 3 *u*m of particle size). The mobile phase utilized consisted of a phosphate buffer solution (0.1 mM, pH 3.2) that contained (in mM) sodium octyl sulfate (0.2), EDTA (0.1) and methanol (15% v/v). The flow rate used was 1.6 ml/min. Statistical analysis of the DA contents was performed with a one-way ANOVA and a post hoc Tukey test, while the motor deficit tests were analyzed using a non-parametric Mann-Whitney's U. In all cases, the level of significance was set at $p \leq 0.05$.

Result

Motor deficit scores showed a significant increase by ~400% in the I30 animals (4.0 ± 1.0; $n = 8$, $P \leq 0.001$) compared to the scores for the S30 group (0.68 ± 0.2; $n = 8$; Figure 1). These results were consistent with the neurological behavior assessments reported by an observer who was blinded to the treatments. This observer qualitatively determined the differences in sensory-motor behaviors between the two groups (Table 1).

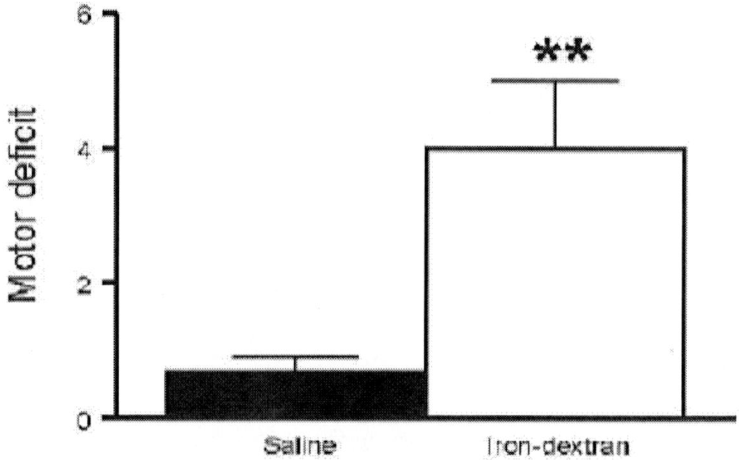

Figure 1. Motor evaluation scores obtained from saline (S30) and injured (I30) groups after iron-dextran or saline solution infusions into the SNc. Thirty days after iron-dextran infusions, the motor deficits were higher in the I30 group than those in the S30 group. Bars represent mean ± S.E.M. Asterisks indicate significant difference (**, P < 0.001) from S30 group.

Table 1.Motor behaviors* after iron-dextran and saline solution infusion

	Groups	
Test	Infusion of Saline solution (S30)	Iron-dextran infusion (I30)
Reaction to touch on either side of trunk	Symmetrical response	Weak response on left side
Climbing wall of wire cage	Weak to normal climbing	Fails to climb
Symmetry of forelimbs (outstretching while held by tail)	Symmetrical outreach	Left side: moves and outreaches than righ side.

*Described by Garcia et al, 2005.

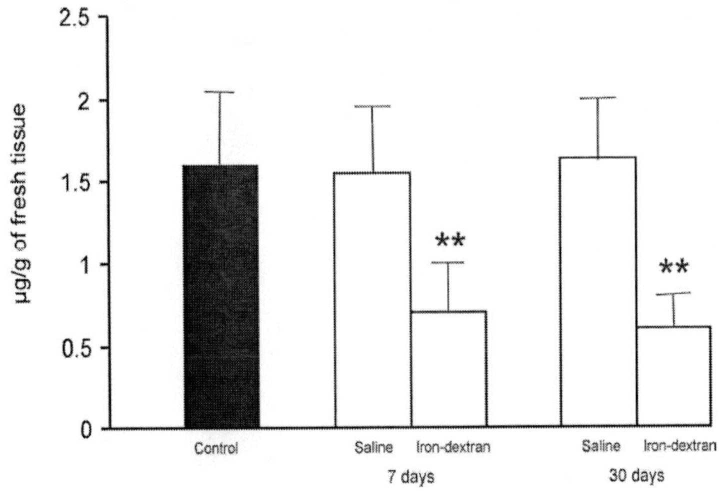

Figure 2. Striatal dopamine (DA) concentration at 7 and 30 days after iron-dextran infusion into the SNc. DA concentrations in the striatum ipsilateral to the injury site at 7 and 30 days post injury were lower in both the I7 and 130 groups than those in the control (C) and sham-operated (S7 and S30) groups. However, there were no differences in DA concentration between the sham-operated (S7 and S30) and control (C) groups. Bars represent mean ± S.E.M. One-way analysis of variance (ANOVA) was used to determine the significance between the groups, followed by a post hoc Tukey test (***P*≤0.01).

a)

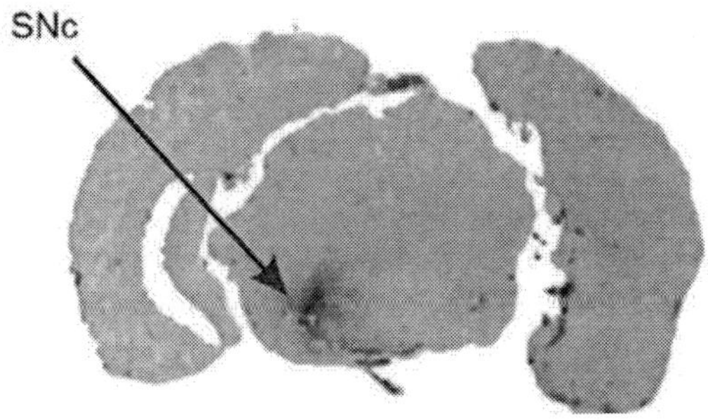

b)

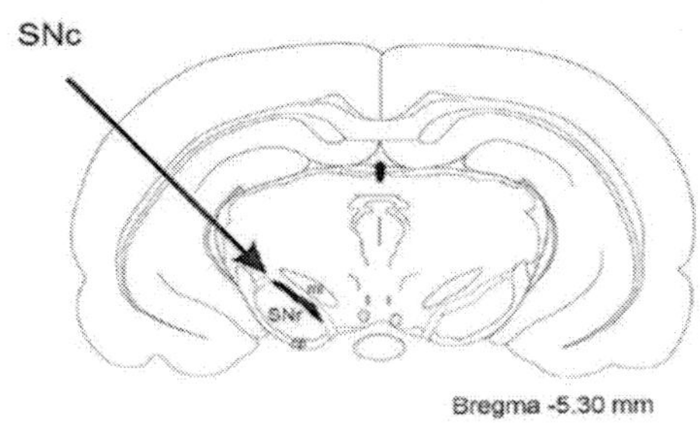

Figure3. Coronal slice showing the extent of the lesion zone into the brain (arrows). (A) Photomicrographs of iron-dextran after infusion in SNc group (n= 6); (B) Schematic representation showing the extent of the lesión, the equivalent schemes taken from the Paxinos and Watson's stereotaxic atlas [17]. Abbreviations: SNc, substantia nigra pars compacta; SNr, substantia nigra, reticular part; ml, medial lemniscus; cp, cerebral peduncle, basal part.

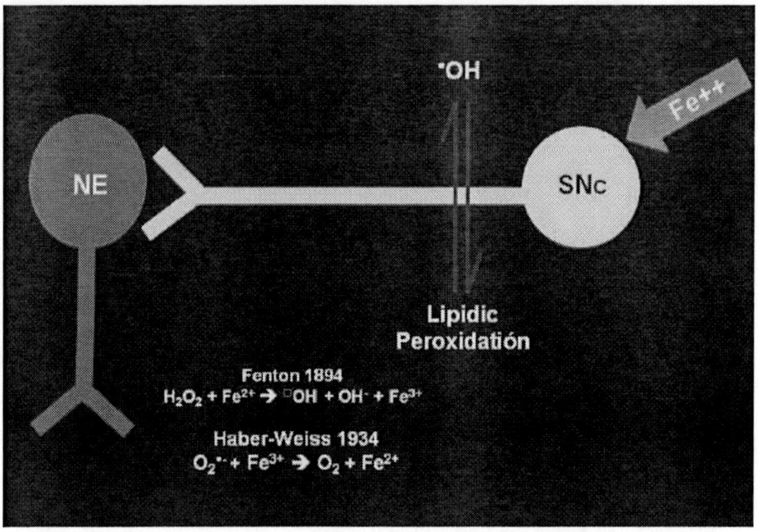

Figure 4 Schematic representation showing Iron catalyzes the formation of free radicals into hydroxyl radicals via Fenton's reaction as possible mechanism of damage.

On the other hand, there were significant decreases in DA concentration in the striatum ipsilateral to the injury site (1.6 ± 0.45; $n = 8$; Figure 2) for animals infused with iron-dextran compared to the DA levels of control groups. There were decreases of ~56% (0.7 ± 0.3 µg/g of fresh tissue; $n = 8$) and ~62% (0.6 ± 0.2; $n = 8$) in DA concentrations for iron-dextran infused animals at 7 and 30 days, respectively. This reduction in DA levels was also reflected between the iron-dextran infused group and the two sham-operated groups (S7 and S30). In contrast, there was no significant difference in terms of DA concentration between the sham-operated and control groups. Furthermore, the striatal DA concentrations in the striatum contralateral to the injury site were not significantly different between the sham-operated (S7 and S30) and injured (I7 and I30) groups (data not shown).

The morphologic analysis was performed in 6 rats. Each rat was deeply anesthetized with sodium pentobarbital (55 mg/kg; ip) and perfused transcardially with 100 ml ice cold 0.1 M sodium phosphate buffer, pH 7.4, followed by 300 ml of 10% formalin in the same buffer. The brains were re-moved after perfusion-fixation. The brain was coronal sectioned and embedding in paraffin in order to proceed with the histological technique. Serial sections of 5 µm were cut and sixteen slides with six sections each were mounted and stained with Cresyl Violet (Figure 3).

Discussion

It is known that Iron levels increase naturally in mature and older brains. Postmortem PD patients can have 25%-100% increased levels of iron in the substantia nigra [10]. Iron catalyzes the formation of free radicals into hydroxyl radicals via Fenton's reaction (Figure 4) [6,10]. Both the hydroxyl radicals and the products of hydroxyl radicals can initiate the propagation of lipid peroxidation by extracting a hydrogen atom from polyunsaturated fatty acids in cell membranes, thus increasing the rates of peroxidation in the brain and contributing to neuronal injury [9,19,22]. Besides peroxidation, free radicals also produce increased levels of free intracellular Ca^{++} [23] and inhibit the Na^{+}-K^{+} ATP-ase [24]. Decreased ATP content and activation of the calcium-dependent proteases have also been reported [25-27].

Our results showed that iron-dextran infusion in the SNc decreased DA concentration in the striatum ipsilateral to the injury site at 7 days post infusion. Lin reported that intranigral infusion of zinc depleted the striatal dopamine content after seven days, and this was enhanced by a concomitant infusion of iron [28]. These authors suggested that the depletion of dopamine was mediated in part by oxidative injury and, subsequently, lipid peroxidation [11,28,29]. It is important to note that these are short-term effects that occur before the onset of neurodegeneration. On the other hand, several long-term effects have been reported by Sengstock et al., who demonstrated that ferric chloride infusion into the SNc induced degeneration at 1-2 months post-injury [11]. Thus, a reduction of striatal dopaminegic metabolism has been reported [30-32]. However, it is possible that an iron-dextran infusion can produce immediate effects on DA content as a result of increased Ca^{++} levels. This may be a cause of long-term dopaminergic neuron loss. The dopaminergic system is particularly vulnerable to free radicals, and Cantuti-Castelvetri et al, have further reported that DA may itself be a source of free radicals [33]. Thus, our results suggest that iron-dextran has the same effects on DA content as infusion of ferrous/ferric iron. Consequently, it is important to assess the early effects of iron on dopaminergic metabolism in order to identify the therapeutic window in rats and to study the mechanisms involved in functional recovery.

It is clear that the long-term effects of iron infusion produce behavioral side effects on sensory-motor performance. We found a dramatic deficit in motor performance at 30 days after iron-dextran infusion and a weak response on the left side as a reaction to touch on the trunk. The last fact suggests that the neuronal loss in SNc also affected other brain regions such as the cortex. It is known that the SNc also sends efferents to the sensorimotor cortex [34], which could be affected by the lack of dopaminergic innervation after iron-dextran infusion.

Although we have discussed the similarities between iron-dextran and ferrous/ferric iron on the levels of DA in the brain, we also expected some differences in their mechanisms that lead to neurodegeneration. There is accumulating evidence suggesting that iron is deposited predominantly in the oligodendrocytes in the brain [35]. However, cell culture studies of nervous tissue showed that neurons could just as easily ingest iron when exposed to a high concentration of iron-dextran. Some of these neurons did not show degenerative changes after exposure to iron-dextran for 10 days, but by 21 days, all soma and axons had degenerated [36]. The difference with ferrous/ferric iron is that these forms are immediately available for free radical formation, while iron-dextran is a more stable form that can be incorporated into the oligodendrocites as well as neurons at higher concentrations [35].

Other reports have suggested that iron-dextran is dissociated into ferrous iron [37]. Miur and Golberg observed a mixture of iron-dextran and ferritin in the cytoplasmic vacuolas of macrophages. These were gradually replaced by vacuoles that contained only ferritin [15]. These observations could in part explain the long-term effects of exposure to iron-dextran. These results supported the changes that we saw with dopamine levels at 30 days and further supported the involvement of these compounds in progressive oxidative injury, neuronal degeneration and death. It has been suggested that a loss of nigral neurons could mediate movement disorders [10]. Our results showed greater motor deficits at 30 days after iron-dextran infusion in the I30 group when compared to the control group. This neurological deficit could be associated with chronic oxidative damage, neuronal degeneration and death in the dopaminergic system [11,28,36,38].

Conclusion

As a long term effect, iron-dextran infusion into the SNc decreased the striatal dopamine concentration ipsilateral to the injury site. This result was consistent with that found in studies of rats with induced Parkinsonism [29]. Thus, iron-dextran infusion into the SNc could be used to study the biochemical basis of Parkinsonism and other dopaminergic neurodegenerative disorders. In addition, this same technique can be used for future animal studies involving antioxidant therapies. This may represent an important step in developing therapeutic strategies in human patients.

References

[1] Groenewegen, H. J. (2003). The basal ganglia and motor control. *Neural Plasticity*, 10:107-120.

[2] Bolam, J. P.; Hanley, J. J.; Booth, P. A. C.; Bevan, M. D. (2000). Synaptic organisation of the basal ganglia. *J. Anat.* 196:527-542.

[3] Arias-Montaño, J. A.; Florán, B.; García, M.; Aceves, J.; Young, J. M. (2001). Histamine H_3 receptor-mediated inhibition of depolarization-induced, dopamine D_1 receptor-dependent release of [^{3}H]-γ-aminobutyric acid from rat striatal slices. *Br. J. Pharmacol.* 133:165-171.

[4] Surmeier, D. J.; Ding, J.; Day, M.; Wang, Z.; Shen, W. (2007). D1 and D2 dopamine-receptor modulation of striatal glutamatergic signaling in striatal medium spiny neurons. *Trends Neurosci.* 30:228-235.

[5] Huff, R. M. (1996). Signal transduction pathways modulated by the D2 subfamily of dopamine receptors. *Cell. Signal.* 8:453-459.

[6] Davies, K. J. (1995). Oxidative stress: the paradox of aerobic life. *Biochem. Soc. Symp.* 61:1-31.

[7] Klein, J. A.; Ackerman, S. L. (2003). Oxidative stress, cell cycle, and neurodegeneration. *J. Clin. Invest.* 111:785-793.

[8] Meredith, G. E.; Sonsalla P.; Chesselet M.-F. (2008). Animal models of Parlinson's disease progression. *Acta Neuropathol.* 115:385-398.

[9] Subbarao, K. V.; Richardson, J. S. (1990). Iron-dependent peroxidation of rat brain: a regional study. *J. Neuroscience Res.* 26: 224-232.

[10] Mosley, R. L.; Benner, E. J.; Kadiu, I.; Thomas, M.; Boska, M. D.; Hasan, K.; Laurie, C. (2006). Gendelman, H. E. Neuroinflammation, oxidative stress and the pathogenesis of Parkinson's disease. *Clin. Neurosci. Res.* 6:261-281.

[11] Sengstock, G. J.; Olanow, C. W.; Dunn, A. J.; Arendash, G. W. (1992). Iron induces degeneration of nigrostriatal neurons. *Brain Res Bull.* 28:645-649.

[12] Thompson, K. J.; Shoham, S.; Connor, J. R. (2001). Iron and neurodegenerative disorders. *Brain Res. Bull.* 2001, 55:155-164.

[13] Gasche, C.; Lomer, M. C. E.; Cavill, I.; Weiss, G. (2004). Iron, anaemia, and inflammatory bowel diseases. *Gut* . 53:1190-1197.

[14] Bueno-Nava, A.; Montes, S.; DelaGarza-Montano, P.; Alfaro-Rodriguez, A.; Ortiz, A.; Gonzalez-Pina, R. (2008). Reversal of noradrenergic depletion and lipid peroxidation in the pons after brain injury correlates with motor function recovery in rats. *Neuroscience Letters*, 443:32-36.

[15] Miur, A. R.; Golberg, L. (1961). Observations on subcutaneous macrophages. Phagocytosis of iron-dextran and ferritin synthesis. Quart. *J. Exp. Physiolo*. 46:289.

[16] Olfert, E. D.; Cross, B. M.; McWilliam, A. A., eds. Guide to the care and use of experimental animals. *Canadian Council on Animal Care*; 1993.

[17] Paxinos, G.; Watson, C. *The Rat Brain in Stereotaxic Coordinates*. Academic Press: New York; 1998.

[18] Garcia, J. H.; Wagner, S.; Liu, K. F.; Hu, X. J. (1995). Neurological deficit and extent of neuronal necrosis attributable to middle cerebral artery occlusion in rats. Statistical validation. *Stroke*. 26:627-35.

[19] Gonzalez-Pina, R.; Bueno-Nava, A.; Montes, S.; Alfaro-Rodríguez, A.; González-Maciel, A.; Reynoso-Robles, R.; Ayala-Guerrero, F. (2006). Pontine and cerebellar norepinephrine content in adult rats recovering from focal cortical injury. *Neurochem. Res*. 31:1443-9.

[20] Pantoni, L.; Bartolini, L.; Pracucci, G.; Inzitari, D. (1998). Interrater agreement on a simple neurological score in rats. *Stroke*. 29:871-872.

[21] González-Piña, R.; Paz, C. (1997). Brain monoamine changes in rats after short periods of ozone exposure. *Neurochem Res*. 22:63-6.

[22] Yoshida, K.; Kaneto, K.; Miyajima, H.; Tokuda, T.; Nakamura, A.; Kato M.; Ikeda, S. I. (2000). Increased lipid peroxidation in the brains of aceruloplasmonemia patients. *J. Neurological Sciences*. 175:91-95.

[23] Braughler, J. M. (1985). Lipid peroxidation-induced inhibition of gamma-aminobutyric acid uptake in rat brain synaptosomes: protection by glucocorticoids. *J. Neurochem*. 44: 1282-1288.

[24] Chan, P. H.; Kerlan, R.; Fishman, R. A. (1983). Reductions of gamma-aminobutyric acid and glutamate uptake and (Na+ + K+)-ATPase activity in brain slices and synaptosomes by arachidonic acid. *J. Neurochem*. 40: 309-316.

[25] Halliwell, B. (1987). Oxidants and human disease: some new concepts. *FASEB J.* 1:358-354.

[26] McConkey, D. J.; Hartzell, P.; Nicotera, P.; Wyllie, A. H.; Orrenius, S. (1988). Stimulation of endogenous endonuclease activity in hepatocytes exposed to oxidative stress. *Toxicol Lett*. 42:123-30.

[27] Cochrane, C. J.; Scraufstatter, I. U.; Hyslop, P.; Jackson, J. (1988). Cellular and biochemical events in oxidants injury. In: Halliwell, B., ed. Oxygen radicals and tissue injury. *FASEB*; 49-54.

[28] Lin, A. M. (2001). Coexistence of zinc and iron augmented oxidative injuries in the nigrostriatral dopaminergic system of SD rats. Free Radic. *Biol. Med.* 30:225-231.

[29] Ben-Shachar, D.; Youdim, M. B. (1991). Intranigral iron injection induced behavioral and bichemical "parkinsonism" in rats. *J. Neurochem*. 57:2133-5.

[30] Lin, A. M.; Yang, C.H.; Chai, C.Y. (1988). Striatal dopamine dynamics are altered following an intranigral infusion of iron in adults rats. Free Radic. *Biol. Med.* 24:988-93.

[31] Sengstock, G. J.; Olanow, C. W.; Dunn, A. J.; Barone, S. Jr.; Arendash, G. W. (1994). Progressive changes in striatal dopaminergic markers, nigral volume, and rotational behavior following iron infusion into the rat substantia nigra. *Exp. Neurol.* 130:82-94.

[32] Paris, I.; Martinez-Alvarado, P.; Perez-Pastene, C.; Vieira, M. N., Olea-Azar, C.; Raisman-Vozari, R.; Cardenas, S.; Graumann, R.; Caviedes, P.; Segura-Aguilar, J. (2005). Monoamine transporter inhibitors and norepinephrine reduce dopamine-dependent iron toxicity in cells derived from the substantia nigra. *J. Neurochem.* 92:1021-32.

[33] Cantuti-Castelvetri, I.; Shukitt-Hale, B.; Joseph, J. A. (2003). Dopamine neurotoxicity: age-dependent behavioral and histological effects. *Neurobiol. Aging.* 24:697-706.

[34] Kandel, E. R.; Schwartz, J. H.; Jessel, T. M. *Principles of neural science*. McGraw-Hill: New York; 2000.

[35] Qian, M. Z.; Wang, Q. (1998). Expression of iron transport proteins and escessive iron accumulation in the brain in neurodegenerative disorders. *Brain Res. Rev.* 27:257-267.

[36] Kristensson, K.; Bornstein, B. M. (1974). Effects of iron-containing substances of nervous tissue in vitro. *Acta Neuropath. (Berl.)* 28: 281-292.

[37] Cox, J. S.; Moss, G. F.; Bremner, I.; Reason, J. (1968). Intravenous iron-dextran: studies on unsaturated iron-binding capacity. *J. Clin. Path.* 21:611-615.

[38] Gregory, A.; Hayflick, S.J. (2005). Neurodegeneration whith brain iron accumulation. *Folia Neuropathol.* 43:286-296.

Index

A

D

E

F

G

H

I

J

K

L

N

O

P

Q

R

S

T

U

V

W

Y

Z